Instructional Course Lectures Hip

Edited by
Thomas Parker Vail, MD
Professor and Chairman
Department of Orthopaedic Surgery
University of California, San Francisco
San Francisco, California

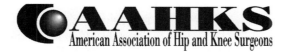

Developed with support from
American Association of Hip and Knee Surgeons

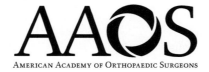

AMERICAN ACADEMY OF ORTHOPAEDIC SURGEONS

Published by the
American Academy
of Orthopaedic Surgeons
6300 North River Road
Rosemont, IL 60018

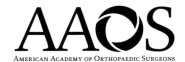

The material presented in the *Instructional Course Lectures Hip* has been made available by the American Academy of Orthopaedic Surgeons for educational purposes only. This material is not intended to present the only, or necessarily best, methods or procedures for the medical situations discussed, but rather is intended to represent an approach, view, statement, or opinion of the author(s) or producer(s), which may be helpful to others who face similar situations.

Some drugs or medical devices demonstrated in Academy courses or described in Academy print or electronic publications have not been cleared by the Food and Drug Administration (FDA) or have been cleared for specific uses only. The FDA has stated that it is the responsibility of the physician to determine the FDA clearance status of each drug or device he or she wishes to use in clinical practice.

The FDA has expressed concern about potential serious patient care issues involved with the use of polymethlymethacrylate (PMMA) bone cement in the spine. A physician might insert the PMMA bone cement into vertebrae by various procedures, including vertebroplasty and kyphoplasty. Orthopaedic surgeons should be alert to possible complications.

Furthermore, any statements about commercial products are solely the opinion(s) of the author(s) and do not represent an Academy endorsement or evaluation of these products. These statements may not be used in advertising or for any commercial purpose.

Some of the authors or the departments with which they are affiliated have received something of value from a commercial or other party related directly or indirectly to the subject of their chapter.

First Edition
Copyright 2007 by the American Academy of Orthopaedic Surgeons
ISBN 10: 0-89203-453-X
ISBN 13: 978-0-89203-453-6
Library of Congress Cataloging-in-Publication Data

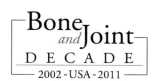

Editorial Board

Contributors

Roy K. Aaron, MD
Professor, Orthopaedics
Department of Orthopaedics
Brown Medical School
Providence, Rhode Island

Matthew S. Austin, MD
Attending Orthopaedic Surgeon
Division of Orthopaedics
Cooper Hospital
University of Medicine and Dentistry of New Jersey
Camden, New Jersey

Diane Back, MBBS, BSc, FRCS Ed (Tr&Orth)
Consultant Orthopaedic Surgeon
Department of Trauma and Orthopaedics
Guy's and St. Thomas' Hospital
London, United Kingdom

Robert L. Barrack, MD
The Charles F. and Joanne Knight Distinguished
    Professor of Orthopaedic Surgery
Washington University School of Medicine
Chief of Orthopedic Surgery Services
Director of Adult Reconstructive Surgery
Barnes-Jewish Hospital
St. Louis, Missouri

Daniel J. Berry, MD
Associate Professor of Orthopedics
Mayo Medical School
Consultant in Orthopedic Surgery
Department of Orthopedic Surgery
Mayo Clinic
Rochester, Minnesota

Hugh Blackley, MD, FRACS
Orthopaedic Department
Auckland Hospital
Auckland, New Zealand

Michael P. Bolognesi, MD
Assistant Professor
Director, Adult Reconstruction
Division of Orthopaedic Surgery
Duke University Medical Center
Durham, North Carolina

Robert B. Bourne, MD, FRCSC
A.D. McLachlin Professor
Chair, Division of Orthopaedic Surgery
Department of Surgery
University of Western Ontario
London Health Sciences Centre, University Campus
London, Ontario, Canada

R. Stephen J. Burnett, MD, FRCSC
Assistant Professor
Washington University School of Medicine
Department of Orthopedic Surgery
Barnes-Jewish Hospital
St. Louis, Missouri

R. Allen Butler, MD
Arthroplasty Fellow
Department of Orthopaedic Surgery
Tulane University School of Medicine
New Orleans, Louisiana

J. W. Thomas Byrd, MD
Orthopaedic Surgeon
Nashville Sports Medicine and Orthopaedic Center
Nashville, Tennessee

John J. Callaghan, MD
The Lawrence and Marilyn Dorr Chair and Professor
Department of Orthopaedics
University of Iowa
Iowa City, Iowa

Mark N. Charles, MD, FRCSC
Fellow
Department of Orthopaedic Surgery
London Health Sciences Centre, University Campus
London, Ontario, Canada

Quanjun Cui, MD, MS
Department of Orthopaedic Surgery
University of Virginia School of Medicine
Charlottesville, Virginia

J. Roderick Davey, MD, FRCSC
Associate Professor, Department of Surgery
University of Toronto
Head, Division of Orthopaedics
Toronto Western Hospital
University Health Network
Toronto, Ontario, Canada

Patrick Duffy, MBBCh, FRCS(Orth)
Department of Orthopaedics
University of British Columbia
Vancouver, British Columbia, Canada

Clive P. Duncan, MD, FRCSC
Professor and Chairman
Department of Orthopaedics
University of British Columbia
Vancouver, British Columbia, Canada

Reinhold Ganz, MD
Professor and Chairman
Department of Orthopaedic Surgery
University of Berne, Inselspital
Berne, Switzerland

Donald S. Garbuz, MD, FRCSC
Assistant Professor
Department of Orthopaedics
University of British Columbia
Vancouver, British Columbia, Canada

Michael J. Gardner, MD
Resident in Orthopaedic Surgery
Hospital for Special Surgery
New York, New York

Andrew J. Glassman, MD
Director, Joint Replacement Surgery
Northern Virginia Community Hospital
Senior Staff Surgeon
The Anderson Clinic
Arlington, Virginia

A. Seth Greenwald, D. Phil. (Oxon)
Director of Orthopaedic Research and Education
Orthopaedic Research Laboratories
Lutheran Hospital
Cleveland Clinic Health System
Cleveland, Ohio

Nelson V. Greidanus, MD, MPH, FRCSC
Assistant Professor
Division of Reconstructive Orthopaedics
University of British Columbia
Vancouver, British Columbia, Canada

Allan E. Gross, MD, FRCSC
Professor of Surgery
University of Toronto
Head, Division of Orthopaedic Surgery
Mount Sinai Hospital
Toronto, Ontario, Canada

Christian Heisel, MD
Research Fellow
Joint Replacement Institute at the Orthopaedic Hospital
Los Angeles, California

Caroline Hing, BSc, MSc, MD, FRCS (Tr&Orth)
Orthopaedic Fellow
Melbourne Orthopaedic Group
Melbourne, Australia

William Hozack, MD
Professor of Orthopaedic Surgery
Rothman Institute
Department of Orthopaedic Surgery
Thomas Jefferson University Medical School
Philadelphia, Pennsylvania

Stephen R. Kantor, MD
Assistant Professor of Orthopaedic Surgery
Dartmouth-Hitchcock Medical Center
Lebanon, New Hampshire

Joseph M. Lane, MD
Professor of Orthopaedic Surgery
Assistant Dean, Medical Students
Weill Medical College of Cornell University
New York, New York

Michael Leunig, MD
Orthopaedic Surgeon
Department of Orthopaedic Surgery
Balgrist University Hospital
Zurich, Switzerland

Jay R. Lieberman, MD
Associate Professor
Department of Orthopaedic Surgery
UCLA Medical Center
Los Angeles, California

Dean G. Lorich, MD
Associate Director
Orthopaedic Trauma Service
Assistant Professor
Weill College of Medicine of Cornell University
Hospital for Special Surgery
New York, New York

Craig R. Mahoney, MD
Fellow
Department of Orthoapedic Surgery
Hospital for Special Surgery
New York, New York

Bassam A. Masri, MD, FRCSC
Professor and Chairman
Department of Orthopaedics
University of British Columbia
Vancouver, British Columbia, Canada

Harry A. McKellop, PhD
Director
The J. Vernon Luck Orthopaedic Research Center
Orthopaedic Hospital
University of California at Los Angeles
Los Angeles, California

William M. Mihalko, MD, PhD
Associate Professor
University of Virginia
Department of Orthopaedic Surgery
Charlottesville, Virginia

Philip A. Mitchell, MD, FRCS (Tr and Orth)
Clinical and Research Fellow
Division of Reconstructive Orthopaedics
University of British Columbia
Vancouver, British Columbia, Canada

Michael A. Mont, MD
Director
Rubin Institute for Advanced Orthopaedics
Sinai Hospital of Baltimore
Baltimore, Mayrland

Bernard F. Morrey, MD
Professor of Orthopaedic Surgery
Adult Reconstruction
Mayo Medical Center
Rochester, Minnesota

Michael R. O'Rourke, MD
Assistant Professor
Department of Orthopaedics and Rehabilitation
University of Iowa
Iowa City, Iowa

Wayne G. Paprosky, MD
Associate Professor
Department of Orthopaedic Surgery
Rush Medical College
Chicago, Illinois

Javad Parvizi, MD, FRCS
Director of Research
Associate Professor of Orthopaedics
Rothman Institute of Orthopaedics
Thomas Jefferson University Medical School
Philadelphia, Pennsylvania

Paul M. Pellicci, MD
Department of Orthopaedic Surgery
Hospital for Special Surgery
New York, New York

William F. Phillips III, MD
Adult Reconstructive Fellow
Arthritis Surgery Center of San Diego
San Diego, California

Amar D. Rajadhyaksha, MD
Fellow
Center for Joint Preservation and Reconstruction
Rubin institute for Advanced Orthopedics
Sinai Hospital of Baltimore
Baltimore, Maryland

Cecil H. Rorabeck, MD, FRCSC
Professor
Department of Orthopaedic Surgery
London Health Sciences Centre
London, Ontario, Canada

Khaled J. Saleh, MD, MSc, FRCSC, FACS
Associate Professor and Division Head,
    Adult Reconstruction
Department of Orthopaedic Surgery
Rothman Institute
Philadelphia, Pennsylvania

Richard F. Santore, MD
Clinical Professor
Department of Orthopaedic Surgery
University of California, San Diego
San Diego, California

Thomas P. Schmalzried, MD
Associate Director
Joint Replacement Institute
Orthopaedic Hospital
Los Angeles, California

Thorsten M. Seyler, MD
Fellow
Rubin Institute for Advanced Orthopedics
Sinai Hospital of Baltimore
Baltimore, Maryland

Peter F. Sharkey, MD
Associate Professor
Department of Orthopaedic Surgery
Thomas Jefferson Medical College
Philadelphia, Pennsylvania

Andrew Shimmin, FAOrthA, FRACS, Dip Anat
Consultant Orthopaedic Surgeon
Melbourne Orthopaedic Group
Melbourne, Australia

Klaus A. Siebenrock, MD
Department of Orthopaedic Surgery
University of Berne, Inselspital
Berne, Switzerland

Mauricio Silva, MD
Research Fellow
Joint Replacement Institute at Orthopaedic Hospital
Los Angeles, California

Scott M. Sporer, MD, MS
Assistant Professor
Department of Orthopaedic Surgery
Rush Medical College
Chicago, Illinois

T. David Tarity, BS
Research Fellow
Rothman Institute of Orthopaedics
Thomas Jefferson University
Philadelphia, Pennsylvania

Thomas R. Turgeon, BSc, MD
Adult Reconstruction Fellow
Arthritis Surgery Center of San Diego
San Diego, California

James R. Urbaniak, MD
Virginia Flowers Baker Chief of Orthopaedic Surgery
Department of Orthopaedic Surgery
Duke University
Durham, North Carolina

Eugene R. Viscusi, MD
Director, Acute Pain Management
Department of Anesthesiology
Thomas Jefferson University
Philadelphia, Pennsylvania

Paul Wong, MD, MSc(Epid), FRCSC
Department of Orthopaedics
Toronto East General Hospital
Toronto, Canada

Ian G. Woodgate, FRACS (Orth)
Orthopaedic Surgeon
Department of Orthopaedic Surgery
St. Vincent's Clinic
Sydney, New South Wales, Australia

Preface

This specialty edition of *Instructional Course Lectures* is dedicated to recent advances in the surgical treatment of hip conditions. Reflected in these articles is the enormous increase in the understanding of both the genesis and development of various hip conditions. Emphasis has been placed on including information that will help the surgeon with both surgical and nonsurgical management of the hip. The value of this volume is that it provides the surgeon with the tools to understand the pathogenesis and natural history of degenerative hip conditions and ultimately to apply appropriate surgical intervention with the benefit of the latest technology.

New information on degenerative hip conditions is based on the development and refinement of long-held beliefs regarding the causes of hip degeneration. The articles in the first section address a range of conditions, from simple surface damage to potentially devastating conditions such as arthrosis, osteoporosis, and osteonecrosis. Deeper understanding of these conditions has breathed life into nonarthroplasty surgical options, particularly continued development in procedures such as arthroscopy and osteotomy. Arthroscopy has enhanced our ability to see and understand intra-articular hip conditions without opening the joint and is now being used in more creative ways to address chondral surface pathology, labral tears, and impingement. Ganz and his colleagues deserve credit for shining new light on dysplasia and impingement by offering a different perspective on the factors that contribute to early hip joint degeneration. These perspectives have led to the application of new procedures such as the periacetabular osteotomy for treatment of dysplasia and open surgical hip dislocation for treatment of impingement.

The second section focuses on the virtual explosion of new technology in primary THA. New technology presents both promise and risks that must be carefully weighed in clinical application. This section will help the surgeon put these new technologies into perspective, differentiating laboratory simulation and clinical reports. As patient expectations have increased and indications for THA have expanded, the imperative of developing better care pathways, as well as longer lasting and better functioning implants, has become acute. New bearing surfaces, more effective pain management, and the re-introduction of procedures such as hip resurfacing are included in the range of options that surgeons can consider for the individual needs of patients.

One unfortunate reality is that with the increased number of primary joint replacements comes the increased burden of complications and revision procedures. Although newer technology holds the promise of lowering revision rates, overall revision rates have been fairly constant for the past 2 decades in North America. The implication of this observation is that problems such as bone loss, dislocation, infection, periprosthetic fracture, and neurovascular complications will need to be addressed. Familiarity with and innovation in managing the above-mentioned complications will help surgeons improve their skill set. The third and fourth sections provide the reader with the latest available information in this critical area of hip arthroplasty.

Recommending and compiling this exceptional collection of contributions has been a pleasure. The commentary by the highly skilled section editors will help place the articles in context and enhance the understanding of the material. My congratulations are extended to the authors, reviewers, and the editors at the AAOS, with gratitude extended personally and on behalf of the many surgeons who will benefit from the commentary and original contributions.

Thomas Parker Vail, MD
Professor and Chairman
Department of Orthopaedic Surgery
University of California, San Francisco

Contents

Section 3 Modern Management of Complications

Section 4 Returning Function Through Revision Surgery

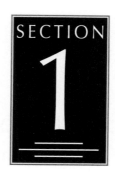

SECTION 1

Preoperative Concerns: Cartilage, Coverage, Deformity, and Degeneration

Preoperative Concerns: Cartilage, Coverage, Deformity, and Degeneration

As healthcare providers treating disorders of the hip, we often are presented with patients who pose a diagnostic therapeutic dilemma. Although surgical options may be quite limited in patients who present with bone-on-bone arthritic changes, how do we best manage those patients in the early stages of the disease? In this series of articles, the experts share their vast experience in tackling some very tough hip problems.

The title of Leunig and associates' article is a little misleading; a more appropriate title would be "Nonarthroplasty Surgical Treatment of Femoroacetabular Impingement" because the article does not address other causes of hip osteoarthritis. Nonetheless, the authors provide a clear, concise explanation of the pathophysiology of hip impingement and why it is a devastating cause of hip osteoarthritis. The article summarizes the vast contribution of the group from Berne, Switzerland, and others, including classification, radiographic assessment, surgical findings, and treatment. Other important points include the significance of failure to diagnose and why physical therapy is often detrimental.

There is no doubt that complete surgical dislocation provides unparalleled access and exposure to perform osteoplasty; however, there is considerable interest among surgeons treating femoroacetabular impingement to perform an adequate débridement in a less invasive manner. Further discussion regarding limited open procedures would have been beneficial (ie, surgical dislocation without trochanteric osteotomy or anterior mini-arthrotomy without dislocation). Questions remain as to what options other than use of implants are feasible for patients with osteoarthritis beyond Tönnis grade 1. Midterm results are promising, but long-term results are needed to determine if the natural history can be changed. The role of hip arthroscopy was given limited coverage in the article, but in fairness, it is a technique in evolution.

This is an extremely important article with current material and should be required reading for any orthopaedic surgeon who treats disorders of the hip.

Santore and associates provide an excellent overview of the types of osteotomies available to treat the conditions that lead to hip osteoarthritis. The historic evolution also is covered, as are the reasons that innovative techniques were developed to overcome shortcomings of more established procedures. A step-by-step description of the technique is not provided, but the copious references can steer the reader to the appropriate original articles. The importance of a thorough physical examination and preoperative planning is stressed as well.

The section on radiographic assessment would have be stronger if the various indices used to quantify dysplasia and coxa valga, such as the center-edge angle and neck-shaft angle, had been included. It is often confusing for surgeons who treat dysplasia to decide between pelvic osteotomy and femoral osteotomy when both the femur and acetabulum are abnormal. Offering more detailed criteria (ie, a center-edge angle less than 15°) may be helpful in the decision-making process. Rotational deformities of the femur must be addressed as well, which is why varus intertrochanteric osteotomies are often referred to as a VRO or varus rotation osteotomy. Although excessive anteversion usually is present in this group of patients, diminished anteversion or, on occasion, femoral retroversion may be present and should be considered during the assessment process. CT or MRI of the hip with cuts through the distal femur can be used to assess femoral version, if necessary.

Although the role of intertrochanteric osteotomy for osteonecrosis was mentioned briefly, a more thorough description of the selection criteria and technique, along with references, would have been helpful.

This article is extremely informative for any surgeon who manages disorders of the hip. The reader should come away with an excellent understanding of the types of hip conditions and the goals of surgical correction.

Thomas Byrd's 2003 article is a thoughtful discourse on issues of patient selection and the disorders that are amenable to arthroscopic treatment. He correctly notes that the best indications are for patients who have significant mechanical symptoms rather than simply vague, diffuse hip pain. He also emphasizes the diagnostic benefit of an intra-articular injection of local anesthetic to confirm the location of the pain source and that labral débridement alone may not provide pain relief. It is crucial to consider the underlying anatomic disorder that leads to labral pathology.

The article indicates that radiographic views such as a false profile view or cross-table lateral may be helpful. Because of the increasing awareness that labral tears and hip osteoarthritis may be caused by very subtle forms of dysplasia and impingement, these views probably should be obtained for all patients with labral pathology or early

osteoarthritis. Also lacking in this article is a discussion of femoroacetabular impingement, which is increasingly becoming accepted as a major cause of damage to the labrum and articular cartilage. A diagnosis of femoroacetabular impingement should not be overlooked because it is hoped that early intervention will delay or perhaps even prevent the progression of osteoarthritis.

Dr. Byrd's article presents a lucid, comprehensive outline of the types of hip conditions that are most appropriate for arthroscopic treatment, but a more updated review will provide important information on techniques that have evolved in the last 4 years.

Lieberman and associates' review of hip osteonecrosis provides an exhaustive review of the etiology, pathophysiology, radiographic assessment, classification system and the variety of surgical options available. Their review is done in a balanced fashion despite the lack of consensus (ie, the choice of core decompression versus bone grafting). The advantages and disadvantages of various treatments are discussed, as are the disparity in outcomes. The importance of etiology, continued steroid use, and patient profile is stressed. Also emphasized are the anatomic considerations: the presence of collapse, the size of the lesion, the

degree of subchondral depression, and the status of the acetabular articular cartilage.

Lacking, however, is a discussion of femoral head insufficiency fracture, a condition that can be confused with osteonecrosis on plain radiographs but has a dramatically different appearance on MRI scans. Understandably, certain implant options such as surface replacement or porous femoral head plugs are not emphasized because these procedures are now just beginning to advance beyond IDE study status in the United States.

Overall, this article is excellent and remains highly applicable 4 years after publication. The treatment algorithm provides a thorough summary with guidelines to choosing the appropriate surgical intervention.

Gardner and associates present a comprehensive review of the etiology, classification, radiographic assessment, and surgical treatment options for osteoporotic femoral neck fractures. Despite a lack of consensus in the treatment of "borderline" patients (ie, displaced fracture in a patient older than age 65 years or a patient with osteoporotic bone), the risks and benefits of the different surgical options are succinctly presented. Outcomes of a variety of studies are presented in such a way that the reader has a good sense of the chance of success in treating various types of femoral neck fractures. Also emphasized is the importance of osteoporosis detection and treatment.

Several topics were not covered, specifically postoperative management, physical therapy, and weight-bearing protocols. Is there any role for nonsurgical treatment (ie, a young patient with an insufficiency stress fracture or a patient with a partially healed impacted femoral neck fracture who is able to walk)? Also beneficial would have been a discussion regarding the treatment of fixation failure, for example, the indications for repeat fixation for valgus intertrochanteric osteotomy.

This article does provides valuable information and guidelines to any surgeon who treats hip fractures. Of particular mention is the excellent examination of the copious and often-confusing pertinent literature.

Siebenrock and colleagues describe the long-term follow-up (minimum 10 years) of an innovative pelvic osteotomy, which was devised as a means to provide a more powerful correction for acetabular dysplasia. The authors detail the lessons and mistakes experienced during the learning curve phase of this operation. Radiographic documentation reveals the corrective power of this osteotomy, which provides greater mobility of the acetabular fragment while maintaining vascularity and pelvic stability. Important prognostic factors came to light: the degree of preoperative osteoarthritis, patient age, the presence of a torn labrum, and the presence of undercorrection. It is reassuring to know that in the absence of significant osteoarthritis and a torn labrum, good and excellent results can approach 90%, even after 10 years. An unfortunate side effect reported iatrogenic femoroacetabular impingement caused by overcorrection. This, along with the increased awareness that femoroacetabular impingement may coexist initially with dysplasia, reinforces the importance of a restrained correction of the socket and the assurance that adequate femoroacetabular clearance is present at normal degrees of hip flexion.

Although the Tönnis classification provides some indication of the degree of preoperative osteoarthritis, it is not nearly as sensitive as MRI. Patients with apparently similar joint space may have vast differences in the integrity of the articular cartilage. Future studies that include evaluation of preoperative MRI scans may provide further prognostic information regarding the incidence of a successful clinical outcome. Also of interest will be a comparison between the long-term results of patients treated after this initial group and their predecessors.

This article presents an honest and informative assessment of the issues and should be studied by any surgeon who performs hip osteotomy. The lessons learned from this landmark article are certainly as important today as they were 6 years ago.

Robert L. Buly, MD
Associate Professor of Clinical
    Orthopaedic Surgery
The Hospital for Special Surgery
Weill Medical College of
    Cornell University
New York, New York

Hip Arthroscopy: Patient Assessment and Indications

J. W. Thomas Byrd, MD

Abstract

Hip arthroscopy is often performed for disorders that in the past have gone unrecognized and untreated. The arthroscope has helped in the understanding of the nature of numerous intra-articular lesions, subsequently leading to improved assessment skills for these often elusive disorders, including interpretation of the history, examination findings, and technical advances in imaging studies. The indications for this procedure have been well defined but continue to evolve. Successful results from arthroscopy are most clearly linked to indications and proper patient selection.

Table 1
Characteristic Hip Symptoms

Groin, anterior, and medial thigh pain

Pain with ambulation

Discomfort sitting with hip flexed

Pain or catching on rising from the seated position

Difficulty entering or exiting an automobile

Difficulty with shoes, socks, or hose

Hip arthroscopy has been instrumental in identifying many previously undiagnosed intra-articular disorders, leading to not only improved clinical assessment of hip problems, but also improved investigational methods overall. This chapter summarizes the current status of investigating hip disorders and the indications for performing hip arthroscopy.

Assessment

The clinical assessment of a patient with a hip problem should determine whether the problem is intra-articular and whether arthroscopic intervention is indicated.[1] It is also important to determine whether a specific traumatic event has occurred because patients whose injuries result from significant trauma are more likely to benefit from arthroscopy.[2] However, if a patient has an insidious onset of symptoms or a minor precipitating episode, the response to arthroscopy, although sometimes favorable, is less predictable. This is because there is likely some underlying predisposition or degenerative process that cannot be completely reversed by arthroscopy. Although patients with mechanical symptoms such as catching, locking, or sharp stabbing are more likely to have a potentially correctable problem, those who simply have pain with activity or, worse yet, aching independent of activity are much less likely to respond favorably to arthroscopic intervention.[3] Patient-reported activities that characteristically exacerbate hip joint disorders are outlined in Table 1.

Although the hip receives innervation from branches of L2 to S1 of the lumbosacral plexus, its principal innervation is the L3 nerve root. This explains why irritation of the hip joint may result in anterior groin pain and pain radiating to the medial thigh, which follows the L3 dermatome. Posterior pain is rarely indicative of hip joint pathology. Even posterior intra-articular lesions will refer pain anteriorly or anterolaterally. Rarely, a hip joint problem will cause posterior pain and can be confirmed when a fluoroscopically guided intra-articular injection of anesthetic temporarily alleviates the pain.

The C-sign is characteristic of hip joint pathology. The patient will grip the hand above the greater trochanter with the thumb over the posterior aspect of the trochanter and cup the fingers into the groin. Although this may suggest that the patient is describing lateral pain, such

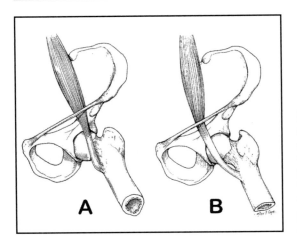

Fig. 1 As the hip is brought from a flexed, abducted, externally rotated position (A) into extension with internal rotation (B), the iliopsoas tendon transiently lodges against the anterior femoral head and capsule or pectineal eminence, creating the audible and palpable clunk.

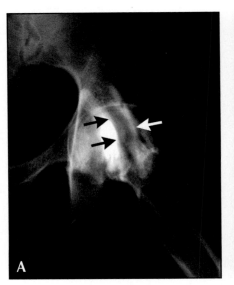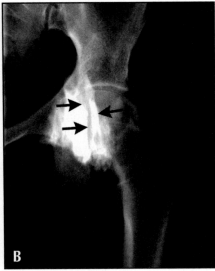

Fig. 2 Iliopsoas bursography silhouettes the tendon (arrows), allowing visual confirmation of the snapping of the tendon as it is brought from flexion abduction and external rotation (A) into extension with internal rotation (B).

Intra-articular lesions can be easily differentiated from external causes of snapping hip. The iliopsoas tendon is commonly mistaken as a source of intra-articular symptoms because the snapping emanates from deep within the anterior groin. With an understanding of the mechanics of snapping hip, however, intra-articular lesions can be easily differentiated. When the hip is brought from a flexed, abducted, externally rotated position into extension with internal rotation, it may produce an audible clunk, which is characteristic of snapping hip and reproducible (Fig. 1). This occurs because the iliopsoas tendon transiently lodges against the anterior capsule or pectineal eminence. For recalcitrant cases, snapping of the iliopsoas tendon can be confirmed by iliopsoas bursography and then by fluoroscopically viewing the tendon flipping back and forth (Fig. 2). Confirmation is dependent on the ability to create the snap while the patient lies supine for imaging. Snapping of the iliotibial band is principally the result of the tensor fascia lata flipping across the greater trochanter. The symptoms are located laterally, and the phenomenon is both visible and palpable. Patients can often stand and voluntarily demonstrate this snapping, which on rare occasions gives the appearance of subluxation of the hip.

Patients with disk pathology of the upper lumbar spine will present with symptoms referred to the anterior groin. These patients may lack the characteristic symptoms associated with lower lumbar disk disease, including low back pain, sciatica, or nerve root traction signs. Hip joint disorders are commonly misdiagnosed as extra-articular problems; therefore, it is important not to overlook referred symptoms when investigating hip pain.[4] Anterior soft-tissue disorders, such as hip flexor or adductor strains, sports hernias, or athletic pubalgia, can usually be identified by localization of symptoms and characteristic provocative examination maneuvers.

as that emanating from the iliotibial band or pain associated with trochanteric bursitis, the C-sign actually demonstrates deep, interior pain from the hip joint.

Log rolling of the hip is the most specific test for intra-articular pathology. Gently rolling the thigh internally and externally moves the articular surface of the femoral head in relation to the acetabulum and capsule but does not stress the surrounding extra-articular structures. More sensitive maneuvers include forced flexion combined with internal rotation

and abduction combined with external rotation. These maneuvers normally cause some discomfort, so it is important to compare the affected hip with the uninvolved hip. When assessing hip pathology, a catching pain, a sharp pain, or possibly even a click will commonly be elicited, symptoms that are somewhat analogous to those elicited by the McMurray test for the knee. Although a click may occasionally be detected, the reproduction of sharp pain is the primary indication of hip joint pathology.

Hip pain can be assessed with radiographs. Standard views consist of an AP pelvic and frog lateral views of the affected hip. The pelvic view film should be centered low to include both hips, allowing comparison for subtle variations and for a survey of the surrounding bony structures. The frog lateral view is really a lateral view of the proximal femur and not a true lateral view of the joint; however, it serves well as a routine screening radiograph. Other views, such as the cross table lateral or false profile, may be helpful in certain circumstances.

High-resolution MRI with a 1.5-T magnet and a surface coil is increasingly reliable for discerning various forms of intra-articular pathology. Studies performed with less powerful magnets or open scanners are unreliable except in detecting obvious pathology such as osteonecrosis. The presence of an effusion, even slight asymmetric fluid accumulation, may be a significant finding because the noncompliant hip capsule does not allow much effusion to develop. Conversely, the absence of an effusion does not preclude the presence of intra-articular pathology because significant joint damage may still be present, even without an accompanying effusion.

MRI with an intra-articular injection of gadolinium as the contrast medium (magnetic resonance arthrography) has demonstrated greater sensitivity and specificity in diagnosing intra-articular disorders than conventional MRI.[5,6] The contrast medium may extrude into areas of tearing of the acetabular labrum or articular surface defects and loose bodies may thereby be identified, artifacts that are often overlooked using conventional MRI. Historically, using a fluoroscopically-guided intra-articular injection of bupivacaine to temporarily alleviate pain has been the single most reliable method to discern whether the source of the pain is intra-articular and thus potentially treatable with arthroscopic intervention. During magnetic resonance arthrography, it is

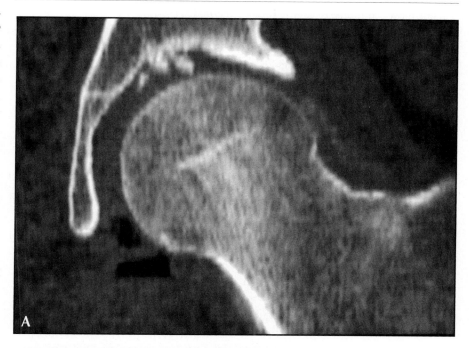

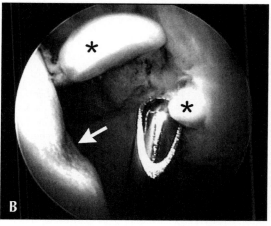

Fig. 3 Lateral impaction injury to the left hip of an 18-year-old man. A, CT with coronal reconstruction demonstrates loose bodies. B, Two loose bodies are evident (*asterisks*) originating from the acetabulum; scoring of the femoral head is evident (*arrow*) as the result of third-body wear.

especially helpful to inject bupivacaine along with gadolinium to obtain information regarding localization of the patient's pain along with imaging information. When bupivacaine is used, it is important for patients to be able to recreate their symptoms prior to the injection so that they can report any relief of symptoms.

CT may be superior to MRI for assessing bony architecture, and radionuclide scanning provides a relatively inexpensive method of assessing the metabolic activity of bone and can provide a survey of surrounding areas.

Indications for Hip Arthroscopy
Loose Bodies

Removal of symptomatic loose bodies represents the clearest indication for hip arthroscopy[7-15] (Fig. 3). The importance of loose body removal has been well documented in the literature, and arthroscopy offers distinct advantages over open approaches, including lower morbidity and faster recovery. Bone fragments can be easily identified with plain films and CT, and radiolucent loose bodies can usually be identified by arthrography combined with CT or MRI.

The most commonly recognized conditions causing loose bodies include trauma, synovial chondromatosis, and osteochondritis dissecans accompanying Legg-Calvé-Perthes disease. Interestingly, in the hip, synovial chondromatosis often presents a very occult clinical picture and may not be well defined, even with current imaging techniques.[12] Removal of fragments in patients with Legg-Calvé-Perthes disease may result in gratifying symptomatic improvement despite accompanying severe joint deformation. Bone fragments may also develop in association with advancing osteoarthritis (Fig. 4). In these cases, the fragments may be inconsequential because the prognosis is determined more by the extent of joint deterioration. Arthroscopy has also been used to remove foreign bodies such as bullets.[16-18]

Labral Lesions

Labral lesions are increasingly being recognized, especially with improvements in high-resolution MRI and magnetic resonance arthrography[8,19-25] (Fig. 5). Débridement of labral lesions can sometimes provide symptom relief, but this outcome is generally not predictable. There is much that remains to be learned regarding the pathophysiology, pathomechanics, and natural history of labral lesions. Normal variants, including a labral cleft, should not be interpreted as traumatic detachment (Fig. 6). The results of débridement are often influenced by the extent of accompanying articular damage or degenerative disease.[2,26] Labral lesions are commonly found in patients with dysplasia (Fig. 7). Although simple débridement of the damaged tissue is often successful, it

may represent just one component in the comprehensive management of dysplasia.[27] An inverted labrum has also been identified as the cause of secondary osteoarthritis.[28] Débridement in such cases may occasionally be beneficial, but the results are usually determined more by the extent of the accompanying arthritis and are often unpredictable.[29]

Degenerative Disease

Arthroscopic débridement has been used in the management of degenerative disease of the hip; however, only 34% to 60% of patients have been reported to show improvement.[30,31] Factors associated with arthroscopic débridement include younger patients with relatively well-preserved joint space and range of motion, a relatively spontaneous onset of symptoms that might suggest the presence of a dislodged fragment, and failure of conservative treatment, especially activity modification. Reasonable expectations of modest improvement are also important to avoid disappointment. Subtle radiographic changes may be indicative of more extensive arthroscopic evidence of degeneration (Fig. 8). Thus, careful scrutiny of the radiographs before counseling patients as to the role of arthroscopy in treatment is important. Santori and Villar,[32] however, found radiographs to be unreliable in detecting early stages of osteoarthritis.

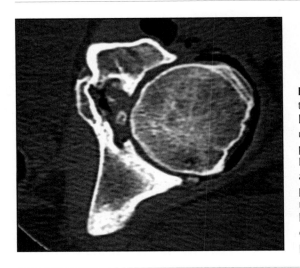

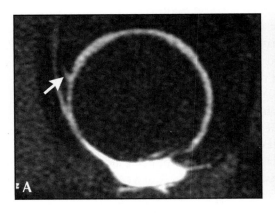

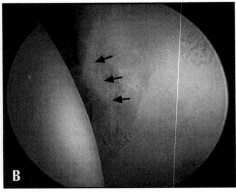

Fig. 4 CT scan with double contrast arthrography of the painful left hip of a 32-year-old man who underwent closed treatment of a posterior acetabular fracture. Bone fragments within the fossa are apparent. However, pain is primarily the result of posttraumatic osteoarthritis characterized by joint space narrowing, subchondral sclerosis, and osteophyte formation.

Fig. 5 Imaging studies of the left hip of a 27-year-old woman whose symptoms are pain and catching. **A,** Sagittal MRI with gadolinium arthrography reveals a tear of the anterior labrum (*arrow*). **B,** Arthroscopic view illustrates the tear of the anterior labrum at the articular labral junction (*arrows*).

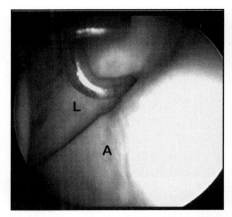

Fig. 6 Arthroscopic view of the right hip from the anterior portal in a 25-year-old woman. Incidentally noted is the separation (probe) between the labrum (L) and the lateral aspect of the bony acetabulum (A).

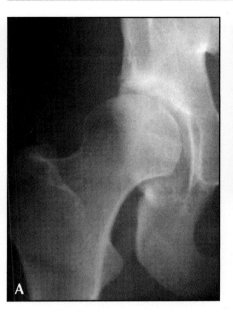

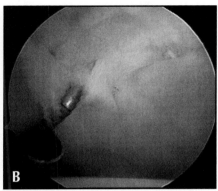

Fig. 7 Imaging studies of the right hip of a 26-year-old woman with spontaneous onset of pain and catching. A, AP radiograph reveals evidence of dysplasia. B, Arthroscopic view demonstrates an inverted lateral labrum with the torn edge reflected by the probe.

Superolateral joint space narrowing is the cardinal radiographic feature indicative of osteoarthritis caused by an inverted labrum[29] (Fig. 9, A). This condition has been implicated in cases of rapidly progressive osteoarthritis. Although an MRI may show evidence of labral pathology, radiographs will often more clearly reflect the degenerative nature of this process. The results of arthroscopy in the presence of labral pathology are no more predictable than those for other causes of degenerative arthritis. Some patients with grade IV articular lesions of the lateral acetabulum and a healthy surrounding articular surface may respond well to microfracture of the subchondral bone (Figs. 9, B through D). Eight to 10 weeks of protected weight bearing is required but, in select cases, microfracture has demonstrated remarkable results.

Chondral Injuries

Traumatic chondral injuries are also being recognized with increasing frequency in young, active adults.[33,34] These occur from a direct blow to the trochanter, such as from a fall. In physically fit individuals without much subcutaneous padding, the force is transferred directly to the hip joint, resulting in acute chondral fragmentation on the medial femoral head or chondronecrosis of the medial acetabulum. This condition is often seen in young adults with high bone density; older adults would more likely sustain a fracture and children would injure the cartilaginous growth plate.

Although investigative studies may not define the nature of the lesion, they may reflect indirect evidence of injury such as effusion or subchondral edema on MRI or increased activity on bone scan (Fig. 10). Removal of these unstable fragments can result in marked symptomatic improvement, but also provide an indicator of potential long-term problems.

Osteonecrosis

Arthroscopy has been used in the assessment and management of patients with osteonecrosis of the femoral head.[3,35,36] Arthroscopic inspection of the integrity of the articular surface has been useful in selecting patients for revascularization procedures, while allowing other coexistent intra-articular pathology to be simultaneously addressed. For end-stage disease, however, arthroscopy as a palliative procedure has been uniformly unsuccessful.[2,37]

Synovial Disease

Arthroscopic synovectomy of the hip can be performed for a variety of conditions, including inflammatory arthritides, synovial chondromatosis, and pigmented villonodular synovitis[2,8,38-40] (Fig. 11). A complete synovectomy cannot be performed, but adequate débridement is often achieved for palliative or therapeutic purposes. Synovectomy for inflammatory disease such as rheumatoid arthritis can be beneficial but should be undertaken cautiously because, like other arthritic disorders, the response to treatment may be dictated by the degree of articular surface erosion.

Synovial disorders of the hip tend to follow either a focal or diffuse pattern. Focal patterns are limited to the area of the pulvinar within the acetabular fossa. Inflammatory processes contained in this region are sometimes quite painful and respond well to débridement, although the exact etiology is not always well understood. Diffuse patterns involve the synovial lining of the capsule.

Arthroscopy can be quite effective in the management of synovial chondromatosis.[10-12] However, diagnosis in the hip can be much more elusive than in

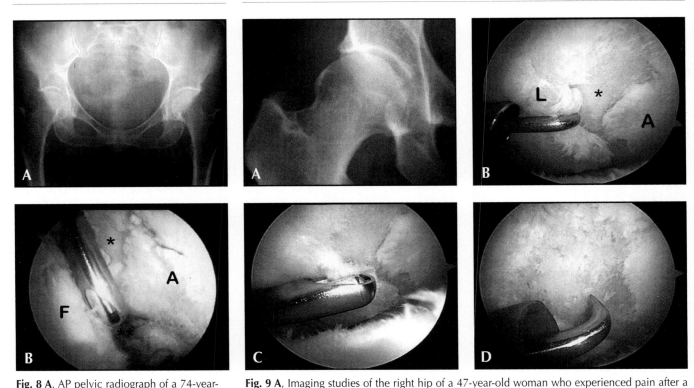

Fig. 8 A, AP pelvic radiograph of a 74-year-old woman with chronic rheumatoid arthritis and recent onset of intractable mechanical left hip pain. Radiographs were reported as superficially normal, with only modest evidence of inflammatory degenerative changes, which was insufficient to solely explain the magnitude of her symptoms. However, subtle, but significant, joint space narrowing is visible. **B,** Arthroscopic view of the left hip from the anterolateral portal reveals extensive articular surface erosion of both the femoral head (F) and acetabulum (A) with areas of exposed bone (*asterisk*) and extensive synovial disease (*double asterisk*).

Fig. 9 A, Imaging studies of the right hip of a 47-year-old woman who experienced pain after a relatively minor injury. **A,** AP radiograph reveals characteristic features of osteoarthritis associated with an inverted labrum: joint space narrowing localized to the superolateral portion of the joint; slight lateral uncovering of the femoral head, suggesting mild acetabular dysplasia; and radius of curvature of the acetabulum intersecting the femoral head at the site of joint space narrowing. **B,** Degenerative tearing of the inverted portion of the labrum is evident (L) adjacent to the grade IV lesion of the acetabulum (*asterisk*), which is surrounded by a relatively healthy acetabular articular surface (A). **C,** Débridement of the torn portion of the labrum and chondroplasty of unstable articular fragments is performed. **D,** The arthroscopic awl is used to create multiple perforations through the subchondral bone for vascular access.

other joints. In many cases, the cartilaginous lesions may not ossify, and only a vague sense of synovial disease or intra-articular lesion may be present on investigative studies.

Ruptured Ligamentum Teres
Lesions of the ligamentum teres have been classified by Gray and Villar.[41] In general, these lesions may be traumatic or degenerative. Traumatic rupture will invariably accompany dislocation, but lesions can also occur in the absence of a dislocation episode[38,42-45] (Fig. 12). These

are often quite painful, with the disrupted fibers catching within the joint, but they respond well to arthroscopy. Indiscriminate débridement of the ligament should be avoided because of its potential contribution to the blood supply of the femoral head; however, resection of the disrupted portion should not create a problem. Degenerative ruptures may also be symptomatic and respond to débridement, but these ruptures frequently accompany more diffuse degenerative disease of the joint.

Impinging Osteophytes
Posttraumatic periacetabular osteophytes or malunited fragments can impinge on

the hip joint, causing pain and restricting motion. This type of osteophyte can be excised and symptoms eliminated by excising a window in the capsule and dissecting peripheral to the joint[8,38] (Fig 13). This procedure requires good visualization and careful orientation to the surrounding extra-articular anatomic structures.

Rim osteophytes on the periphery of the femoral head may occasionally be large enough to block motion, and cause impingement and pain. As with posttraumatic periacetabular osteophytes, excision may similarly improve the symptoms; however, in general, débridement of degenerative osteophytes is unproductive because the cause of pain is more com-

Instability

Thermal capsular shrinkage can be done in the hip. More thermal energy is needed because of the thick capsule. The procedure is reserved for patients with instability resulting from an incompetent capsule with normal joint geometry. In the absence of any true joint instability, the sensation of subluxation can be caused by many factors; therefore, thermal capsular shrinkage should be undertaken with caution. Patient compliance is also imperative to achieve a successful result. Currently, patients with hyperlaxity, usually resulting from a collagen disorder such as Ehlers-Danlos syndrome, are the most likely candidates for this technique.

Joint Sepsis

Numerous articles support the role of arthroscopic lavage and débridement in the treatment of joint sepsis of the hip.[46-49] Arthroscopy, therefore, offers an attractive alternative to the potential morbidity associated with an open procedure. Patient selection may be a factor as preferable outcomes are more likely for patients with an acute process who receive early intervention. These parameters especially apply for infection in the presence of a total hip arthroplasty.[49]

Problems Following Total Hip Arthroplasty

Case reports detail using arthroscopy to successfully remove entrapped material following total hip arthroplasty.[50-52] Arthroscopy may also have a role in the management of disease accompanying polyethylene wear debris associated with total hip arthroplasty. However, there are relatively few hip prosthesis problems that are treatable with arthroscopic intervention.[8,38] Hyman and associates[49] have reported successful arthroscopic management of eight consecutive patients with late, acutely infected total hips.

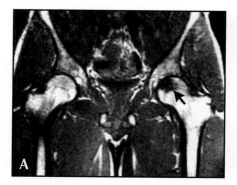
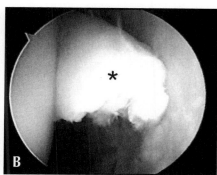

Fig. 10 Imaging studies of the left hip of a 20-year-old man who plays collegiate basketball. He had painful catching following a fall with lateral impaction of the joint. **A,** MRI revealed extensive signal changes in the medial aspect of the femoral head (*arrow*), characterizing the subchondral injury associated with a fall. **B,** A full-thickness chondral flap lesion (*asterisk*) associated with the injury is identified; excision resulted in complete alleviation of symptoms allowing advancement to a professional career.

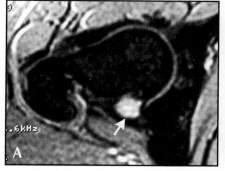
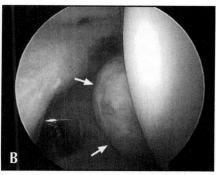

Fig. 11 **A,** CT scan of the right hip of an 18-year-old woman with a 2-year history of ill-defined hip pain, suggesting the presence of a posterior intra-articular cyst (*arrow*). **B,** Arthroscopy reveals a nodular form of pigmented villonodular synovitis (*arrows*); excision resulted in resolution of symptoms.

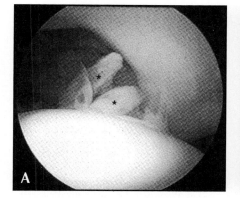
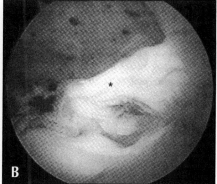

Fig. 12 **A,** Arthroscopy of the right hip of a 19-year-old woman with persistent mechanical pain following a dashboard injury reveals rupture of the ligamentum teres (*asterisks*) silhouetted by the pulvinar. **B,** A close-up view further defines the magnitude of the rupture (*asterisk*).

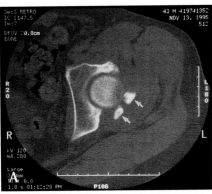
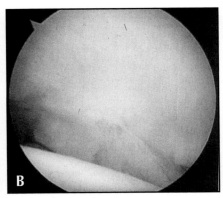
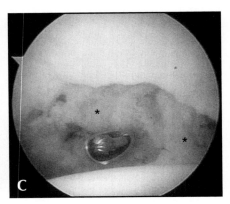

Fig. 13 CT scan and arthroscopic views of the left hip of a 46-year-old man with residual pain, 18 months following closed treatment of a posterior fracture dislocation. **A,** CT scan demonstrates two large fragments (*arrows*) posterior to the joint impinging on the femoral head. **B,** Arthroscopic view from the anterior portal looking posteriorly reveals that the fragments obscured from view by the overlying healed capsule (C), reside outside the joint and scar which is evident between the posterior acetabulum (A) and the femoral head (F). **C,** Dissecting through the capsule, the two fragments have been exposed (*asterisks*) and are being excised with a burr.

Unresolved Hip Pain

Arthroscopy has been used to identify many formerly unrecognized but treatable causes of hip pain, which has done much to stimulate advancements among other noninvasive investigational tools, such as CT and MRI. As various imaging methods continue to improve, the role of diagnostic arthroscopy in the assessment and treatment of hip problems should diminish, but recent literature still supports its role.[53,54] Although diagnostic arthroscopy is often considered for patients with idiopathic hip pain, it is usually used when there is at least a high degree of suspicion that the problem is intra-articular and potentially treatable with arthroscopic intervention.

Open Procedures

Arthroscopy has been used effectively in conjunction with, or as a prelude to, select open procedures, such as pinning for slipped capital femoral epiphysis, revascularization for osteonecrosis, osteotomy, or in association with miniarthrotomy.[55-58]

Summary

Arthroscopy has expanded understanding of intra-articular hip disorders and improved clinical assessment skills and investigative technology. The indications for arthroscopy continue to evolve. Understanding the technical aspects of performing this procedure is important for carrying out the operation as safely as possible. However, proper patient selection remains the most important factor in assuring successful results.

References

1. Byrd JWT: Investigation of the symptomatic hip: Physical examination, in Byrd JWT (ed): *Operative Hip Arthroscopy.* New York, NY, Thieme, 1998, pp 25-41.

2. Byrd JW, Jones KS: Prospective analysis of hip arthroscopy with a 2-year follow-up. *Arthroscopy* 2000;16:578-587.

3. O'Leary JA, Berend K, Vail TP: The relationship between diagnosis and outcome in arthroscopy of the hip. *Arthroscopy* 2001;17:181-188.

4. Byrd JW, Jones KS: Hip arthroscopy in athletes. *Clin Sports Med* 2001;20:749-761.

5. Leunig M, Werlen S, Ungersbock A, Ito K, Ganz R: Evaluation of the acetabular labrum by MR arthrography. *J Bone Joint Surg Br* 1997;79:230-234.

6. Czerny C, Hofmann S, Neuhold A, et al: Lesions of the acetabular labrum: Accuracy of MR imaging and MR arthrography in detection and staging. *Radiology* 1996;200:225-230.

7. Byrd JW: Hip arthroscopy for posttraumatic loose fragments in the young active adult: Three case reports. *Clin J Sport Med* 1996;6:129-134.

8. Byrd JWT: Indications and contraindications, in Byrd JWT (ed): *Operative Hip Arthroscopy.* New York, NY, Thieme, 1998, pp 7-24.

9. Sampson TG, Glick JM: Indications and surgical treatment of hip pathology, in McGinty JB, Caspari RB, Jackson RW, Poehling GG (eds): *Operative Arthroscopy,* ed 2. Philadelphia, PA, Lippincott-Raven, 1996, pp 1067-1078.

10. Okada Y, Awaya G, Ikeda T, Tada H, Kamisato S, Futami T: Arthroscopic surgery for synovial chondromatosis of the hip. *J Bone Joint Surg Br* 1989;71:198-199.

11. Witwity T, Uhlmann RD, Fischer J: Arthroscopic management of chondromatosis of the hip joint. *Arthroscopy* 1988;4:55-56.

12. McCarthy JC, Bono JV, Wardell S: Abstract: Is there a treatment for synovial chondromatosis of the hip joint? *Arthroscopy* 1997;13:409-410.

13. Bowen JR, Kumar VP, Joyce JJ III, Bowen JC: Osteochondritis dissecans following Perthes' disease: Arthroscopic-operative treatment. *Clin Orthop* 1986;209:49-56.

14. Medlock V, Rathjen KE, Montgomery JB: Abstract: Hip arthroscopy for the late sequelae of Perthes disease. *Arthroscopy* 1999;15:552-553.

15. Epstein HC: Posterior fracture-dislocations of the hip: Comparison of open and closed methods of treatment in certain types. *J Bone Joint Surg Am* 1961;43:1079-1098.

16. Goldman A, Minkoff J, Price A, Krinick R: A posterior arthroscopic approach to bullet extraction from the hip. *J Trauma* 1987;27:1294-1300.

17. Glick JM: Hip arthroscopy, in McGinty JB, Caspari RB, Jackson RW, Poehling GG (eds): *Operative Arthroscopy.* New York, NY, Raven Press, 1991, pp 663-676.

18. Cory JW, Ruch DS: Arthroscopic removal of a .44 caliber bullet from the hip. *Arthroscopy* 1998;14:624-626.

19. Altenberg AR: Acetabular labrum tears: A cause of hip pain and degenerative arthritis. *South Med J* 1977;70:174-175.

20. Byrd, JW: Labral lesions: An elusive source of hip pain: Case reports and literature review. *Arthroscopy* 1996;12:603-612.

21. Santori N, Villar RN: Acetabular labral tears: Result of arthroscopic partial limbectomy. *Arthroscopy* 2000;16:11-15.

22. Ikeda T, Awaya G, Suzuki S, Okada Y, Tada H: Torn acetabular labrum in young patients: Arthroscopic diagnosis and management. *J Bone Joint Surg Br* 1988;70:13-16.

23. Lage LA, Patel JV, Villar RN: The acetabular labral tear: An arthroscopic classification. *Arthroscopy* 1996;12:269-272.

24. Suzuki S, Awaya G, Okada Y, Maekawa M, Ikeda T, Tada H: Arthroscopic diagnosis of ruptured acetabular labrum. *Acta Orthop Scand* 1986;57:513-515.

25. Ueo T, Suzuki S, Iwasaki R, Yosikawa J: Rupture of the labra acetabularis as a cause of hip pain detected arthroscopically, and partial limbectomy for successful pain relief. *Arthroscopy* 1990;6:48-51.

26. Farjo LA, Glick JM, Sampson TG: Hip arthroscopy for acetabular labral tears. *Arthroscopy* 1999;15:132-137.

27. Byrd JWT, Jones KS: Results of hip arthroscopy in the presence of dysplasia. *Arthroscopy* 2001;17(suppl 1):1.

28. Harris WH, Bourne RB, Oh I: Intra-articular acetabular labrum: A possible etiological factor in certain cases of osteoarthritis of the hip. *J Bone Joint Surg Am* 1979;61:510-514.

29. Byrd JW, Jones KS: Abstract: Inverted acetabular labrum and secondary osteoarthritis: Radiographic diagnosis and arthroscopic treatment. *Arthroscopy* 2000;16:417.

30. Farjo LA, Glick JM, Sampson TG: Abstract: Hip arthroscopy for degenerative joint disease. *Arthroscopy* 1998;14:435.

31. Villar RN: Abstract: Arthroscopic debridement of the hip: A minimally invasive approach to osteoarthritis. *J Bone Joint Surg Br* 1991;73(suppl 2):170-171.

32. Santori N, Villar RN: Arthroscopic findings in the initial stages of hip osteoarthritis. *Orthopaedics* 1999;22:405-409.

33. Byrd JWT: Low velocity lateral impact injury to the hip: A source of occult hip pathology. *J South Orthop Assoc* 1997;6:151.

34. Byrd JW: Lateral impact injury: A source of occult hip pathology. *Clin Sports Med* 2001;20:801-805.

35. Hunter DM, Ruch DS: Hip arthroscopy. *J South Orthop Assoc* 1996;5:243-250.

36. Sekiya JK, Ruch DS, Hunter DM, et al: Hip arthroscopy in staging avascular necrosis of the femoral head. *J South Orthop Assoc* 2000;9:254-261.

37. Glick JM: Hip arthroscopy using the lateral approach. *Instr Course Lect* 1988:37;223-231.

38. Byrd JWT: Arthroscopy of select hip lesions, in Byrd JWT (ed): *Operative Hip Arthroscopy*. New York, NY, Thieme, 1998, pp 153-170.

39. Danzig LA, Gershuni DH, Resnick D: Diagnosis and treatment of diffuse pigmented villonodular synovitis of the hip. *Clin Orthop* 1982;168:42-47.

40. Gondolph-Zink B, Puhl W, Noack W: Semiarthroscopic synovectomy of the hip. *Int Orthop* 1988;12:31-35.

41. Gray AJ, Villar RN: The ligamentum teres of the hip: An arthroscopic classification of its pathology. *Arthroscopy* 1997;13:575-578.

42. Delcamp DD, Klaaren HE, Pompe van Meerdervoort HF: Traumatic avulsion of the ligamentum teres without dislocation of the hip: Two case reports. *J Bone Joint Surg Am* 1988;70:933-935.

43. Barrett IR, Goldberg JA: Avulsion fracture of the ligamentum teres in a child: A case report. *J Bone Joint Surg Am* 1989;71:438-439.

44. Ebraheim NA, Savolaine ER, Fenton PJ, Jackson WT: A calcified ligamentum teres mimicking entrapped intraarticular bony fragments in a patient with acetabular fracture. *J Orthop Trauma* 1991;5:376-378.

45. Kashiwagi N, Suzuki S, Seto Y: Arthroscopic treatment for traumatic hip dislocation with avulsion fracture of the ligamentum teres. *Arthroscopy* 2001;17:67-69.

46. Blitzer CM: Arthroscopic management of septic arthritis of the hip. *Arthroscopy* 1993;9:414-416.

47. Bould M, Edwards D, Villar RN: Arthroscopic diagnosis and treatment of septic arthritis of the hip joint. *Arthroscopy* 1993;9:707-708.

48. Chung WK, Slater GL, Bates EH: Treatment of septic arthritis of the hip by arthroscopic lavage. *J Pediatr Orthop* 1993;13:444-446.

49. Hyman JL, Salvati EA, Laurencin CT, Rogers DE, Maynard M, Brause DB: The arthroscopic drainage, irrigation, and debridement of late, acute total hip arthroplasty infections: Average 6-year follow-up. *J Arthroplasty* 1999;14:903-910.

50. Nordt W, Giangarra CE, Levy IM, Habermann ET: Arthroscopic removal of entrapped debris following dislocation of a total hip arthroplasty. *Arthroscopy* 1987;3:196-198.

51. Shifrin LZ, Reis ND: Arthroscopy of a dislocated hip replacement: A case report. *Clin Orthop* 1980;146:213-214.

52. Vakili F, Salvati EA, Warren RF: Entrapped foreign body within the acetabular cup in total hip replacement. *Clin Orthop* 1980;150:159-162.

53. Baber YF, Robinson AH, Villar RN: Is diagnostic arthroscopy of the hip worthwhile? A prospective review of 328 adults investigated for hip pain. *J Bone Joint Surg Br* 1999;81:600-603.

54. Dorfmann H, Boyer T: Arthroscopy of the hip: 12 years of experience. *Arthroscopy* 1999;15:67-72.

55. Futami T, Kasahara Y, Suzuki S, Seto Y, Ushikubo S: Arthroscopy for slipped capital femoral epiphysis. *J Pediatr Orthop* 1992;12:592-597.

56. Hawkins RB: Arthroscopy of the hip. *Clin Orthop* 1989;249:44-47.

57. Ruch DS, Satterfield W: The use of arthroscopy to document accurate position of core decompression of the hip. *Arthroscopy* 1998;14:617-619.

58. Sekiya JK, Wojtys EM, Loder RT, Hensinger RN: Hip arthroscopy using a limited anterior exposure: An alternative approach for arthroscopic access. *Arthroscopy* 2000;16:16-20.

Periacetabular Osteotomy: The Bernese Experience

Klaus A. Siebenrock, MD
Michael Leunig, MD
Reinhold Ganz, MD

Introduction

The periacetabular osteotomy (PAO) developed in 1983 provides the ability to reorient severe dysplastic acetabula in adults and adolescents with closed physes. Advantages of this technique are: the fragment has great mobility as a result of cuts close to the acetabulum; pelvic stability is maintained because the posterior column is preserved, requiring less fixation of the acetabular fragment; and the shape of the true pelvis essentially is preserved. The first PAO was performed in April 1984. Since then more than 700 PAOs have been performed at our institution. Increasing experience over time has led to some changes in assessment and surgical technique. Surgical exposure of the outer iliac wing has been limited. More emphasis is placed on balancing the anterior and posterior coverage of the femoral head at reorientation of the acetabulum. Intraoperative joint revision is done routinely with specific attention to potential impingement of the anterosuperior femoral head-neck junction against the acetabular rim. This area now is trimmed, usually after acetabular reorientation.

Improved understanding of this rather complex pathology will increase patients' benefit from a joint-preserving procedure that can be judged only after many years and even decades. For that reason, the results of the first 75 PAOs, reported in the original description of this technique[1] in 1988, have been analyzed 10 years or more after initial surgery.

Patients and Methods

Seventy-five PAOs were performed in 63 patients between April 1984 and December 1987. The male to female ratio was 1:3.4, and the average age of the patients was 29.3 years (13 to 56 years). An underlying neurologic disease was found in six hip joints, a posttraumatic acetabular deficiency was found in two, and a proximal femoral focal dysplasia was seen in another two. Twenty-three hips (31%) had undergone previous surgery for dysplasia (Table 1). Thirty-seven hips (50%) were classified as group III dysplasia according to Severin,[2] representing dysplastic hips without subluxation of the femoral head. Thirty-three hips (44%) were classified as group IV with femoral head subluxation, four hips (5%) represented group V with a secondary acetabululm, and one hip (1%) was classified as group II dysplasia. All patients had pain at time of surgery,

Table 1	
Previous surgeries on 23 affected hip joints	
Previous Surgery	**Number of Hip Joints**
Intertrochanteric osteotomies (IO)	9
Combined pelvic osteotomy and IO	8
Pelvic osteotomies	4
Shelfplasty and IO	2
(Reproduced with permission from Siebenrock KA, Schöll E, Lottenbach M, Ganz R: Bernese periacetabular osteotomy. *Clin Orthop* 1999;363:9-20.)	

and in 55 patients (73%) ambulation was restricted.

Radiographic evaluations were performed on a standard anteroposterior (AP) pelvis view and a false profile view according to Lequesne and de Sèze.[3] Dysplasia was measured using the lateral center edge (LCE) angle according to Wiberg,[4] the anterior center edge (ACE) angle according to Lequesne and de Sèze,[3] and the acetabular index described by Tönnis[5] for the obliquity of the acetabular roof. Lateralization of the femoral head was measured by the distance between the medial edge of the femoral head and the ilioischial line. The distance was measured before and after surgery and compared with normal contralateral hips. Instances of Shenton's line were recorded pre- and postoperatively. At the time of surgery radiographs were graded for osteoarthritis according to the criteria of Tönnis.[5] Grade 1 is represented by a widened sclerosis zone and minimal osteophytes, grade 2 by a moderate loss of joint width and cysts, and grade 3 by

Table 2
Preoperative and postoperative radiographic variables

Variable	Preoperative	Postoperative
Mean LCE angle	6° (–24° to 25°)	34° (10° to 55°)
Mean ACE angle	4° (–20° to 24°)	26° (12° to 50°)
Acetabular index	26° (12° to 50°)	6° (–15° to 18°)
Lateralization	16 mm (6 to 30 mm)	10 mm (–9 to 24 mm)
Shenton's line intact	39%	62%

(Reproduced with permission from Siebenrock KA, Schöll E, Lottenbach M, Ganz R: Bernese periacetabular osteotomy. *Clin Orthop* 1999;363:9-20.)

Table 3
D'Aubigne score[6] before and after surgery

Points	Preoperative (n = 58)	Postoperative (n = 58)
Total*	14.6 (7 to 17)	16.3 (12 to 18)
Pain*	3.9 (2 to 5)	5.3 (3 to 6)
Ambulation*	4.9 (1 to 6)	5.6 (4 to 6)
Motion	5.8 (4 to 6)	5.4 (3 to 6)

* Differences statistically significant ($P < 0.0001$)

(Reproduced with permission from Siebenrock KA, Schöll E, Lottenbach M, Ganz R: Bernese periacetabular osteotomy. *Clin Orthop* 1999;363:9-20.)

degenerative findings with a joint space less than 1 mm.

The clinical evaluation included recording of pain level, ambulatory status, and range of motion. The results for the three subgroups scored according to the system of D'Aubigné and Postel[6] and the overall evaluation were recorded. The impingement test, which is performed in forced flexion, internal rotation, and adduction,[7] was used to test for an acetabular rim lesion, usually represented by an anterosuperior labral and adjacent cartilage lesion. Surgery was performed using the technique described earlier by the senior author.[1] After reorientation of the acetabulum, an intraoperative radiograph was taken routinely. Thereby, an additional intertrochanteric osteotomy was judged to be necessary to improve joint congruency in 16 hips. An abduction osteotomy was performed in 13 hips, an adduction osteotomy in 2, and an extension osteotomy in 1. In 7 of

the 13 abduction osteotomies, this was done to reverse the effect of a previous adduction osteotomy. Surgery time averaged 3.5 hours (range 2 to 5 hours), blood loss averaged 2,000 cc (range 750 to 4,500 cc), and a mean of four red blood cell units were required (range 1 to 11 units).

Minimum follow-up (10 years) could be obtained in 71 cases (95%) at an average of 11.3 years (range 10 to 13.8 years). One patient with bilateral osteotomy (2.5%) died during the observation period 6 years after the PAO. Two patients (2.5%) were lost to follow-up early after the osteotomy.

Radiographic Results
The LCE and ACE angles and the acetabular index improved significantly after surgery. Shenton's line was interrupted preoperatively in 40 of 66 available radiographs (61%) and postoperatively in 25 cases (38%). Preoper-

ative lateralization of the femoral head averaged 16 mm on the affected side (range 6 to 30 mm) compared to 11 mm on the unaffected hips (range –3 to +18 mm) and to 10 mm (range –9 to +24 mm) postoperatively. All these differences were statistically significant with a P value between 0.001 and 0.0001. The results are summarized in Table 2.

Fifty-eight (82%) of the 71 hips that underwent surgery had a preserved hip joint at an average follow-up of 11.3 years. Thirteen hips were revised subsequently to either a total hip arthroplasty (12 hips) or a hip fusion. These procedures were performed at an average of 6.1 years (range 1 to 13.2 years) after the PAO. In 4 of these hips, total hip replacement was done after an interval of 10 years or more.

Clinical Results
The average D'Aubigné score increased from 14.6 points (range 7 to 17) preoperatively to 16.3 points (range 12 to 18 points) at last follow-up in the 58 preserved hip joints ($P < 0.0001$). There was a significant improvement in pain and ambulation. The range of motion decreased in most hips, especially for flexion and internal rotation (Table 3). In 6 of the 58 hips, the D'Aubigné score was less than 15 points, ranging from 12 to 14 points. Thus, a total of 52 (73%) of the 71 surgically corrected hip joints were preserved and rated clinically as good or excellent (Fig. 1).

Osteoarthritis
The immediately preoperative radiographs from 55 patients with a preserved hip joint were available and could be graded for osteoarthritis (OA). In 27 hips (49%), there were no signs of OA and 46 (84%) had no or grade 1 OA. At last follow-up, 44 hips (80%) had no or grade 1 OA (Table 4). In 14 hips (25%), there was progression of degenerative signs including 10 hips with progression from no to grade 1 OA. Each of four hips had a radio-

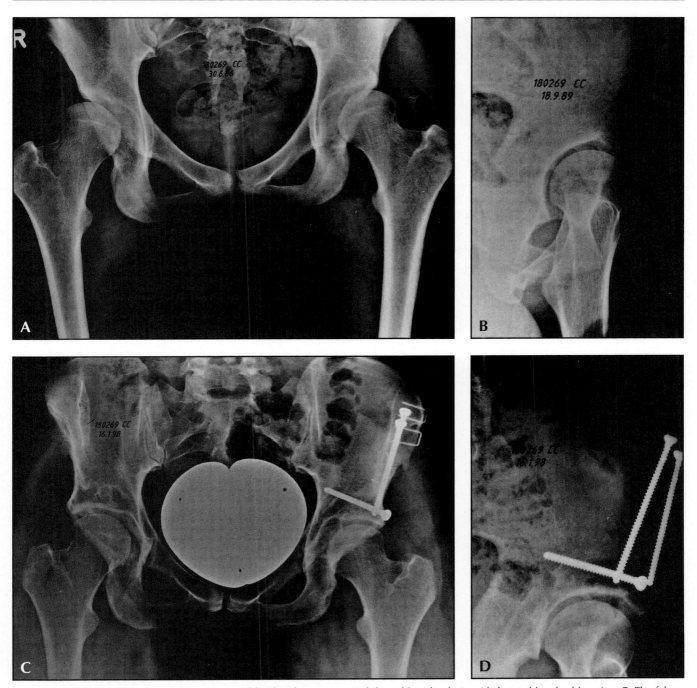

Fig. 1 A, AP radiograph obtained from a 17-year-old girl with symptomatic bilateral hip dysplasia with femoral head subluxation. **B,** The false-profile view of the left side, showing severely deficient anterior coverage. AP pelvic radiograph (**C**) and false-profile view (**D**) 9 and 12 years after surgery with an excellent clinical result on both sides.

graphic improvement of one grade. Complete preoperative radiographic documentation was available in 11 of 13 patients with nonpreserved hip joints. Six (55%) of these hip joints had grade

2 OA prior to surgery (Table 5). Five (10%) of a total of 51 hips with no or grade 1 OA were not preserved, whereas, six (46%) of a total of 13 hips joints with grade 2 OA were replaced at

last follow-up. A statistically significant correlation with an unsatisfactory clinical outcome in patients with advanced OA after a PAO has been reported. At a mean follow-up of 4 years, eight of nine

Table 4
Tönnis[5] grading of OA before surgery and at last follow-up in 55 patients with preserved hip joints

OA	Grade 0	Grade 1	Grade 2	Grade 3
(n=55)*				
Preoperative	27 (49%)	19 (34%)	7 (13%)	2 (4%)
Last follow-up	18 (33%)	26 (47%)	8 (15%)	3 (5%)

*Three cases with incomplete radiographs are not included

(Reproduced with permission from Siebenrock KA, Schöll E, Lottenbach M, Ganz R: Bernese periacetabular osteotomy. *Clin Orthop* 1999;363:9-20.)

Table 5
Tönnis[5] grading of OA before surgery in 11 patients with replaced hip joints

OA	Grade 0	Grade 1	Grade 2	Grade 3
(n=11)*				
Preoperative	1 (9%)	4 (36%)	6 (55%)	—

*Two cases with incomplete radiographs are not included

(Reproduced with permission from Siebenrock KA, Schöll E, Lottenbach M, Ganz R: Bernese periacetabular osteotomy. *Clin Orthop* 1999;363:9-20.)

patients with grade 3 OA had a Harris hip score of less than 70 points.[8]

Labral Lesions

Labral lesions were detected in 15 hips (21%) during joint revision surgery, although arthrotomy was not done routinely in the early period. A positive impingement test on the initial physical examination, which was present in 27 (38%) of 71 hip joints, has been found over the years to be closely correlated with acetabular rim pathology[7] and detectable labral lesions on magnetic resonance arthrography.[9] The 15 hip joints with labral lesions detected by arthrotomy were correlated with a significantly worse outcome. The labral lesions were left untreated in 12 hips in the present series. Resuturing the torn labrum in 2 cases failed and led to joint revision with later resection of the labrum.

Additional Intertrochanteric Osteotomy

A simultaneous intertrochanteric osteotomy was performed in 16 hips (21%) as a second step after the PAO. The decision was predominantly based on the intraoperative radiographs after the acetabular correction was performed, although it was possible to suspect additional benefit from an intertrochanteric osteotomy on preoperative radiographs. Intraoperative imaging routinely included an AP pelvis view. An abduction or adduction view was taken to simulate the effects of an additional intertrochanteric osteotomy in hips with insufficient joint congruency, joint space width, or femoral head coverage, despite adequate acetabular correction. Thirteen of the 16 hips underwent an abduction osteotomy. An adduction osteotomy was performed in two hips and an extension osteotomy in one. Seven of the 13 abduction osteotomies, however, were performed to reverse the effects of former adduction osteotomies.

Prognostic Factors

The Wilcoxon signed rank sum test was used to evaluate the significance of differences between preoperative and postoperative clinical and radiographic variables. Patient groups with different variables (eg, preoperative OA, labral tear) were compared using the Mann-Whitney U-test. Logistic regression analysis of the different variables was used to detect independent factors that might indicate prognostic relevance. Significant variables predicting negative outcome were older age at surgery ($P > 0.0001$), presence and grade of OA ($P < 0.0001$), and presence of a labral lesion ($P < 0.001$). A low ACE angle after correction and an acetabular index after correction outside of the range of 0° to 10° were also correlated to less favorable outcome ($P < 0.0058$).

Complications

All major complications in these series occurred during the first 18 osteotomies. They included an intra-articular osteotomy in two hips. In one patient, the joint was replaced by a total hip arthroplasty 19 months later. A fair result was seen in the other patient who died in a traffic accident 6 years later. Three hips underwent a re-osteotomy. In two hips, this was due to loss of correction with too-early weight bearing, and in one it was due to too extensive lateralization of the fragment. Dorsal subluxation of the femoral head occurred in 3 hips, with lack of posterior coverage postoperatively. In two of these hips, a subsequent dorsal shelfplasty was performed. One transient femoral nerve palsy was observed in this series. There was no damage to major blood vessels. Significant heterotopic ossifications with restricted motion occurred in four patients (5.6%). Subsequent successful resection of ectopic bone was performed in two of them. In one patient nonunion of an osteotomy site was seen at the pubis with a large gap after an extreme correction. Consolidation did not occur despite subsequent autogenous bone grafting. All subsequent surgeries are listed in Table 6. An extensive study about the complications in 508 PAOs was performed by Hussell and associates.[10]

Discussion

The study represents the results in a heterogenous, predominantly adult patient group with variable features and degrees of hip dysplasia, including patients with underlying neurologic pathology, a high number of previous surgeries (31%), advanced OA changes (23%), and four patients (5%) with a false acetabulum. It also represents the early learning curve with a new surgical technique, which is underlined by the fact that the major complications occurred in the first 18 osteotomies. Nevertheless, the results after a minimal follow-up of 10 years are encouraging, with 87% of hip joints lasting over a minimal period of ten years and 82% of the hip joints preserved at the last follow-up. A good to excellent clinical result was seen in 73% of the hips at that time.

Comparison with the results of other reconstructive techniques for hip dysplasia in adults is difficult because there are only a few results with a 10-year or longer follow-up. The single osteotomy described by Salter[11] may be efficient for minor corrections in childhood, but does not have the potential for correct spatial reorientation in major deficiencies in adults.[12] This lack also exists for the osteotomies in which the pubic or ischial cuts are distant from the acetabululm.[13,14] After acetabular reorientation with the triple osteotomy, according to Tönnis and associates[5,15] the LCE angle still was less than 20° in up to 26%, and the ACE angle measured less than 20° in up to 39% of the hips with Severin grade 3 or 4 dyslpasia.[5,15] Good to excellent results were seen in 85% at an average follow-up of 7.7 years, rated by a different scoring system. Thirty-six percent of the patients were younger than 18 years old. Younger age is a significant prognostic factor for favorable outcome, as has been shown in the present study and by other authors.[15-19]

Spherical or dial osteotomies have been described by several authors.[18,20,21]

Ninomiya[22] reported on 41 patients with a rotational acetabular osteotomy at a mean follow-up of 7.9 years. Corrected angles showed a large variation with a postoperative LCE angle ranging from –20° to 50° and an acetabular index ranging from –15° to 35°. Twenty-nine percent showed progression of OA, and good/excellent results were described in 76%. Recently published long-term results for 145 hips with an average follow-up of 13 years, showed good and excellent results in 68%.[23] Marked progression of OA was seen in 26.5% of 68 hip joints after spherical reorientation according to Schramm and associates[24] at a follow-up ranging from 2 to 25 years (mean 11.2 years). The Chiari technique and its modifications rely on the formation of secondary fibrocartilage in the weight-bearing zone.[25] The correction potential is limited in regard to balancing anterior and posterior coverage. Postoperative LCE and ACE angles vary considerable according to the applied techniques, with a correction of the LCE angle to an average of 25° to 41°.[16,26,27] After a minimal follow-up of 10 years, progression of OA was in the range of 20% to 79%, varying with different osteotomy angles and levels and age of the patients. Good to excellent results were reported in the range of 55% to 75%, defined by different

criteria and also varying with the surgical technique; typically there were better results in very young patients.[16,19,26]

Compromised blood supply and osteonecrosis of the acetabular fragments after performing a PAO was a concern in the early period. However, anatomic studies have shown that this technique can be applied safely.[1,28] In the present series, persistent sclerotic density of the supra-acetabular region in a single case was interpreted as partial osteonecrosis of the acetabular fragment. This was seen in one of the two hip joints with an intra-articular osteotomy and occurred in the patient who died 6 years later. Modifications of the surgical exposure of the outer iliac wing, with less muscle stripping, further decreased the risk for compromised acetabular blood supply and the postoperative recovery time of this muscle group without ectopic ossifications. The abductor muscles are no longer detached from the outer iliac wing but are tunnelled at the level of the horizontal part of the iliac osteotomy. A blunt retractor protecting the soft tissues is inserted in a posterior direction through this tunnel into the greater sciatic notch. For many years, no routine prophylaxis against heterotopic ossifications has been given. In a series of more than 500 PAOs, revision for resection of heterotopic ossification was necessary in less than 1%.[10]

Table 6
Subsequent surgeries after periacetabular osteotomy

Type	Description	Number of Hips
Major surgeries	Revision of hip joint	2
	Shelfplasty	2
	Reosteotomy	3
	Total hip arthroplasty (+1 hip fusion)	13
Minor surgeries	Screw removal from pelvis	14
	Additional removal of femoral plate	7
	Intertrochanteric osteotomy	5
	Resection of heterotopic ossification	2
	Bone grafting of pubis	1
Total	(38 patients)	49

(Reproduced with permission from Siebenrock KA, Schöll E, Lottenbach M, Ganz R: Bernese periacetabular osteotomy. *Clin Orthop* 1999;363:9-20.)

The need for an additional intertrochanteric osteotomy depends on several factors, including extrusion index of the femoral head, abnormal femoral anteversion angles, and a deformed femoral head and signs of OA.[7,29] The most significant predictive factor, however, was a previous adduction osteotomy.[29] Adduction osteotomies alone are insufficient for correction of hip dysplasia in most cases, because only the usually less-involved femoral side is addressed. Over the years there has been an essential decrease in the number of combined intertrochanteric osteotomies and PAOs. This decrease may partially be due to the decreased number of corrections attempted through an intertrochanteric osteotomy alone. In addition, our increased experience with acetabular corrections and the awareness of negative effects caused by overcorrection, especially by creating an overabundant anterosuperior coverage, have led to a more restrictive attitude toward additional intertrochanteric osteotomies.

Advanced OA changes are correlated with unfavorable clinical results for the PAO and other reconstructive procedures.[8,16-19] The decision for performing a joint-perserving procedure has to be based on the sum of all the patient's individual, clinical, and radiographic variables, taking into account, especially, the patient's age and treatment alternatives. The hips of the two patients with grade 3 OA in the current study were preserved at last follow-up. In adolescents and young adults, total hip arthroplasty does not represent a sound procedure for a painful hip, because it implies bony reconstruction of the socket, shorter prosthesis survival and subsequent increasingly complex surgeries in an active young population.[30-35]

Over the years it has become evident that labral lesions and acetabular rim fractures as consequences of an overload to the dysplastic rim[7] are more frequently encountered than had been expected. Clinical examination and more frequent indications for MR arthrography provide very sensitive tests for detection of acetabular rim lesions that could be verified by routine intraoperative capsulotomy.[9] A labral lesion in the dysplastic hip indicates the onset of an anterolateral migration of the femoral head, leading to pressure-point loading and more rapid degeneration of the acetabular cartilage.[7,36] Degeneration and thinning of adjacent cartilage next to a labral lesion in dysplastic hips also was demonstrated recently by an magnetic resonance arthrography study.[37]

In patients with long-standing symptoms, intra-articular degenerative changes are frequently far more advanced than had been believed. Conventional radiography is insufficient to demonstrate these changes and, to our minds, depicts only degenerative changes in a stage that probably should no longer be called early. Reorientation of the acetabular fragment reduces the load on the acetabular rim and torn labrum. Resection of the labrum initially may be necessary only in extended lesions, and refixation of an osseous acetabular rim lesion seems beneficial in large lesions.[38,39] The present study underlined the clinical importance of resection and refixation, revealing a significantly worse outcome in the presence of a labral lesion. Regarding only the 48 hip joints of the present study with no or grade 1 OA and without a known labral lesion, a good or excellent outcome was found in 42 hip joints (88%). Unfavorable prognosis due to rapid progression of OA in dysplastic hips with a labral tear has also been observed earlier.[36]

The study also revealed an unexpected finding that led to the awareness of the potential danger of a critically limited clearance after reorientation. This problem is caused by overcorrection or, more frequently, by the shape of the anterior head-neck junction with little or no offset in many dysplastic hips. At last follow-up, 17 (29%) of the 58 patients with a preserved hip joint had a positive impingement test, which was a new finding in 7 of them. Impingement of the femoral head and neck against the anterosuperior acetabular rim with new labral lesions after correction could be identified in 5 patients undergoing hip-joint revision for newly developed impingement signs.[40] As a consequence, routine arthrotomy during a PAO now includes visual control of hip joint motion and impingement. Impingement in flexion and internal rotation with adequate acetabular correction can be remedied by trimming the anterosuperior head and neck until a range of motion necessary for daily activities is obtained. Furthermore, a lateral approach to the hip joint for performing a simultaneous PAO and joint revision with femoral head subluxation has been developed. This procedure is reserved for hips with a pathologic morphology of the proximal femur such as a short neck and/or hips in which the head diameter does not essentially exceed the neck diameter. These hips are associated with increased risk for impingement during flexion and rotation.

The understanding of an optimal correction has considerably improved over time, especially with regard to evaluation of the anterior coverage from an AP pelvis view taken during surgery. Developmental hip dysplasia, however, does not represent a unique entity but, rather, a pathoanatomic situation with a wide variance in shape and orientation of the acetabulum including retroversion and potential abnormal morphologies of the proximal femur.[12,41] The range between insufficient, normal, and overcoverage is rather small and is influenced by a multitude of factors. Isolated, radiographically measured angles may be less helpful than the combined evaluation of all radiographic parameters together. It is a balancing of the maloriented horseshoe-shaped acetabular cartilage over the femoral head that leads to an optimal use of a limited area of hyaline cartilage for weight bearing. Improvements in surgical technique, introduction of magnetic resonance arthrography, routine joint inspection, and eventual trimming of the anterosuperior femoral head and neck, together with an improved understanding of what is believed to be an optimal correction should further decrease wrong indications, unfavorable outcome, and complications.

References

1. Ganz R, Klaue K, Vinh TS, Mast JW: A new periacetabular osteotomy for the treatment of hip dysplasias: Technique and preliminary results. *Clin Orthop* 1988;232:26-36.

2. Severin E: Contribution to the knowledge of congenital dislocation of the hip joint: Late results of closed reduction and arthrographic studies of recent cases. *Acta Chir Scand* 1941;63(suppl):7-142.

3. Lequesne M, de Sèze S: Le faux profil du bassin. Nouvelle incidence radiographique pour l'étude de la hanche: Son utilité dans les dysplasies et les differentes coxopathies. *Rev Rhum Mal Osteoartic* 1961;28:643-652.

4. Wiberg G: Studies on dysplastic acetabula and congenital subluxation of the hip joint: With special reference to the compliction of osteoarthritis. *Acta Chir Scand* 1939;58(suppl): 5-135.

5. Tönnis D (ed): *Congenital Dysplasia and Dislocation of the Hip in Children and Adults.* Berlin, Germany, Springer-Verlag, 1987.

6. D'Aubigné RM, Postel M: Functional results of hip arthroplasty with acrylic prosthesis. *J Bone Joint Surg Am* 1954;36:451-475.

7. Klaue K, Durnin CW, Ganz R: The acetabular rim syndrome: A clinical presentation of dysplasia of the hip. *J Bone Joint Surg Br* 1991;73:423-429.

8. Trousdale RT, Ekkernkamp A, Ganz R, Wallrichs SL: Periacetabular and intertrochanteric osteotomy for the treatment of osteoarthrosis in dysplastic hips. *J Bone Joint Surg Am* 1995;77:73-85.

9. Leunig M, Werlen S, Ungersböck A, Ito K, Ganz R: Evaluation of the acetabular labrum by MR arthrography. *J Bone Joint Surg Br* 1997;79:230-234.

10. Hussell JG, Rodriguez JA, Ganz R: Technical complications of the Bernese periacetabular osteotomy. *Clin Orthop* 1999;363:81-92.

11. Salter RB: Innominate osteotomy in the treatment of congential dislocation and subluxation of the hip. *J Bone Joint Surg Br* 1961;43:518-539.

12. Murphy SB, Kijewski PK, Millis MB, Harless A: Acetabular dysplasia in the adolescent and young adult. *Clin Orthop* 1990;261:214-223.

13. Steel HH: Triple osteotomy of the innominate bone. *J Bone Joint Surg Am* 1973;55:343-350.

14. Sutherland DH, Moore M: Clinical and radiographic outcome of patients treated with double innominate osteotomy for congenital hip dysplasia. *J Pediatr Orthop* 1991;11:142-148.

15. Tönnis D, Arning A, Bloch M, Heinecke A, Kalchschmidt K: Triple pelvic osteotomy: Part B. *J Pediatr Orthop* 1994;3:54-67.

16. Calvert PT, August AC, Albert JS, Kemp HB, Catterall A: The Chiari pelvic osteotomy: A review of the long-term results. *J Bone Joint Surg Br* 1987;69:551-555.

17. Millis MB, Murphy SB, Poss R: Osteotomies about the hip for the prevention and treatment of osteoarthritis. *J Bone Joint Surg Am* 1995;77:626-647.

18. Wagner H: Osteotomies for congenital hip dislocation, in *The Hip: Proceedings of the Fourth Open Scientific Meeting of the Hip Society.* St Louis, MO, CV Mosby, 1976, pp 45-66.

19. Windhager R, Pongracz N, Schönecker W, Kotz R: Chiari osteotomy for congenital dislocation and subluxation of the hip: Results after 20 to 34 years follow-ups. *J Bone Joint Surg Br* 1991;73:890-895.

20. Eppright RH: Abstract: Dial osteotomy of the acetabulum in the treatment of dysplasia of the hip. *J Bone Joint Surg Am* 1975;57:1172.

21. Ninomiya S, Tagawa H: Rotational acetabular osteotomy for the dysplastic hip. *J Bone Joint Surg Am* 1984;66:430-436.

22. Ninomiya S: Rotational acetabular osteotomy for the severly dysplastic hip in the adolescent and adult. *Clin Orthop* 1989;247:127-137.

23. Nakamura S, Ninomiya S, Takatori Y, Morimoto S, Umeyama T: Long-term outcome of rotational acetabular osteotomy: 145 hips followed for 10-23 years. *Acta Orthop Scand* 1998;69:259-265.

24. Schramm M, Pitto RP, Bär K, Meyer M, Rohn E, Hohmann D: Prophylaxis of secondary osteoarthrosis with spherical osteotomy in residual acetabular dysplasia: Analysis of predictive factors of success. *Arch Orthop Trauma Surg* 1999;119:418-422.

25. Chiari K: Beckenosteotomie zur Pfannendachplastik. *Wein Med Wochenschr.* 1953;103:707-709.

26. Lack W, Windhager R, Kutschera HP, Engel A: Chiari pelvic osteotomy for osteoarthritis secondary to hip dysplasia. *J Bone Joint Surg Br* 1991;73:229-234.

27. Matsuno T, Ichioka Y, Kaneda K: Modified Chiari pelvic osteotomy: A long-term follow-up study. *J Bone Joint Surg Am* 1992;74:470-478.

28. Damsin JP, Lazennec JY, Gonzales M, Guerin-Surville H, Hannoun L: Arterial supply of the acetabulum in the fetus: Application to periacetabular surgery in childhood. *Surg Radiol Anat* 1992;14:215-221.

29. Hersche O, Casillas M, Ganz R: Indications for intertrochanteric osteotomy after periacetabular osteotomy for adult hip dysplasia. *Clin Orthop* 1998;347:19-26.

30. Booth RE Jr: The closing circle: Limitations of total joint arthroplasty. *Orthopedics* 1994;17: 757-759.

31. Buckwalter JA, Lohmander S: Operative treatment of osteoarthrosis: Current practice and future development. *J Bone Joint Surg Am* 1994;76:1405-1418.

32. Chandler HP, Reineck FT, Wixson RL, McCarthy JC: Total hip replacement in patients younger than thirty years old: A five-year follow-up study. *J Bone Joint Surg Am* 1981;63: 1426-1434.

33. Dorr LD, Takei GK, Conaty JP: Total hip arthroplasties in patients less than forty-five years old. *J Bone Joint Surg Am* 1983;65: 474-479.

34. Istrup DM, Nolan DR, Beckenbaugh RD, Coventry MB: Factors influencing the results in 2012 total hip arthroplasties. *Clin Orthrop* 1973;95:250-262.

35. Kavanagh BF, Ilstrup DM, Fitzgerald RH Jr: Revision total hip arthroplasty. *J Bone Joint Surg Am* 1985;67:517-526.

36. Dorrell JH, Catterall A: The torn acetabular labrum. *J Bone Joint Surg Br* 1986;68:400-403.

37. Hasegawa Y, Fukatsu H, Matsuda T, Iwase T, Iwata H: Magnetic resonance imaging in osteoarthrosis of the dysplastic hip. *Arch Orthop Trauma Surg* 1996;115:243-248.

38. Mast JW, Mayo KA, Chosa E, Berlemann U, Ganz R: The acetabular rim fracture: A variant of the acetabular rim syndrome. *Semin Arthroplasty* 1997;8:97-101.

39. Pitto RP, Klaue K, Ganz R: Labrum lesions and acetabular dysplasia in adults. *Z Orthop Ihre Grenzgeb* 1996;134:452-456.

40. Myers SR, Eijer H, Ganz R: Anterior femoroacetabular impingement after periacetabular osteotomy. *Clin Orthop* 1999;363: 93-99.

41. Reynolds D, Lucas J, Klaue K: Retroversion of the acetabulum: A cause of hip pain. *J Bone Joint Surg Br* 1999;81:281-288.

Pelvic and Femoral Osteotomy in the Treatment of Hip Disease in the Young Adult

Richard F. Santore, MD
Thomas R. Turgeon, BSc, MD
William F. Phillips III, MD
Stephen R. Kantor, MD

Abstract

Osteotomies of the pelvis and upper femur play a useful and enduring role in the overall management of posttraumatic and developmental conditions of the hip. Rotational osteotomies of the pelvis have supplanted intertrochanteric osteotomies for treatment of most dysplasia-related conditions. In particular, the Bernese (Ganz) periacetabular osteotomy with lateral muscle sparing has emerged as the most effective and widely used pelvic osteotomy. Other methods, such as the Tönnis juxta-articular and triple innominate, also can be successful. These procedures have a risk profile that demands respect for the possible occurrence of significant complications and outcomes that are not uniformly excellent. Once significant arthritis is present, total hip arthroplasty is the procedure of choice in most instances.

On the femoral side, the effectiveness of valgus osteotomy for femoral neck nonunion is unquestioned. Precollapse osteonecrosis is not a contraindication. Limb-length inequalities, malrotations, and displacements of posttraumatic deformities can be uniquely benefited by intertrochanteric osteotomy. Grade II slipped capital femoral epiphysis, Legg-Calvé-Perthes disease, and osteonecrosis sometimes can be effectively treated with intertrochanteric osteotomy.

All osteotomies should be planned and performed in a manner that anticipates the possible need for future conversion to total hip replacement.

Despite advances in artificial hip replacement technology, osteotomies continue to play a vital role in the management of hip pathology in young adults. Wear debris and osteolysis remain prevalent in total hip replacement (THR) and are particularly problematic for young patients who have a long life expectancy and increased activity levels. These factors are associated with higher failure rates in these patients.[1-12] THR in patients younger than 45 years of age should be considered as a last resort. Timely correction of anatomic abnormalities with osteotomy may prevent or postpone hip arthroplasty for many years. Once arthritis is present, an osteotomy may serve as a bridge to carry the patient safely into the age range for which THR has a better rate of success.

Patient Evaluation
History
It is important to determine the extent of antecedent trauma and prior treatment during the clinical evaluation. Patients may have vague anterior groin or lateral hip pain that has long been misdiagnosed as a "groin pull" or muscle strain before a subtle dysplasia is confirmed. Additionally, patients may sense locking, snapping, weakness, instability, or limping.[13] They may report difficulties with athletic performance and endurance. Sudden sharp or catching groin pain can be the result of acetabular rim syndrome.[14] Architectural abnormalities and consequent instability of the hip lead to failure of the supporting structures around the anterosuperior or lateral acetabular margin, which commonly is associated with labral tears in the affected region, principally in the anterolateral acetabular region.

When considering an osteotomy,

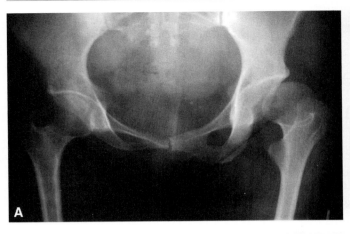

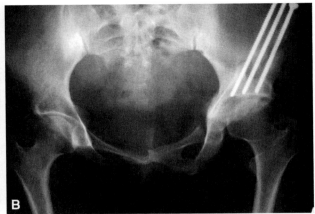

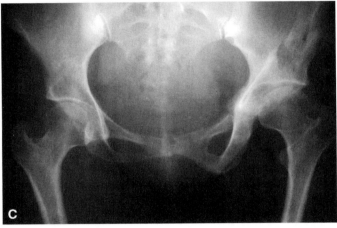

Figure 1 Upright AP radiographs of the pelvis of a 30-year-old woman with neuromuscular dysplasia caused by childhood polio. In such patients, alternatives to THR are particularly appealing because of the risk of recurrent dislocation after THR. **A,** Preoperative radiograph. **B,** Postoperative radiograph following periacetabular osteotomy. Note the delayed union of the pubic osteotomy. **C,** Radiograph following hardware removal. Note the union of all three osteotomy sites.

the patient's goals and expectations should be realistic. A social history, including consideration of lifestyle and occupation, is important. Patients whose jobs involve heavy labor have a poorer prognosis after osteotomy than those with more sedentary jobs and lifestyles.[15] In patients with irreversible preoperative articular cartilage damage, participation in running and impact sports on a regular basis following osteotomy is not recommended. However, when intervention (such as an osteotomy) occurs before arthritic changes develop, the patient may engage in unrestricted activities.

Physical Examination

Determination of hip range of motion in all planes and documentation of contractures is an important first step in the examination of the affected hip. Provocative tests are useful to confirm suspected labral pathology, especially in instances of dysplasia.[14,16,17] These tests include the apprehension test of hip extension-external rotation and the impingement test of flexion-adduction-internal rotation.[17-23] The position of maximal comfort for the hip with the patient at rest and while standing should be identified and correlated with radiographic findings. Passive abduction should be pain free in any patient being considered for a rotational pelvic osteotomy or varus intertrochanteric osteotomy (ITO). Conversely, passive adduction should be very comfortable for a patient who is a potential

candidate for valgus ITO. Gait assessment, abductor strength testing against gravity and resistance, and actual and apparent limb-length measurement must be performed. Careful examination of the spine, ipsilateral knee, and contralateral hip should be done to assess for other sources of pain. A general health assessment, noting the degree of fitness or presence of obesity, is also important.

Radiographic Assessment

Supine and weight-bearing AP radiographic views of the pelvis as well as AP and frog-lateral views of the involved hip are an important base for assessment (Figures 1 through 3). The false profile radiograph provides the best plain radiographic

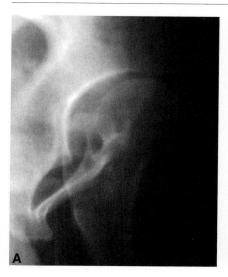

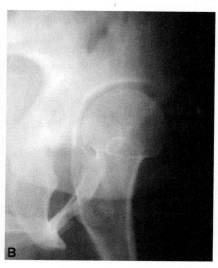

Figure 2   **A,** False profile radiograph of the patient in Figure 1. **B,** Postoperative radiograph following periacetabular osteotomy and subsequent hardware removal. Note the improved concentric reduction of the femoral head relative to **A.**

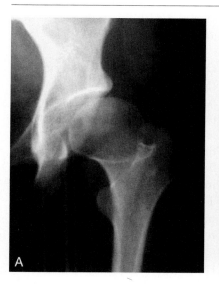

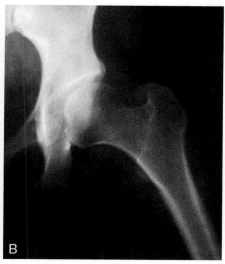

Figure 3   Radiographs of the same patients shown in Figure 1. **A,** AP view of the left hip. **B,** AP view of the left hip with the hip in abduction and internal rotation. Note the concentric reduction and congruency on the abducted view.

documentation of the anterior acetabular coverage of the femoral head,[24] and it provides a true lateral view of the proximal femur (Figure 2, *A*).

The AP abduction-internal rotation view demonstrates articular congruency and simulates the corrected joint position of a typical lateral and anterior coverage-enhancing rotational pelvic osteotomy (Figure 3, *B*). The persistence of fixed subluxation on this view is a contraindication to rotational pelvic osteotomy. AP views of the hip with the femur in abduction and adduction demonstrate the adequacy of motion in the required plane and allow assessment of the joint space before varus and valgus ITO, respec-

tively. An AP radiograph with the hip in adduction and flexion approximates the position of the joint after a valgus-extension ITO. Because the mechanical axis of the lower extremity will be changed after femoral osteotomy, a full-length standing radiograph is useful to plan proposed changes.

Most dysplastic hips are associated with an increase in acetabular anteversion; however, almost one in six dysplastic hips will have some degree of retroversion.[25] An unrecognized retroverted acetabulum could be made worse as a result of incorrect routine anterior repositioning at the time of surgery. Li and Ganz[25] at the University of Bern called attention to the role of iatrogenic retroversion following periacetabular osteotomy. On the AP view of the pelvis or hip, the anterior and posterior walls of the acetabulum can be identified. The crossover sign is identified as the shadows become more perpendicular to each other, signifying increased acetabular retroversion.

Gadolinium arthrogram MRI is useful in assessing labral pathology.[22,26] MRI also is essential in the evaluation of osteonecrosis.[10]

A three-dimensional CT scan is used routinely in some centers as a preoperative planning tool for pelvic osteotomies.[27,28] The images, and sometimes additional three-dimensional plastic models, can provide a more detailed understanding of coverage deficiencies. In addition, such studies are useful in instances of suspected acetabular retroversion. CT scans usually are not necessary to determine which patients are appropriate for surgery. Most decisions regarding reconstructive surgery of the hip can be made on the basis of high-quality plain radiographs.

Patient Selection and Timing

Age is one of the key issues when a patient is considered for an osteotomy around the hip joint. Osteotomy rarely is indicated in patients older than age 60 years. However, physiologic age, life expectancy, status of the joint cartilage, and lifestyle are more relevant factors than chronological age alone.

In general, results are most predictable when osteotomies are performed for correctable biomechanical abnormalities in joints with mild or no arthritis. Good range of motion also correlates with a better long-term outcome for hip osteotomies.[29,30] Failure to follow these principles may yield good results, but the risk of failure is increased after a limited number of years. The risks of increased stiffness, pain, or other modes of clinical failure increase with the degree of preoperative degenerative changes.[31-38]

The ideal candidate for an osteotomy is highly motivated and has realistic expectations of outcome. Absolute contraindications to osteotomy include severe joint stiffness ($< 60°$ flexion), severe osteopenia, inflammatory arthritis, and active infection. Overweight status with a body mass index (BMI) between 27 and 30 should be considered a relative contraindication, and obesity (BMI > 30) is a nearly absolute contraindication. Patients must be willing to abstain from smoking for 3 months postoperatively. Additional relative contraindications include moderate joint stiffness (flexion 60° to 90°), moderate arthritis, and neuropathic arthropathy.[39]

Surgical management should be directed to the site of the major deformity or condition. Pelvic procedures should be used when acetabular pathology predominates, with femoral procedures reserved for femoral con-

ditions. When major deformities are present on both sides of the joint, combined femoral and pelvic surgeries can be considered. These surgeries may be done in a staged manner or with the patient under a single anesthetic. If deformity exists on both sides of the joint, or if the major deformity is on the acetabular side, femoral osteotomy alone is either contraindicated or a secondary option.[31]

Preoperative Planning

Careful planning must be undertaken before surgery and is as important as the surgery itself. Issues that should be planned preoperatively include osteotomy level, angulation, acetabular rotation, possible wedge resection, limb-length adjustment, displacement, effect on mechanical axis alignment, fixation choices, bone grafting, and compatibility with future THR. All relevant preoperative planning drawings or computer printouts should be brought to the operating room and posted for easy reference during the procedure. Careful planning reduces errors and converts a complex procedure to a more straightforward technical exercise.

Reconstructive Pelvic Osteotomies

The reconstructive osteotomies of the pelvis described below reorient the acetabulum relative to the femoral head. Concentric reduction must be demonstrated before consideration for surgery. Presence of a false acetabulum is a contraindication.

Single Innominate Osteotomy (Salter)

The Salter innominate osteotomy cuts the ileum just proximal to the anterior inferior iliac crest[40] (Figure 4). The osteotomy is wedged open,

and the fragment hinges on the symphysis pubis. The acetabulum is redirected, increasing the lateral coverage of the dysplastic acetabulum.[41] The degree of anterior correction is limited by the symphysis pubis and the other soft-tissue connections to the fragment. The use of full-thickness iliac crest bone graft is associated with donor site morbidity.

Wedge and Salter[41] reported good pain relief in 16 of 18 adult patients at 6-year follow-up. Bohm and Weber[42] reported a cumulative survival rate of 79% at 12 years in 69 hips, with the patient's age at surgery and grade of preoperative coxarthrosis affecting the clinical outcome. McCarthy and associates[43] reported two conversions to THR and one salvage osteotomy in 28 patients followed for a mean of 5.9 years.

Double Innominate Osteotomy (Sutherland)

A modification of the Salter innominate osteotomy, the Sutherland osteotomy cuts the pubis adjacent to the pubic symphysis, resecting a 0.7-cm to 1.4-cm segment of bone in addition to the iliac cut (Figure 4). The fragment should be moved in a medial, posterior, and proximal direction.[44]

A total of 25 patients in Sutherland and Greenfield's[44] series were followed for an average of 22 months. Radiographic follow-up indicated medialization of the femoral head with adequate correction. One patient was converted to THR within this short follow-up period because of persistent hip pain.

Triple Innominate Osteotomy (Steel)

The triple innominate osteotomy of Steel is performed by transecting the ischial tuberosity in addition to osteotomies of the pubic ramus and

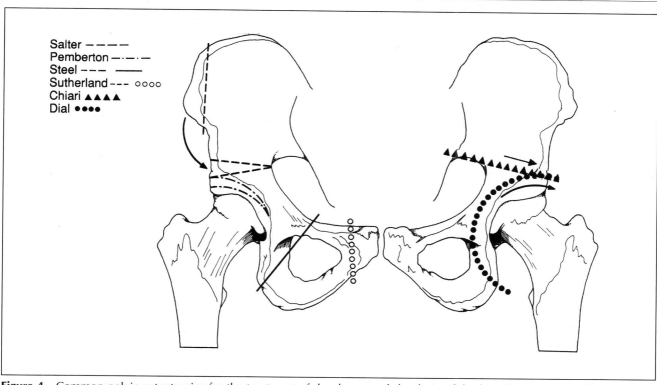

Figure 4 Common pelvic osteotomies for the treatment of developmental dysplasia of the hip. (Reproduced with permission from Stefko RM, Erickson MA: Pediatric orthopaedics, in Miller MD, Brinker MR (eds): *Review of Orthopaedics*, ed 3. Philadelphia, PA, WB Saunders, 2000, p 177.)

the ileum (Figure 4). Peters and associates[45] followed 50 adult osteotomy patients (60 hips) for an average of 9 years, reporting a 27% failure rate. A strong correlation was found between radiographic progression of arthritis and failure of the osteotomy. Patients who underwent conversion of the Steel osteotomy to THR were compared with a control group of primary THR patients who had similar preoperative findings. Harris hip scores were reported to be lower in the patients with previous osteotomy compared with the control group at an average follow-up of 36 and 28 months, respectively.[46] Unlike the Bernese periacetabular osteotomy, the Steele osteotomy can be done in children whose triradiate cartilage growth centers are open.

Spherical/Rotational Acetabular Osteotomy (Wagner, Tagawa, Eppright)

Because of limitations of the other available pelvic osteotomies, Wagner[47] developed the spherical osteotomy. However, high-grade corrections required concomitant Chiari-type pelvic transection. In the Steele triple osteotomy, soft-tissue attachments act as a leash, restricting the degree of correction attainable. Disruption of the posterior column also leads to fragment instability, requiring no weight bearing postoperatively. By making the bone cuts closer to the joint and not disrupting the posterior column, large corrections could be accomplished without losing the stability afforded by the intact pelvic ring.[47] The spherical and rotational osteotomies

create a hemispheric osteotomy about the acetabulum that allows greater freedom in corrective joint positioning (Figure 4). The inner cortical table of the pelvis and the posterior column remain intact. Proximity to the joint makes intra-articular penetration and osteonecrosis of the acetabular segment ever-present risks.

Ninomiya and Tagawa[48] reported on 45 hips in 41 patients at an average follow-up of 4.5 years. Seventy percent of their patients were pain free, with the rest reporting only mild pain. Osteonecrosis of the acetabular fragment occurred in one patient and intra-articular penetration with subsequent joint degeneration in two others. Nakamura and associates[49] reported on a study of 145 osteotomies in 131 patients with a mean follow-up of 13 years. When minimal or no arthritis was identified on preoperative radiographs, 90 of 112 patients (80%) had good to excellent results. When moderate to severe arthritis was identified preoperatively, 9 of 33 hips (27%) had good to excellent results. Yano and associates[50] reported that results were satisfactory in 41 of 50 osteotomies at 3.3 years.

Multiple limitations of these techniques have been noted. Because blood is supplied to the acetabular fragment by only the hip capsular vessels, intra-articular pathology cannot be addressed by arthrotomy at the time of surgery without increasing the risk of osteonecrosis. During the surgical exposure, the abductors are damaged, slowing rehabilitation and making patients more likely to limp. The quadrilateral plate remains intact, preventing medialization of the fragment. Finally, the brittle bone of the dysplastic pelvis increases the risk of fracture of the acetabular fragment during the procedure.[51]

Tönnis Juxta-Articular Triple Osteotomy

To reduce the degree of soft-tissue attachment to the mobile segment, Tönnis and associates[52] described this modification of the triple osteotomy. A greater correction of the acetabular deformity can be achieved by making the three osteotomies closer to the acetabulum than is possible with the Steele osteotomy (Figure 5).

Kooijman and Pavlov[53] reported that 47 of 51 hips (92%) in 43 patients were pain free and maintained improved hip range of motion at 4 years after surgery. At 10 years, the percentage of patients with minimal to no pain had declined to 58%. Despite the increased reports of pain,

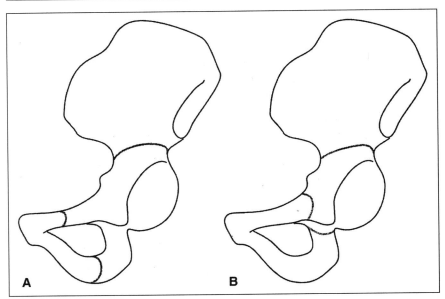

Figure 5 Site of iliac, pubic, and ischial osteotomies in the various triple innominate osteotomy procedures. **A,** Steele osteotomy. **B,** Tönnis osteotomy (Reproduced with permission from Rab GT: Surgery for developmental dysplasia of the hip, in Chapman MW (ed): *Chapman's Orthopaedic Surgery*, ed 3. Philadelphia, PA, Lippincott Williams and Wilkins, 2001, p 4255.)

81% of patients were still believed to be improved clinically compared with their preoperative status.[36]

Bernese Periacetabular Osteotomy

Because of the limitations of the previously described procedures, Ganz and associates[54] described the Bernese periacetabular osteotomy. The polygonal osteotomy is performed through a single anterior incision and allows for large, multiplanar corrections in skeletally mature patients (Figure 6). The integrity of the posterior column is maintained, enabling patients to start range-of-motion exercises early and better preserving the anatomy of the true pelvis. Because the soft-tissue attachment is increased relative to the spherical osteotomies, the blood supply provides sufficient perfusion to maintain fragment viability, even when hip arthrotomy, which allows for management of intra-articular pa-

thology during the procedure, is done at the same time. Modification of the original procedure so that dissection occurs solely on the medial aspect of the ileum protects the abductors and tensor muscles.[55,56] With the osteotomy complete and adequately released, the surgeon should be able to freely move the acetabular segment in all planes, allowing medialization and correction of version. Arthrotomy may be performed to confirm that no intra-articular osteotomy extension or instrument penetration have occurred and to address any anterior intra-articular pathology. The extent of arthrotomy can be minimized by preceding the osteotomy with hip arthroscopy, which can be done with the patient under the same anesthetic and can be used to more effectively manage labral and other intra-articular pathology in many patients. Final positioning of the acetabular fragment is performed with fluoroscopic guidance, followed by defini-

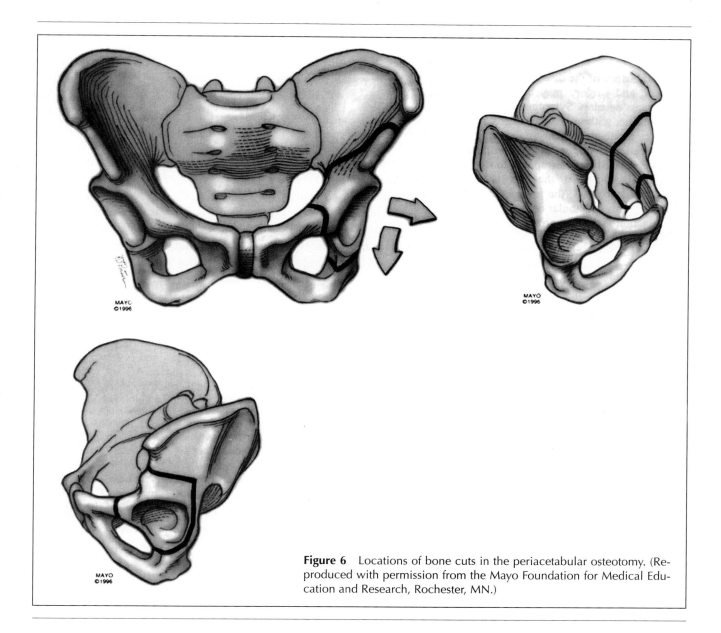

Figure 6 Locations of bone cuts in the periacetabular osteotomy. (Reproduced with permission from the Mayo Foundation for Medical Education and Research, Rochester, MN.)

tive internal fixation. A bone graft substitute can be placed within the ischial and pubic ramus osteotomies to fill the remaining diastasis (Figures 1 through 3).

Assessment at 4 years of the initial cohort of 75 patients who underwent the Bernese periacetabular osteotomy indicated improvement in the average Harris hip scores from 62 to 86.[31] Of the 14% of the patients who had undergone revision to THR at the time of follow-up,

56% had end-stage arthritis before the osteotomy, whereas 97% of the patients with little to no arthritis had a good or excellent score. Murphy and associates[51] found that 3.7% of 135 patients had arthritic progression and required conversion to THR at a mean of 3.9 years. As in the previous studies, all of the patients requiring revision had advanced arthritis preoperatively.

The Bernese periacetabular osteotomy is a technically challenging

procedure. Davey and Santore[57] reported on the learning curve of the procedure, noting a reduction in the major complication rate from 17% in the first 35 patients to 2.9% in the next 35 patients. The complications of the first 508 consecutive osteotomies performed by Ganz have also been reported.[58] Nerve injuries were the most common complication reported, with 30% of hips having a lateral femoral cutaneous nerve injury and 1% and 0.6% affected by sciatic and femoral nerve injury, respectively. Intra-articular extension of the osteotomy or intraoperative fracture of the acetabular fragment was the next most frequent complication affecting 3% of hips. In 13 of 508 hips (3%), arthritis subsequently developed and the patients were treated using primary THR. Overcorrection was reported in 1.4% of hips. Inadequate immobilization with loss of fixation resulting in undercorrection was found in 0.7% of hip. Osteonecrosis was seen in 0.6% of hips and Brooker grade 4 ossification was observed in 1%. All patients had resection of the heterotopic bone.

Salvage Pelvic Osteotomies

Salvage osteotomies support the femoral head by providing a buttress superior to the hip capsule. With time, the inner layer of the hip capsule undergoes metaplasia to fibrocartilage. It is this fibrocartilage that articulates with the femoral head rather than hyaline cartilage. When a congruent acetabulum can be redirected over the femoral head, a reconstructive osteotomy should be used. However, if incongruity of the femoral head and acetabulum is present or dysplasia with degenerative changes is too advanced for reconstruction, salvage may be indicated. Fixed subluxation of the hip is not a contraindication to salvage pelvic osteotomy.

The Shelf Arthroplasty

A variety of shelf arthroplasties have been described, dating as far back as 1891.[59] The principle behind all shelf arthroplasties is the use of local bone to augment the deficient lateral margin of the acetabulum. This bone provides a buttress that reduces the stress on the deficient native acetabulum. The bone is fixed to the ileum just proximal to the hip capsule by a variety of techniques, depending on the shelf arthroplasty procedure used.

Using revision to THR or the patient's desire for revision surgery as indicators of failure, Love and associates[60] reported a failure rate of 16% in 33 adolescents at a mean follow-up of 11 years. Thirteen percent of the patients deemed to have successful results reported moderate pain, necessitating analgesics and limitation of daily activities. Residual limp was identified in 44% of the patients. Using hip replacement as an end point, Migaud and associates[61] reviewed 56 shelf arthroplasties and found a survival rate of 37% at 20 years. Hamanishi and associates[62] found that patients younger than age 30 years had better clinical outcomes than those age 30 years and older at 10-year follow-up. Nishimatsu and associates[32] reported 119 patients with a mean follow-up of 23.8 years. A good clinical result was obtained in 87% of patients, and there was minimal to no radiographic evidence of arthritis at the time of surgery as opposed to 51% of patients with evidence of moderate to severe arthritis. Despite these clinical results, only 11 of the 119 patients underwent additional hip surgery. The articulation with fibrocartilage and the imperfect congruity of the joint limit the results of shelf arthroplasty. Poor postoperative abductor function is not addressed and frequently is exacerbated by the exposure required to perform the procedure. In addition, lateral subluxation may persist, and pathologic lateralization of the proximal femur remains unaddressed.

Chiari Medial Displacement Osteotomy

Recognizing the limitations of the shelf arthroplasty, Chiari[63] proposed the use of the ileum to buttress the femoral head. A curved osteotomy angled slightly from distal to proximal through the isthmus of the ileum is made just proximal to the hip capsule (Figure 4). Medialization of the caudal fragment creates support for prevention of subluxation. Hip joint reactive forces and the stress on the abductor muscles are also improved.

Windhager and associates[64] noted that only 9% of 236 hips required revision at a minimum follow-up of 20 years. Of the remaining patients, 88% could walk for more than 1 hour, but 93 of 213 patients (43%) had pain with ambulation. Within the first 10 years after surgery, 95% of the patients reported being pain free. In contrast, Migaud and associates[61] reported a survival rate of 68% among 89 patients at 18 years using THR as the end point. Macnicol and associates[65] reported a 5.3% revision rate to THR at a minimum follow-up of 20 years. Rozkydal and Kovanda[66] reported that 59 of 130 hips (45%) had undergone or were scheduled for THR at a mean follow-up of 22 years. Even among the failed procedures, a favorable result lasted for 17.6 years on average before the need for revision. Ohashi and associates[33] reviewed 103 osteotomies with a mean follow-up of 17.1 years and found that differences in survivorship curves were significantly related to the severity of the preoperative arthritis, the shape of the femoral head, and the level of the osteotomy.

Pelvic Osteotomies and Pregnancy

Because the prevalence of dysplastic hips is greater among women and the pelvic osteotomy is frequently the preferred treatment in women of childbearing age, there has been concern about how these procedures could affect childbirth. The Salter,

Sutherland, and Chiari osteotomies have been found to reduce the intertuber-ischial diameter. The Chiari osteotomy also narrows the pelvis at the pelvic brim.[67] These findings were contradicted by Kusswetter and Magers[68] who reported that the birth canal was not altered by the Chiari osteotomy but was narrowed by the Salter osteotomy. Loder and associates[69] reported the Salter, Sutherland, and Steel osteotomies all narrowed both the inlet and outlet of the pelvis. Because of these alterations, discussion of the possible need for cesarean section for future pregnancies is recommended before undertaking these procedures.

As stated previously, the posterior column remains intact with the periacetabular osteotomy, and the true pelvis is not altered. To date, there is no indication that the Bernese periacetabular osteotomy or the rotational osteotomies should prevent women from proceeding with normal vaginal delivery.

Femoral Osteotomy

Femoral osteotomies continue to provide valuable management options in the care of young adults with hip pathology. By using appropriately directed femoral procedures, biomechanical forces, cartilage loading, and limb-length discrepancies can all be improved. The two broad categories of femoral osteotomies are varus and valgus, referring to the final geometry of the proximal femur. In addition to varus and valgus angulation, rotation, length, and coronal plane abnormalities also can be corrected.

Varus Intertrochanteric Osteotomy

Isolated varus ITO for dysplasia rarely is performed except for situations in which a high neck-shaft an-

gle is combined with an ipsilateral long leg in the presence of mild dysplasia. Some patients with early osteoarthritis and certain patients with osteonecrosis (flexion or flexion-varus) may also benefit.[70] A minimum of 15° of passive abduction preoperatively is required to achieve a satisfactory result. Although medial displacement of the femoral shaft has been suggested to be vital to the success of the procedure, experience has shown that results do not depend on this step.[71-73] Future placement of a femoral arthroplasty stem should be the most important consideration in planning the osteosynthesis of an ITO. Excessive medial displacement of the distal fragment is strongly contraindicated. A 90° osteotomy plate generally provides excellent fixation.

In a patient with equal limb lengths preoperatively, limb shortening is the principal drawback of varus ITO, especially if a full wedge is resected. Use of an opening wedge technique results in less shortening, but is associated with a longer time to achieve union. A Trendelenburg gait is common and may persist permanently in up to 30% of patients.[29,74] Lateral and/or distal transfer of the greater trochanter may be required to improve abductor function. Prominence of the greater trochanter resulting from varus positioning can be undesirable and can predispose patients to bursitis over the plate and trochanter.

Iwase and associates[34] did follow-up studies on 110 hips with dysplasia more than 20 years after ITO with nearly equal numbers of varus and valgus osteotomies. Varus osteotomy was selected for early coxarthrosis (mean age, 25 years). Using the end point of a Harris hip score of less than 70 or salvage sur-

gery, the 10- and 15-year survival rates for varus osteotomy were 89% and 87%, respectively. The younger age range in this series was almost certainly a factor in the excellent long-term outcomes, which included 82% good to excellent 20-year results for varus osteotomies. Morscher's summary[15] of the large Swiss series reported the varus ITO results separately, with nearly 90% good to excellent long-term outcomes.

Valgus Intertrochanteric Osteotomy

Femoral neck nonunions continue to be the most common indication for a valgus ITO. By increasing the compressive forces, the osteotomy increases the probability of union, thus avoiding hemiarthroplasty.[75,76] Proximal femoral deformity may also be corrected using the valgus ITO (Figure 7). Valgus ITOs also may be useful in limb-length inequality (lengthening up to 3 cm), adult sequelae of Legg-Calvé-Perthes disease, and slipped capital femoral epiphysis. Additionally, osteonecrosis with a geographically small superolateral area of necrosis or collapse sometimes may respond favorably to a flexion-valgus osteotomy. In most instances, the goal is to move healthier articular cartilage into the weight-bearing zone of the acetabulum and to relieve impingement.

Adding extension to the osteotomy improves anterior coverage of the femoral head and reduces the clinical effects of fixed flexion contractures. Extension reduces a major source of pain and impingement and relaxes the stress of hyperlordosis on the lumbar spine. Reliable fixation usually is achieved using a high-angled blade plate; however, in the senior author's experience, 90° blade plates may be used in patients with

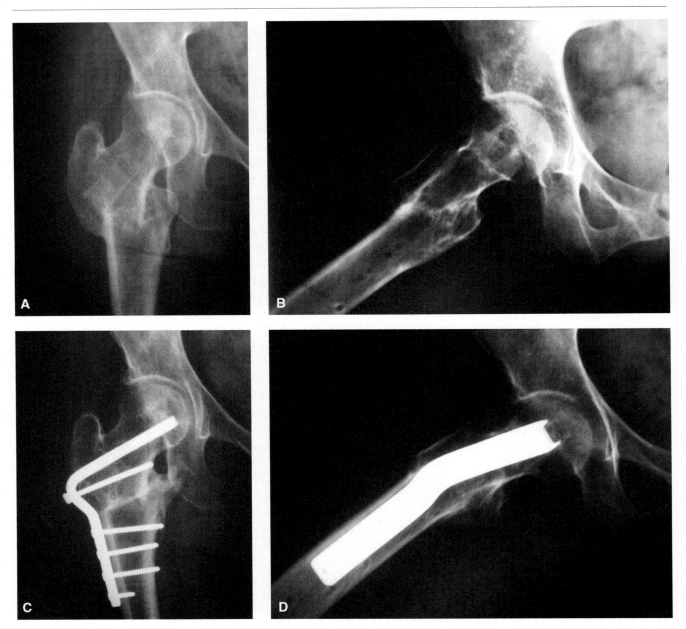

Figure 7 **A,** AP hip radiograph of a 53-year-old woman with malunion that includes displacement in the frontal and sagittal planes, malrotation, and limb lengthening of 20 mm. **B,** Frog-lateral radiograph demonstrating posterior displacement of the femoral shaft distal to the fracture. **C,** AP hip radiograph after multiplane corrective osteotomy including shortening. The leg lengths are now equal. **D,** Frog-lateral radiograph after corrective osteotomy. Note the reversal of displacement of the femoral shaft at the osteotomy site and the extension component.

small bone.

The results of valgus ITO for femoral neck nonunions have been reported in several studies. Marti and associates[1] found a 94% union rate among 50 patients. Seven of the 50 had undergone hip arthroplasty by 7-year follow-up. Weber and Cech[77] reported on 41 patients with femoral neck pseudarthroses. Of those adults with no femoral head necrosis, 91% healed, with 61% achieving normal function. Only 54% of the 13 adult patients with osteonecrosis experi- enced healing and revascularization of the femoral head, with the other patients having a poor outcome. Five osteotomies were performed in ado- lescents, with 4 of 5 patients (80%) having good or excellent results.

Maistrelli and associates[29] reported the results of 277 valgus-extension osteotomies with 67% good or excellent results at a minimum follow-up of 11 years. Better results were associated with patients younger than age 40 years at the time of surgery (76% good or excellent). Good results were obtained in 68% of patients whose degree of preoperative flexion was 60° or more, and in only 31% whose degree of flexion was less than 60°. Multiple surgeons have recommended a minimum bi-plane correction of 20° to obtain reported results.[29,78-81] At a mean follow-up of 11 years, Santore and Bombelli[74] reported on 45 patients with 75% good to excellent results after 35 valgus and 10 varus ITOs. In contrast to other reports, increased age and hip stiffness were not associated with poorer outcomes.

Historically, the most common indication for ITO was for the adult sequelae of developmental dysplasia of the hip. Isolated ITO now is indicated only occasionally because of the success of rotational acetabular procedures. A valgus-extension osteotomy is indicated with superolateral arthritis in young patients. This group had the best results in Bombelli and associates' series[78,79] as well as those of others.[82,83]

Several studies have evaluated the role of valgus ITO in the young patient with more advanced osteoarthritis. Long-term studies have reported good to excellent results for between 63% and 86% of patients, with a minimum follow-up of 10 years.[29,34,83] These ITOs, when planned and performed carefully, have not been shown to compromise future conversion to THR.[84]

Despite the heterogeneous groups with incomplete subtyping of morphologies reported in most of the literature, similar results have emerged over time. There is a con-

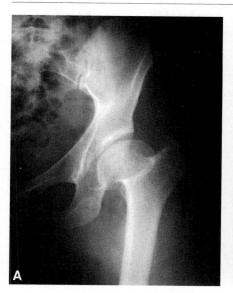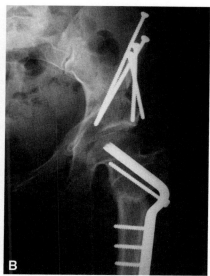

Figure 8 **A,** AP radiograph of the hip of a 41-year-old woman who was treated as a child for developmental dysplasia of the hip with closed reduction and casting. Note the residual dysplasia of the acetabulum, coxa magna, femoral neck shortening, and high-riding greater trochanter. **B,** Radiograph following combined valgus intertrochanteric and periacetabular corrective osteotomies performed under a single anesthetic.

sensus that at 10 years or more after surgery, 70% to 80% of patients continue to have satisfactory results following an appropriate valgus ITO and have not required conversion to THR.[15,29,82,84-88]

Combined Pelvic and Femoral Osteotomy
Frequently, pathology is found on both sides of the hip joint. An isolated femoral or pelvic osteotomy can be considered if the deformity is minimal on one of the two sides. However, when significant pathology exists on both sides of the joint, surgical procedures should be used for both the acetabulum and the femur (Figure 8). Selection of the appropriate procedure for each side of the joint should be based on the same criteria used in selecting an isolated procedure, and consideration should be given to the placement of the additional incision.

Summary
Osteotomies continue to play a vital role in the surgical treatment of hip pathology in the young adult. Each osteotomy should be planned and performed with consideration of the possible need for future conversion to THR. For this reason, routine removal of internal fixation implants is recommended. Appropriate use of both pelvic and femoral osteotomies can relieve pain and improve function on a lasting basis.

References
1. Marti RK, Schuller HM, Raaymakers EL: Intertrochanteric osteotomy for non-union of the femoral neck. *J Bone Joint Surg Br* 1989;71:782-787.

2. Sullivan PM, MacKenzie JR, Callaghan JJ, Johnston RC: Total hip arthroplasty with cement in patients who are less than fifty years old: A sixteen to twenty-two-year follow-up study. *J Bone Joint Surg Am* 1994;76:863-869.

3. Sochart DH, Porter ML: The long-term

results of Charnley low-friction arthroplasty in young patients who have congenital dislocation, degenerative osteoarthrosis, or rheumatoid arthritis. *J Bone Joint Surg Am* 1997;79:1599-1617.

4. Ranawat CS, Atkinson RE, Salvati EA, Wilson PD Jr: Conventional total hip arthroplasty for degenerative joint disease in patients between the ages of forty and sixty years. *J Bone Joint Surg Am* 1984;66:745-752.

5. Mont MA, Maar DC, Krackow KA, Jacobs MA, Jones LC, Hungerford DS: Total hip replacement without cement for non-inflammatory osteoarthrosis in patients who are less than forty-five years old. *J Bone Joint Surg Am* 1993;75:740-751.

6. Halley DK, Wroblewski BM: Long-term results of low-friction arthroplasty in patients 30 years of age or younger. *Clin Orthop Relat Res* 1986;211:43-50.

7. Dorr LD, Luckett M, Conaty JP: Total hip arthroplasties in patients younger than 45 years: A nine- to ten-year follow-up study. *Clin Orthop Relat Res* 1990;260:215-219.

8. Dorr LD, Takei GK, Conaty JP: Total hip arthroplasties in patients less than forty-five years old. *J Bone Joint Surg Am* 1983;65:474-479.

9. Chandler HP, Reineck FT, Wixson RL, McCarthy JC: Total hip replacement in patients younger than thirty years old: A five-year follow-up study. *J Bone Joint Surg Am* 1981;63:1426-1434.

10. Callaghan J: Results of primary total hip arthroplasty in young patients. *Instr Course Lect* 1994;43:315-321.

11. Buckwalter JA, Lohmander S: Operative treatment of osteoarthrosis: Current practice and future development. *J Bone Joint Surg Am* 1994;76:1405-1418.

12. Booth RE Jr: The closing circle: Limitations of total joint arthroplasty. *Orthopedics* 1994;17:757-759.

13. MacDonald SJ, Hersche O, Rodriguez J, Ganz R: The Bernese periacetabular osteotomy for the treatment of adult hip dysplasia. *Chir Organi Mov* 1997;82:143-154.

14. Klaue K, Durnin CW, Ganz R: The acetabular rim syndrome: A clinical presentation of dysplasia of the hip. *J Bone Joint Surg Br* 1991;73:423-429.

15. Morscher E: Intertrochanteric osteotomy in osteoarthritis of the hip, in Riley L (ed): *The Hip: Proceedings of the Eighth Open Scientific Meeting of the Hip Society.* St. Louis, MO, Mosby, 1980, pp 24-46.

16. Chandler H, Reineck F, Wixson R: Total hip replacement in patients younger than thirty years old: A five-year follow-up study. *J Bone Joint Surg Am* 1981;63:1426-1434.

17. Dorrell JH, Catterall A: The torn acetabular labrum. *J Bone Joint Surg Br* 1986;68:400-403.

18. Allen WC, Cope R: Coxa saltans: The snapping hip revisited. *J Am Acad Orthop Surg* 1995;3:303-308.

19. Altenberg AR: Acetabular labrum tears: A cause of hip pain and degenerative arthritis. *South Med J* 1977;70:174-175.

20. Byrd JW: Labral lesions: An elusive source of hip pain case reports and literature review. *Arthroscopy* 1996;12:603-612.

21. Czerny C, Hofmann S, Neuhold A, et al: Lesions of the acetabular labrum: Accuracy of MR imaging and MR arthrography in detection and staging. *Radiology* 1996;200:225-230.

22. Leunig M, Werlen S, Ungersbock A, Ito K, Ganz R: Evaluation of the acetabular labrum by MR arthrography. *J Bone Joint Surg Br* 1997;79:230-234.

23. McCarthy JC: Hip arthroscopy: Applications and technique. *J Am Acad Orthop Surg* 1995;3:115-122.

24. Lequesne M, de Seze S: False profile of the hip: A new radiographic incidence for the study of the hip. Its use in dysplasias and different coxopathies. *Rev Rhum Mal Osteoartic* 1961;28:643-652.

25. Li PL, Ganz R: Morphologic features of congenital acetabular dysplasia: One in six is retroverted. *Clin Orthop Relat Res* 2003;416:245-253.

26. Ikeda T, Awaya G, Suzuki S, Okeda Y, Tada H: Torn acetabular labrum in young patients: Arthroscopic diagnosis and management. *J Bone Joint Surg Br* 1988;70:13-16.

27. Klaue K, Wallin A, Ganz R: CT evaluation of coverage and congruency of the hip prior to osteotomy. *Clin Orthop Relat Res* 1988;232:15-25.

28. Millis MB, Murphy SB: Use of computed tomographic reconstruction in planning osteotomies of the hip. *Clin Orthop Relat Res* 1992;274:154-159.

29. Maistrelli GL, Gerundini M, Fusco U, Bombelli R, Bombelli M, Avai A: Valgus-extension osteotomy for osteoarthritis of the hip: Indications and long-term results. *J Bone Joint Surg Br* 1990;72:653-657.

30. Handelsman JE: The Chiari pelvic sliding osteotomy. *Orthop Clin North Am* 1980;11:105-125.

31. Trousdale RT, Ekkernkamp A, Ganz R, Wallrichs SL: Periacetabular and intertrochanteric osteotomy for the treatment of osteoarthrosis in dysplastic hips. *J Bone Joint Surg Am* 1995;77:73-85.

32. Nishimatsu H, Iida H, Kawanabe K, Tamura J, Nakamura T: The modified Spitzy shelf operation for patients with dysplasia of the hip: A 24-year follow-up study. *J Bone Joint Surg Br* 2002;84:647-652.

33. Ohashi H, Hirohashi K, Yamano Y: Factors influencing the outcome of Chiari pelvic osteotomy: A long-term follow-up. *J Bone Joint Surg Br* 2000;82:517-525.

34. Iwase T, Hasegawa Y, Kawamoto K, Iwasada S, Yamada K, Iwata H: Twenty years' followup of intertrochanteric osteotomy for treatment of the dysplastic hip. *Clin Orthop Relat Res* 1996;331:245-255.

35. Nakamura N, Sugano N, Masuhara K, Ohzono K, Takaoka K: Bone scintigraphy as an indicator for dome osteotomy of the pelvis: Comparison between scintigraphy, radiography and outcome in 57 hips. *Acta Orthop Scand* 1996;67:138-142.

36. de Kleuver M, Kooijman MA, Pavlov PW, Veth RP: Triple osteotomy of the pelvis for acetabular dysplasia: Results at 8 to 15 years. *J Bone Joint Surg Br* 1997;79:225-229.

37. Reynolds DA: Chiari innominate osteotomy in adults: Technique, indications and contra-indications. *J Bone Joint Surg Br* 1986;68:45-54.

38. Calvert PT, August AC, Albert JS, Kemp HB, Catterall A: The Chiari pelvic osteotomy: A review of the long-term results. *J Bone Joint Surg Br* 1987;69:551-555.

39. Trousdale RT, Cabanela ME: Lessons learned after more than 250 periacetabular osteotomies. *Acta Orthop Scand* 2003;74:119-126.

40. Salter RB: Innominate osteotomy in the treatment of congenital dislocation and subluxation of the hip. *J Bone Joint Surg Br* 1961;43:518.

41. Wedge JH, Salter RB: Innominate osteotomy: Its role in the arrest of secondary degenerative arthritis of the hip in the adult. *Clin Orthop Relat Res* 1974;98:214-224.

42. Bohm P, Weber G: Salter's innominate osteotomy for hip dysplasia in adolescents and young adults: Results in 58 patients (69 osteotomies) at 4-12 years. *Acta Orthop Scand* 2003;74:277-286.

43. McCarthy JJ, Fox JS, Gurd AR: Innominate osteotomy in adolescents and adults who have acetabular dysplasia. *J Bone Joint Surg Am* 1996;78:1455-1461.

44. Sutherland DH, Greenfield R: Double innominate osteotomy. *J Bone Joint Surg Am* 1977;59:1082-1091.

45. Peters CL, Fukushima BW, Park TK, Coleman SS, Dunn HK: Triple innominate osteotomy in young adults for the treatment of acetabular dysplasia: A 9-year follow-up study. *Orthopedics* 2001;24:565-569.

46. Peters CL, Beck M, Dunn HK: Total hip arthroplasty in young adults after failed triple innominate osteotomy. *J Arthroplasty* 2001;16:188-195.

47. Wagner H: Experiences with spherical acetabular osteotomy for the correction of the dysplastic acetabulum, in Weil UH (ed): *Progress in Orthopaedic Surgery: Acetabular Dysplasia: Skeletal Dysplasia in Childhood*, ed 2. New York, NY, Springer, 1978, pp 131-145.

48. Ninomiya S, Tagawa H: Rotational acetabular osteotomy for the dysplastic hip. *J Bone Joint Surg Am* 1984;66:430-436.

49. Nakamura S, Ninomiya S, Takatori Y, Morimoto S, Umeyama T: Long-term outcome of rotational acetabular osteotomy: 145 hips followed for 10-23 years. *Acta Orthop Scand* 1998;69:259-265.

50. Yano H, Sano S, Nagata Y, et al: Modified rotational acetabular osteotomy (RAO) for advanced osteoarthritis of the hip joint in the middle-aged person: First report. *Arch Orthop Trauma Surg* 1990;109:121-125.

51. Murphy SB, Millis MB, Hall JE: Surgical correction of acetabular dysplasia in the adult: A Boston experience. *Clin Orthop Relat Res* 1999;363:38-44.

52. Tonnis D, Behrens K, Tscharani F: A new technique of triple osteotomy for turning dysplastic acetabula in adolescents and adults. *Z Orthop Ihre Grenzgeb* 1981;119:253-265.

53. Kooijman MA, Pavlov PW: Triple osteotomy of the pelvis: A review of 51 cases. *Clin Orthop Relat Res* 1990;255:133-137.

54. Ganz R, Klaue K, Vinh TS, Mast JW: A new periacetabular osteotomy for the treatment of hip dysplasias: Technique and preliminary results. *Clin Orthop Relat Res* 1988;232:26-36.

55. Pogliacomi F, Stark A, Vaienti E, Wallensten R: Periacetabular osteotomy of the hip: The ilioinguinal approach. *Acta Biomed Ateneo Parmense* 2003;74:38-46.

56. Murphy SB, Millis MB: Periacetabular osteotomy without abductor dissection using direct anterior exposure. *Clin Orthop Relat Res* 1999;364:92-98.

57. Davey JP, Santore RF: Complications of periacetabular osteotomy. *Clin Orthop Relat Res* 1999;363:33-37.

58. Hussell JG, Rodriguez JA, Ganz R: Technical complications of the Bernese periacetabular osteotomy. *Clin Orthop Relat Res* 1999;363:81-92.

59. König F: Osteoplastische Behandlung der kongenital Hüftgelenkluxation. *Verh Deutsch Ges Chir* 1891;20:75-80.

60. Love BR, Stevens PM, Williams PF: A long-term review of shelf arthroplasty. *J Bone Joint Surg Br* 1980;62:321-325.

61. Migaud H, Chantelot C, Giraud F, Fontaine C, Duquennay A: Long-term survivorship of hip shelf arthroplasty and Chiari osteotomy in adults. *Clin Orthop* 2004;418:81-86.

62. Hamanishi C, Tanaka S, Yamamuro T: The Spitzy shelf operation for the dysplastic hip: Retrospective 10 (5-25) year study of 124 cases. *Acta Orthop Scand* 1992;63:273-277.

63. Chiari K: Medial displacement osteotomy of the pelvis. *Clin Orthop Relat Res* 1974;98:55-71.

64. Windhager R, Pongracz N, Schonecker W, Kotz R: Chiari osteotomy for congenital dislocation and subluxation of the hip: Results after 20 to 34 years follow-up. *J Bone Joint Surg Br* 1991;73:890-895.

65. Macnicol MF, Lo HK, Yong KF: Pelvic remodelling after the Chiari osteotomy: A long-term review. *J Bone Joint Surg Br* 2004;86:648-654.

66. Rozkydal Z, Kovanda M: Chiari pelvic osteotomy in the management of developmental hip dysplasia: A long term follow-up. *Bratisl Lek Listy* 2003;104:7-13.

67. Winkelmann W: The narrowing of the bony pelvic cavity (birth canal) by the different osteotomies of the pelvis. *Arch Orthop Trauma Surg* 1984;102:159-162.

68. Kusswetter W, Magers H: Changes in the pelvis after the Chiari and Salter osteotomies. *Int Orthop* 1985;9:139-146.

69. Loder RT, Karol LA, Johnson S: Influence of pelvic osteotomy on birth canal size. *Arch Orthop Trauma Surg* 1993;112:210-214.

70. Millis MB, Murphy SB, Poss R: Osteotomies about the hip for the prevention and treatment of osteoarthrosis. *Instr Course Lect* 1996;45:209-226.

71. DePalma AF, Rothman RH, Klemek JS: Osteotomy of the proximal femur in degenerative arthritis. *Clin Orthop Relat Res* 1970;73:109-115.

72. Miegel RE, Harris WH: Medial-displacement intertrochanteric osteotomy in the treatment of osteoarthritis of the hip: A long-term follow-up study. *J Bone Joint Surg Am* 1984;66:878-887.

73. Reigstad A, Gronmark T: Osteoarthritis of the hip treated by intertrochanteric osteotomy: A long-term follow-up. *J Bone Joint Surg Am* 1984;66:1-6.

74. Santore RF, Bombelli R: Long-term follow-up of the Bombelli experience with osteotomy for osteoarthritis: Results at 11 years. *Hip* 1983;106-128.

75. Blount W: Blade plate internal fixation for high femoral osteotomies. *J Bone Joint Surg Am* 1943;25:319.

76. Blount W: Proximal osteotomies of the femur. *Instr Course Lect* 1952;9:1.

77. Weber B, Cech O: *Pseudoarthrosis*. Bern, Switzerland, Hans Huber, 1976.

78. Bombelli R, Gerundini M, Aronson J: The biomechanical basis for osteotomy in the treatment of osteoarthritis of the hip: Results in younger patients. *Hip* 1984;18-42.

79. Bombelli R, Santore RF, Poss R: Mechanics of the normal and osteoarthritic hip: A new perspective. *Clin Orthop Relat Res* 1984;182:69-78.

80. Aronson J, Schatzker J: *The Intertrochanteric Osteotomy*. Berlin, Germany, Springer-Verlag, 1984.

81. Brand RA: Hip osteotomies: A biomechanical consideration. *J Am Acad Orthop Surg* 1997;5:282-291.

82. Gotoh E, Inao S, Okamoto T, Ando M: Valgus-extension osteotomy for advanced osteoarthritis in dysplastic hips: Results at 12 to 18 years. *J Bone Joint Surg Br* 1997;79:609-615.

83. Langlais F, Roure JL, Maquet P: Valgus osteotomy in severe osteoarthritis of the hip. *J Bone Joint Surg Br* 1979;61:424-431.

84. Iwase T, Hasegawa Y, Iwasada S, Kitamura S, Iwata H: Total hip arthroplasty after failed intertrochanteric

valgus osteotomy for advanced osteoarthrosis. *Clin Orthop Relat Res* 1999;364:175-181.

85. Pauwels F: *Biomechanics of the Normal and Diseased Hip*. Berlin, Germany, Springer-Verlag, 1976.

86. Poss R: The role of osteotomy in the treatment of osteoarthritis of the hip. *J Bone Joint Surg Am* 1984;66:144-151.

87. Schneider R: Intertrochanteric osteotomy in osteoarthritis of the hip joint, in Schatzker J (ed): *The Intertrochanteric Osteotomy*. New York, NY, Springer-Verlag, 1984.

88. Schneider R: Results of intertrochanteric osteotomies in patients with coxarthrosis 12-15 years after surgery, in Weil H (ed): *Joint Preserving Procedures of the Lower Extremities: Progress in Orthopaedic Surgery*. Berlin, Germany, Springer-Verlag, 1980.

Nonarthroplasty Surgical Treatment of Hip Osteoarthritis

Michael Leunig, MD
Javad Parvizi, MD
Reinhold Ganz, MD

Abstract

The two conditions that give rise to osteoarthritis of the hip are dysplasia and nondysplasia. Dysplasia, commonly associated with anterolateral acetabular deficiency, may lead to osteoarthritis in 40% of patients in the United States with this condition. In a distinct category of patients with so-called idiopathic arthritis, there is no apparently identifiable cause for osteoarthritis. There is emerging evidence that subtle morphologic abnormalities around the hip, resulting in femoroacetabular impingement, may often be a contributing factor to osteoarthritis in young patients.

Biomechanical causes of hip osteoarthritis generally include concentric or eccentric overload.[1] In the dysplastic hip, a maloriented articular surface with a decreased contact area results in eccentric overload of the anterosuperior area and promotes the development of early hip osteoarthritis.[2-4] Although this vertical overload provides a satisfactory explanation for the onset of hip osteoarthritis in the dysplastic acetabulum, it fails to provide a convincing explanation for the development of osteoarthritis in a group of young patients with normal skeletal structures and normal intra-articular pressure. Hence, alternative mechanisms may be responsible for the development of osteoarthritis in these patients.

Based on clinical experience, it is now known that in many instances of idiopathic arthritis, predisposing factors in the form of femoroacetabular impingement exist that are not easily recognized using traditional diagnostic modalities.[5-8] Reduced joint clearance resulting in repetitive contact between the prosthetic femoral neck and the edge of the acetabular component is a well-recognized problem in total hip replacement.[9-11] A similar mechanism of repetitive impingement in the constrained native hip may also result in chondral and/or labral lesions. This theory implies that in some patients the presence of aberrant morphology involving the proximal femur and/or the acetabulum results in abnormal contact between the femoral neck and the acetabular rim during terminal motion of the hip. This abnormal contact, in turn, can lead to development of lesions in the labrum and the adjacent acetabular cartilage. These early chondral and labral lesions continue to progress and result in degenerative joint disease if the underlying cause of impingement is not addressed.

Femoroacetabular Impingement

The concept of femoroacetabular impingement is not entirely novel. Stulberg and associates[12] are credited with introducing the term "pistol grip" deformity to describe the abnormal morphologic features of the femoral head and neck on AP radiographs of patients with early idiopathic osteoarthritis. Although this term was introduced to describe the radiologic appearance of morphologic abnormality, it did not elucidate the underlying mechanisms resulting in early osteoarthritis. An abnormal anatomic relationship between the femoral head and neck has also been suggested by other authors as a possible cause for osteoarthritis.[3,4,13,14] Several investigators suggested subclinical displacement of the femoral epiphysis as a risk factor for osteoarthritis and have used the terms "head-tilt" or "post-slip" to describe the deformity resulting from mildly slipped capital femoral epiphysis.[3,7,12,15] In a small series of consecutive patients,[16,17] evidence has been reported to support the notion of an anterior metaphyseal femoroacetabular impingement in patients with slipped capital femoral epiphysis.[13] Similar configurations may result from femoral neck fractures in which the fracture malunited in a retroverted position,[18] from morphologic deviations (residual childhood diseases such as Legg-Calvé-Perthes disease), and from surgical interventions such as femoral osteotomies that lead to a reduction of the joint clearance. Most patients with femoroacetabular impingement, however, typically lack a history of detected predisposing factors.

In addition to deviations at the proximal femur, a variety of morphologic changes of the acetabulum may predispose patients to femoroacetabular impingement, including acetabular retroversion, coxa profunda, and protrusio acetabuli, as well as some posttraumatic deformities. Retroversion of the acetabulum has been described as a posterior orientation of the acetabular opening.[19] A retroverted acetabulum may occur alone[20] or as part of complex acetabular developmental deformities.[3] It results in a prominent anterolateral acetabular overcoverage, creating an obstacle for flexion and internal rotation, predisposing patients to femoroacetabular impingement. Problems may be more pronounced if the prominent acetabular edge impinges against a proximal femur with an insufficient femoral head

and neck offset, as seen in patients with hips with a pistol grip deformity.[12,21] Finally, coxa profunda and protrusio acetabuli predispose patients to femoroacetabular impingement by increasing the relative depth of the acetabulum.[22,23]

Cam Femoroacetabular Impingement
Based on the skeletal morphology and the pattern of chondral and labral injuries observed during surgical dislocation of the hip, two distinct types of femoroacetabular impingement have been distinguished: cam femoroacetabular impingement and pincer femoroacetabular impingement. Cam femoroacetabular impingement (alteration of the femoral head-neck junction) is caused by the entry of an abnormal femoral head with increasing radius into the acetabulum during forceful motion, especially flexion.[7,24] The resulting shear forces produce an outside-in abrasion of the acetabular cartilage and/or its avulsion from the labrum and the subchondral bone in a relatively constant location (the anterosuperior rim area). Chondral avulsion, in turn, can lead to tear or detachment of the primarily uninvolved labrum.

Pincer Femoroacetabular Impingement
Pincer femoroacetabular impingement is the result of linear contact between the acetabular rim and the femoral head-neck junction. The femoral head may be normal in morphology, and the abutment is the result of acetabular abnormality. The acetabular abnormality may be generalized, as in patients with a deep socket, or localized anteriorly over coverage, as in patients with acetabular retroversion. The first structure to fail in this situation may

be the acetabular labrum. Continued impact of abutment results in degeneration of the labrum, with intrasubstance ganglion formation. Ossification of the rim leads to further deepening of the acetabulum and worsening of the overcoverage. The persistent abutment (usually anterior) can lead to chronic leverage of the head in the acetabulum and over time can result in contrecoup chondral damage of the posteroinferior head and/or acetabulum, resulting in central joint space narrowing. Cam and pincer femoroacetabular impingement are also discussed in chapters 14 and 36.

Assessment of Femoroacetabular Impingement
Pincer femoroacetabular impingement is more common in middle-aged females with morphologic abnormality of the acetabulum. Chondral lesions in pincer femoroacetabular impingement may remain limited to a small rim area of the acetabulum over a long period and are therefore more benign. This is in contrast to deep and extensive chondral lesions that are seen with cam femoroacetabular impingement, which is more common in young males with morphologic abnormality involving the femoral head-neck junction. Two sets of observations made during surgical dislocation of the hip have furnished the evidence in support of the theory that chondral injury can lead to labral tear and not the reverse, as has been suggested by some surgeons who perform arthroscopic examination of the hip.[25] First, labral tears or detachments occur at the articular and not the capsular margin. Second, chondral damage is frequently observed without labral tears in patients who are in the early stages

of femoroacetabular impingement. Labral tears not associated with chondral injuries are only observed in patients with early pincer femoroacetabular impingement. Labral tears noted during arthroscopic examination of the hip (particularly those in the anterosuperior region of the acetabulum)[25] most likely represent femoroacetabular impingement. Although some of these patients may have a medical history and clinical examination evidence that suggest a traumatic etiology and seem to confirm the presence of labral tears, experience has shown that it is the underlying femoroacetabular impingement, however subtle, that leads to the labral lesion as part of a more extensive process. This premise is supported by the observation that most labral tears noted during hip arthroscopy are also associated with chondral damage.[25]

Clinical Assessment

Femoroacetabular impingement usually occurs in active young adults and begins with slow onset of groin pain that often is preceded by a minor traumatic event. During the initial stages of the disease, the pain is intermittent and may be exacerbated by excessive demands on the hip, such as that from athletic activities or prolonged walking. The pain is often present after sitting for a prolonged period. Frequently, these symptoms are considered to be of muscular origin and are treated with physical therapy, including stretching. Pain medication and chondroprotective drugs are commonly administered. Based on the presence of normal pelvic radiographs, these patients are sometimes subjected to extensive diagnostic workup and inappropriate surgical modalities,[26-28] including tenotomy,[29] laparoscopy,[30,31] laparotomy,[32] lumbar spine

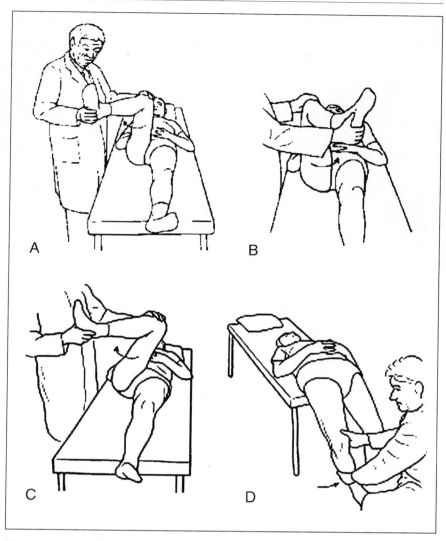

Figure 1 Internal rotation (**A**) and external rotation (**B**) in flexion. The patient is placed supine with the hip flexed to 90°. Rotation is assessed in neutral abduction. In the impingement test, flexion, internal rotation, and adduction (**C**) test for the anterior femoroacetabular impingement, whereas extension and external rotation (**D**) test for posterior femoroacetabular impingement.

decompression,[33] and inguinal hernia repair.[34] More detailed clinical investigation almost always reveals an internal rotation, which is limited. Thus, the leading symptoms of femoroacetabular impingement are pain with motion and limited internal rotation, whereas overall hip function is almost unaffected according to established scores (Figure 1).

Radiographic Assessment

Conventional radiography is indispensable for the assessment of hip biomechanics; however, it may be insufficient to detect borderline femoral alterations leading to femoroacetabular impingement.[8] To better delineate alterations of intra-articular structures within the hip that are not readily detectable using conventional radiography, improve-

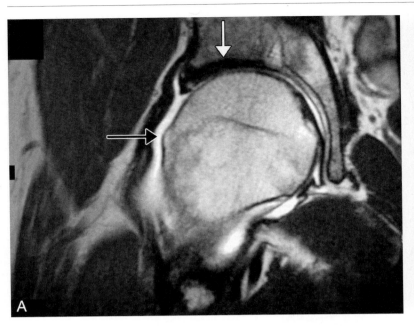
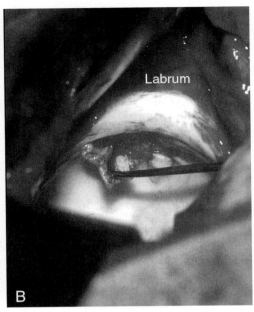

Figure 2 **A,** MRA of femoroacetabular impingement using radial sequencing (proton density weighted sequence) shows a normal size labrum and an undersurface tear (*white arrow*) caused by the anterior femoral prominence (*black arrow*). **B,** Intraoperative photograph shows the corresponding acetabular full-thickness cartilage damage, whereas the labral substance initially remains uninvolved, which indicates that the cartilage is avulsed from the labrum and not the labrum from the cartilage. (Reproduced with permission from Leunig M, Podeszwa D, Beck M, Werlen S, Ganz R: Magnetic resonance arthrography of labral disorders in dysplasia and impingement hips. *Clin Orthop* 2004;418:74-80.)

ments in current techniques of MRI and magnetic resonance arthrography (MRA) have been developed.[35,36] Small flexible surface coils are used to selectively show the hip to be examined, gadolinium is applied intra-articularly, radial imaging sequences are obtained that are perpendicular to the true plane of the acetabulum (Figure 2). Based on these modifications, an undistorted image of each aspect of the acetabular rim can be obtained, with regions of special interest defined and pathologies identified, which may possibly be related to morphologies of the acetabulum and the proximal end of the femur. Noninvasive or minimally invasive protocols have also been developed to determine the femoral head-neck offset,[7] the femoral head-neck contour,[24] and the extension of the lateral physeal scar.[37]

Findings from MRA indicate that the anterosuperior acetabulum may represent the initial fatiguing site of the hip under both impingement conditions. The capability of MRA to depict these differences in labral pathologies suggests that this method can be a helpful diagnostic tool to define the most appropriate treatment strategy in patients with conventional radiographic signs of developmental dysplasia of the hip who actually have femoroacetabular impingement.[38]

Treatment Options

Appropriate management of patients with femoroacetabular impingement commences with a trial of conservative treatment, which may include activity modification, restriction of athletic activities, and reduction of excessive motion and demand on the hip. A trial of non-

steroidal anti-inflammatory medications may be appropriate to relieve pain of acute onset, but doing so may also mask the symptoms of the underlying destructive process. Physical therapy, with emphasis on improving passive range of motion or stretching, is not beneficial but rather it is counterproductive. Although conservative management is likely to be temporarily successful in some patients, the young age of these patients and their high activity levels and athletic ambitions usually jeopardize patient compliance.

Recognition of the detrimental effect of femoroacetabular impingement has prompted the development of novel joint-preserving surgical approaches[39] that are aimed at delivering timely treatment and decelerating the degenerative process set forth by the impingement. For this new joint-preserving surgical approach, a safe technique for surgical dislocation of the hip was required.[5] This technique was developed based on the exact topographic knowledge of the course of the blood supply to the femoral head. This joint-preserving approach is also discussed in chapter 36.

Vascular Supply of the Femoral Head

The primary and only necessary source for the blood supply to the head of the femur is the deep branch of the medial femoral circumflex artery. It is endangered with posterior approaches to the hip and pelvis because the short external rotators are divided. The anatomy of the medial femoral circumflex artery and its branches have been studied based on dissections of 24 cadaver hips after injection of neoprene latex into the femoral or internal iliac arteries (Figure 3). The most important findings were that the deep branch of the medial femoral circumflex artery crosses the obturator externus muscle posteriorly while it runs anteriorly to the short external rotators, the posterior femoral neck contains no vessels feeding the femoral neck, and the deep branch of the medial femoral circumflex artery is not stretched or ruptured during hip dislocation as long as the external rotators (especially the obturator externus muscle) are intact.

Technique of Surgical Dislocation

Based on the findings of blood supply studies, a technique for surgical dislocation (Figure 4) of the hip was developed.[5] This technique is discussed in detail in chapter 14.

It combines different aspects of approaches reported previously and consists of an anterior dislocation through a posterior approach with a

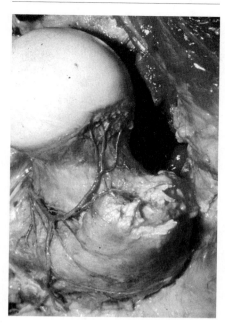

Figure 3 Intraoperative photograph showing the course of the deep branch of the medial femoral circumflex artery along the posterior part of the greater trochanter before its terminal branches enter the femoral head. (Reproduced with permission from Ganz R, MacDonald SJ: Indications and modern technique of proximal femoral osteotomies in adults. *Semin Arthroplasty* 1997;8:38-50.)

trochanteric flip osteotomy.[40] The external rotator muscles are not divided, and the medial femoral circumflex artery is protected by the intact obturator externus. Early experience using this approach in 213 consecutive hips over 7 years, including hips of 19 patients who underwent simultaneous intertrochanteric osteotomy, has been assessed. Minimal morbidity was associated with the technique (no osteonecrosis), and it has been shown to allow for the treatment of a variety of conditions that may not respond well to other methods, including arthroscopy. Surgical dislocation gives new insight into the pathogenesis of some hip disorders and the possibil-

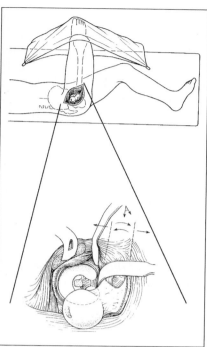

Figure 4 Schematic representation of the surgical dislocation of the hip. As shown in the inset, the exposure provides full access to the acetabulum, femoral neck, and femoral head. The sites and the cause of impingement can be identified accurately and appropriate treatment can be delivered by this technique of joint-preserving surgery. (Reproduced with permission from Lavigne M, Parvizi J, Beck M, Siebenrock KA, Ganz R, Leunig M: Anterior femoroacetabular impingement: Part I: Technique of joint preserving surgery. *Clin Orthop Relat Res* 2004;418:61-66.)

ity of preserving the hip with techniques such as transplantation of cartilage.

In one study, laser Doppler flowmetry with a high-energy (20-mW) laser was used to confirm perfusion of the femoral head intraoperatively in 32 hips during surgical dislocation.[41] During subluxation or dislocation, blood flow was impaired when the posterosuperior femoral neck was allowed to rest on the posterior acetabular rim. A pulsatile signal returned when the hip was reduced or was taken out of extreme positions when dislocated. After the final reduction, the signal amplitudes were first slightly lower than the initial value (on average 12%), but they were restored to initial levels within 30 minutes. Most of the signal changes can be explained by compromising of the extraosseous branches of the medial femoral circumflex artery and are reversible. These findings suggest that perfusion of the femoral head is maintained after dislocation if specific surgical precautions are followed.

Femoroacetabular Impingement Osteoplasty

Surgical treatment of femoroacetabular impingement focuses on improving the clearance for hip motion and alleviation of femoral abutment against the acetabular rim. The type of treatment modality proposed depends on various factors, but it is mainly determined by the underlying morphologic abnormality giving rise to femoroacetabular impingement. A combination of anatomic aberrations or causal factors often may coexist. Recognition and appropriate addressing of all these factors is necessary to ensure successful outcome. The surgical dislocation of the hip provides a full 360° view of the femoral head and the acetabulum for inspection. The site of impingement is identified, and the joint surfaces are examined for the presence of any lesions. Hip arthroscopy seems to be an attractive procedure for the treatment of femoroacetabular impingement.[42,43] Snow and associates[44] described the use of this technique to treat femoroacetabular impingement in patients with femoral head deformities caused by Legg-Calvé-Perthes disease. Femoroacetabular impingement-free range of motion of the

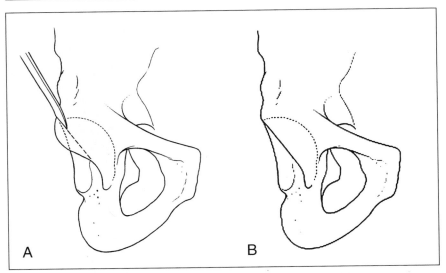

Figure 5 Schematic representation of a resection osteoplasty of the excessive anterior rim of the acetabulum before (**A**) and after (**B**) the osteoplasty removes the site of anterior impingement. (Reproduced with permission from Lavigne M, Parvizi J, Beck M, Siebenrock KA, Ganz R, Leunig M: Anterior femoroacetabular impingement: Part I: Technique of joint preserving surgery. *Clin Orthop Relat Res* 2004;418:61-66.)

hip improved after débridement of the anterior femoral head that was hinging on the anterior acetabular rim during hip flexion.[45] Although débridement or reattachment of labral tears may be done with arthroscopy, the constrained hip renders access to the underlying cause of impingement technically challenging if not impossible.

On the acetabular side, the local or global overcoverage can be addressed by resection osteoplasty of the excessive acetabular rim (Figure 5), by reorientation of a retroverted acetabulum,[19] or by a periacetabular osteotomy.[45] The acetabular depth, in particular the posterior wall, and the status of the acetabular articular cartilage determines which of the aforementioned options is elected. In patients with relatively intact acetabular cartilage and lack of posterior overcoverage, reverse periacetabular osteotomy is preferred. In contrast, in patients with relative posterior overcoverage or a chondral lesion of the

acetabular area to be reoriented, excision osteoplasty is preferred.

On the femoral side, the clearance of the femoral neck during flexion can be improved by resection osteoplasty of the prominent anterior neck or nonspherical femoral head (Figure 6), which optimizes the femoral head-neck offset or the sphericity of the head. Although infrequent, reorientation of the proximal femur with a flexion-valgus intertrochanteric osteotomy[46] also can be done to reduce femoroacetabular impingement in patients with decreased anteversion or varus position of the femoral neck. Relative femoral neck lengthening with trochanteric advancement presents another technique for increasing clearance.

It has been theorized that with the surgical elimination of cam or pincer type femoroacetabular impingement, further osteoarthritis of the hip can be prevented or delayed. To assess the potential of this approach, 19 consecutive young adults

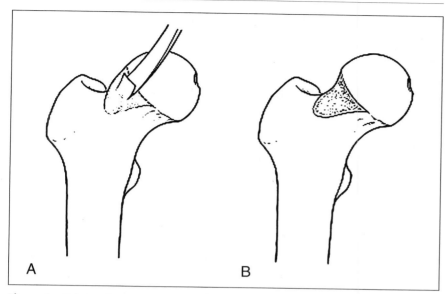

Figure 6 Schematic representation of a resection osteoplasty of the femoral head-neck junction before (**A**) and after (**B**) the osteoplasty recreates the normal concave contour of the femoral neck. (Reproduced with permission from Lavigne M, Parvizi J, Beck M, Siebenrock KA, Ganz R, Leunig M: Anterior femoroacetabular impingement: Part I: Technique of joint preserving surgery. *Clin Orthop Relat Res* 2004;418: 61-66.)

were prospectively followed-up after surgical treatment of femoroacetabular impingement for an average of 5 years.[47] The condition of most hips was rated as excellent to good, with pain scores having improved considerably. In stable hips without subluxation of the femoral head into the acetabular cartilage defect, no additional joint space narrowing occurred. This exploratory study, therefore, indicated that surgical dislocation combined with offset optimization may yield good results in patients with early degenerative changes not exceeding grade I osteoarthritis. However, results may be potentially unsatisfactory in patients with advanced degenerative changes and those with extensive articular cartilage damage.

Summary

Through extensive clinical observations with more than 600 surgical dislocations of the hip, it has been observed that femoroacetabular impingement results in lesions of the joint and acts as an initiator for early degenerative disease of the hip in patients with idiopathic osteoarthritis. These observations provided the impetus for devising novel therapeutic modalities that have helped achieve relief of symptoms and improvement in function. These surgical procedures are less likely to be successful in patients presenting late who have evidence of extensive articular cartilage injuries. These patients have often been misdiagnosed or have been subjected to a prolonged period of conservative treatment. Early recognition of femoroacetabular impingement and timely delivery of care is likely to have a considerable impact on the natural history of the disease, delaying the onset of end-stage osteoarthritis in young, active patients.

References

1. Pauwels F (ed): *Biomechanics of the Normal and Diseased Hip: Theoretical Foundation, Technique and Results of Treatment. An Atlas.* Berlin, Germany, Springer Verlag, 1976.

2. Murphy SB, Kijewski PK, Millis MB, et al: Acetabular dysplasia in the adolescent and young adult. *Clin Orthop* 1990;261:214-223.

3. Murray RO: The aetiology of primary osteoarthritis of the hip. *Br J Radiol* 1965;38:810-824.

4. Solomon L: Patterns of osteoarthritis of the hip. *J Bone Joint Surg Br* 1976;58:176-183.

5. Ganz R, Gill TJ, Gautier E, Ganz K, Krügel N, Berlemann U: Surgical dislocation of the adult hip: A technique with full access to femoral head and acetabulum without the risk of avascular necrosis. *J Bone Joint Surg Br* 2001;83:1119-1124.

6. Ganz R, Parvizi J, Beck M, Leunig M, Nötzli H, Siebenrock KA: Femoro-acetabular impingement: An important cause of early osteoarthritis of the hip. *Clin Orthop Relat Res* 2003;417:112-120.

7. Ito K, Minka MA II, Leunig M, Werlen S, Ganz R: Femoroacetabular impingement and the cam-effect: A MRI-based quantitative anatomical study of the femoral head-neck offset. *J Bone Joint Surg Br* 2001;83:171-176.

8. Locher S, Werlen S, Leunig M, Ganz R: Inadequate detectability of early stages of coxarthrosis with conventional roentgen images. *Z Orthop Ihre Grenzgeb* 2001;139:70-74.

9. Iida H, Kaneda E, Takada H, Uchida K, Kawanabe K, Nakamura T: Metallosis due to impingement between the socket and the femoral neck in a metal-on-metal bearing total hip prosthesis: A case report. *J Bone Joint Surg Am* 1999;81:400-403.

10. Kobayashi S, Takaoka K, Tsukada A, Ueno M: Polyethylene wear from femoral bipolar neck-cup impingement as a cause of femoral prosthetic loosening. *Arch Orthop Trauma Surg* 1998;117:390-391.

11. Yamaguchi M, Akisue T, Bauer TW, Hashimoto Y: The spatial location of impingement in total hip arthroplasty. *J Arthroplasty* 2000;15:305-313.

12. Stulberg SD, Cordell LD, Harris WH, Ramsey PL, MacEwen GD: Unrecognized childhood disease: A major

cause of idiopathic osteoarthritis of the hip, in Hip T (ed): *Proceedings of the Third Meeting of the Hip Society*, 1975, pp 212-228.

13. Rab GT: The geometry of slipped capital femoral epiphysis: Implications for movement, impingement, and corrective osteotomy. *J Pediatr Orthop* 1999;19:419-424.

14. Tonnis D, Heinecke A: Acetabular and femoral anteversion: Relationship with osteoarthritis of the hip. *J Bone Joint Surg Am* 1999;81:1747-1770.

15. Goodman DA, Feighan JE, Smith AD, Latimer B, Buly RL, Cooperman DR: Subclinical slipped capital femoral epiphysis: Relationship to osteoarthrosis of the hip. *J Bone Joint Surg Am* 1997;79:1489-1497.

16. Leunig M, Casillas MM, Hamlet M, et al: Slipped capital femoral epiphysis: Early mechanical damage to the acetabular cartilage by a prominent femoral metaphysis. *Acta Orthop Scand* 2000;71:370-375.

17. Leunig M, Fraitzl CR, Ganz R: Early damage to the acetabular cartilage in slipped capital femoral epiphysis: Therapeutic consequences. *Orthopade* 2002;31:894-899.

18. Eijer H, Myers SR, Ganz R: Anterior femoroacetabular impingement after femoral neck fractures. *J Orthop Trauma* 2001;15:475-481.

19. Reynolds D, Lucas J, Klaue K: Retroversion of the acetabulum: A cause of hip pain. *J Bone Joint Surg Br* 1999;81:281-288.

20. Dora C, Zurbach J, Hersche O, Ganz R: Pathomorphologic characteristics of posttraumatic acetabular dysplasia. *J Orthop Trauma* 2000;14:483-489.

21. Harris WH: Etiology of osteoarthritis of the hip. *Clin Orthop* 1986;213:20-33.

22. Gekeler J: Coxarthrosis with a deep acetabulum (proceedings). *Z Orthop Ihre Grenzgeb* 1978;116:454.

23. Klaue K, Durnin CW, Ganz R: The acetabular rim syndrome: A clinical presentation of dysplasia of the hip. *J Bone Joint Surg Br* 1991;73:423-429.

24. Notzli HP, Wyss TF, Stoecklin CH, Schmid MR, Treiber K, Hodler J: The contour of the femoral head-neck junction as a predictor for the risk of anterior impingement. *J Bone Joint Surg Br* 2002;84:556-560.

25. McCarthy JC, Noble PC, Schuck MR, Wright J, Lee J: The role of labral lesions to development of early degenerative hip disease. *Clin Orthop* 2001;393:25-37.

26. Ekberg O, Persson NH, Abrahamsson PA, Westlin NE, Lilja B: Longstanding groin pain in athletes: A multidisciplinary approach. *Sports Med* 1988;6:56-61.

27. Fricker PA: Management of groin pain in athletes. *Br J Sports Med* 1997;31:97-101.

28. Gibbon WW: Letter. *Lancet* 1999;353:1444-1445.

29. MacDonald SJ, Garbuz D, Ganz R: Clinical evaluation of the symptomatic young adult hip. *Semin Arthroplasty* 1997;8:3-9.

30. Azurin DJ, Go LS, Schuricht A, McShane J, Bartolozzi A: Endoscopic preperitoneal herniorrhaphy in professional athletes with groin pain. *J Laparoendosc Adv Surg Tech A* 1997;7:7-12.

31. Eames NW, Deans GT, Lawson JT, Irwin ST: Herniography for occult hernia and groin pain. *Br J Surg* 1994;81:1529-1530.

32. Gray FJ: Letter. *Med J Aust* 1992;156:366.

33. Yukawa Y, Kato F, Kajino G, Nakamura S, Nitta H: Groin pain associated with lower lumbar disc herniation. *Spine* 1997;22:1736-1739.

34. Malycha P, Lovell G: Inguinal surgery in athletes with chronic groin pain: The sportsman's hernia. *Aust N Z J Surg* 1992;62:123-125.

35. Leunig M, Werlen S, Ungersbock A, Ito K, Ganz R: Evaluation of the acetabular labrum by MR arthrography. *J Bone Joint Surg Br* 1997;79:230-234.

36. Locher S, Werlen S, Leunig M, Ganz R: Arthro-MRI mit radiärer Schnittsequenz zur Darstellung der präradiologischen Hüftpathologie. *Z Orthop Ihre Grenzgeb* 2002;140:52-57.

37. Siebenrock KA, Wahab K, Werlen S, Kalhor M, Leunig M, Ganz R: Abnormal extension of the femoral head epiphysis as a cause of cam impingement. *Clin Orthop* 2004;418:54-60.

38. Leunig M, Podeszwa D, Beck M, Werlen S, Ganz R: Magnetic resonance arthrography of labral disorders in dysplasia and impingement hips. *Clin Orthop* 2004;418:74-80.

39. Gautier E, Ganz K, Krugel N, Gill T, Ganz R: Anatomy of the medial femoral circumflex artery and its surgical implications. *J Bone Joint Surg Br* 2000;82:679-683.

40. Mercati E, Guary A, Myquel C, Bourgeon A: A postero-external approach to the hip joint: Value of the formation of a digastric muscle. *J Chir (Paris)* 1972;103:499-504.

41. Notzli HP, Siebenrock KA, Hempfing A, Ramseier LE, Ganz R: Perfusion of the femoral head during surgical dislocation of the hip: Monitoring by laser Doppler flowmetry. *J Bone Joint Surg Br* 2002;84:300-304.

42. Glick JM: Hip arthroscopy using the lateral approach. *Instr Course Lect* 1988;37:223-231.

43. Ide T, Akamatsu N, Nakajima I: Arthroscopic surgery of the hip joint. *Arthroscopy* 1991;7:204-211.

44. Snow SW, Keret D, Scarangella S, Bowen JR: Anterior impingement of the femoral head: A late phenomenon of Legg-Calve-Perthes' disease. *J Pediatr Orthop* 1993;13:286-289.

45. Siebenrock KA, Schoeniger R, Ganz R: Anterior femoro-acetabular impingement due to acetabular retroversion: Treatment with periacetabular osteotomy. *J Bone Joint Surg Am* 2003;85-A:278-286.

46. Ganz R, MacDonald SJ: Indications and modern technique of proximal femoral osteotomies in adults. *Semin Arthroplasty* 1997;8:38-50.

47. Beck M, Leunig M, Parvizi J, Boutier V, Wyss D, Ganz R: Anterior femoro-acetabular impingement: Part II. Clinical midterm results. *Clin Orthop Relat Res* 2004;418:37-73.

Osteonecrosis of the Hip: Management in the 21st Century

Jay R. Lieberman, MD
Daniel J. Berry, MD
Michael A. Mont, MD
Roy K. Aaron, MD
John J. Callaghan, MD
Amar D. Rajadhyaksha, MD
James R. Urbaniak, MD

Abstract

Osteonecrosis of the femoral head is a progressive condition that often leads to collapse of the femoral head. The ultimate goal in the treatment for osteonecrosis of the hip is preservation of the femoral head. However, the condition is difficult to treat because it is associated with a number of different diseases, and the etiology and natural history of the condition have not been definitively determined. The delineation of new information regarding the etiology, pathogenesis, and natural history of osteonecrosis is ongoing. Core decompression, vascularized and nonvascularized bone grafting procedures, and arthroplasty procedures play an important role in treatment.

Osteonecrosis, also known as avascular necrosis or aseptic necrosis, is a disease of impaired osseous blood flow. The term aseptic necrosis had been commonly used in the past to distinguish osteonecrosis related to nonseptic causes from that related to septic causes. It commonly affects patients in the third, fourth, or fifth decade of life. Three hundred thousand to 600,000 people have osteonecrosis of the femoral head in the United States. The

development of osteonecrosis can have a major impact on an individual's lifestyle. Because so many of the patients are young when they are diagnosed, they often need to alter their work and leisure activities. The ultimate goal of treating osteonecrosis of the hip is preservation of the femoral head. However, this is difficult because the condition is associated with a number of different diseases and neither the etiology nor the natural history has been definitively determined. The diagnosis of osteonecrosis accounts for 5% to 12% of total hip replacements performed.[1]

Etiology and Risk Factors

It is difficult to obtain an understanding of the etiologic factors in osteonecrosis because the clinical composition of medical centers varies widely and because, for the most part, reported etiologic associations are based not on prospective studies but rather on cross-sectional and case-control studies. Osteonecrosis can be associated with traumatic or nontraumatic conditions. Because osteonecrosis eventually develops in only a relatively small percentage of patients with any of these conditions,[2] recent attention has been focused on understanding underlying predispositions to the development of osteonecrosis when challenged by environmental factors. Current interest is centering on genetic mutations leading to hypercoagulability, which results in microthrombosis and osteonecrosis when challenged by environmental (epigenetic) events. Patients with so-called idiopathic osteonecrosis most likely have some type of coagulation abnormality that has not been identified.

Traumatic Osteonecrosis Osteonecrosis of the femoral head caused by trauma almost always involves a displaced fracture of the femoral neck or a hip dislocation. The prevalence of osteonecrosis after hip dislocation has been reported to be 10% to 25% in various series.[2-4] The duration of dislocation may be related to the eventual development of osteonecrosis, with the prevalence of osteonecrosis associated with dislocations of more than 12 hours in duration being double that associated with dislocations that are reduced more promptly.[5] Displaced fractures of the femoral neck have been associated with a 15% to 50% prevalence of osteonecrosis, depending on fracture type, time until reduction, and accuracy of reduction.[6-8] It is presumed that both hip dislocations and femoral neck fractures are associated with mechanical interruption of the circulation to the femoral head.

Nontraumatic Osteonecrosis A variety of etiologic associations with osteonecrosis have been proposed and have been more or less convincingly demonstrated. They include corticosteroid intake, excessive alcohol use, hemoglobinopathies, and dysbarisms. Osteonecrosis has been associated with a variety of other medical conditions, including Gaucher's disease, intraosseous lipid deposition, hypersensitivity reactions, Shwartzman reaction, and conditions associated with thromboplastin release, including pregnancy, malignant tumors, and inflammatory bowel disease.

In cross-sectional studies, 10% to 30% of the cases of osteonecrosis have been associated with corticosteroid administration. However, the few prospective longitudinal studies that can be found in the literature have indicated that osteonecrosis may occur in only 8% to 10% of patients exposed to corticosteroid therapy.[9] With some diseases, it is difficult to separate the effects on bone of corticosteroids from those of the underlying diseases, including mineralization defects and osteoporosis associated with renal and liver failure and vasculitis associated with systemic lupus erythematosus. Evidence linking corticosteroids and osteonecrosis is largely circumstantial and is based on the association of

osteonecrosis with corticosteroid therapy in a number of respiratory and rheumatic conditions and in patients who have undergone organ transplantation as well as on the fact that patients with Cushing's disease have a somewhat higher prevalence of osteonecrosis.[10]

Finally, the dose of corticosteroids necessary to induce osteonecrosis is not known. Dose has been expressed as mean daily dose, peak dose, cumulative dose, and duration of exposure. In the few studies examining the relationship of corticosteroid dose with osteonecrosis, the mean daily or peak dose, rather than the cumulative dose or duration of therapy, appeared to be associated with osteonecrosis.[11,12] Higher doses, even for shorter duration, present greater risks. Doses of corticosteroids of more than 20 mg/day appear to be associated with a higher risk of osteonecrosis. The risk of osteonecrosis associated with corticosteroids may be particularly high in patients undergoing renal transplantation, possibly because of an association of underlying mineralization defects and structural weakening of the cancellous bone. A meta-analysis of 22 studies of steroid-associated osteonecrosis revealed a 4.6-fold increase in the rate of osteonecrosis for every 10 mg/day increase in mean daily dose.[9]

Excessive alcohol intake has been identified as an etiologic factor in osteonecrosis, but difficulties have been encountered in defining the term excessive. The true prevalence of alcohol-associated osteonecrosis has been difficult to determine because most reports are cross-sectional. One prospective study[13] suggested that an intake of more than 400 mL of alcohol per week increased the relative risk of osteonecrosis 9.8-fold. The relative risk increased from 2.7 for less than 4,000 drink-years (with drink-years defined as weekly alcohol consumption multiplied by the number of years of drinking) to 9.0 for 10,000 drink-years.[13,14]

Osteonecrosis has been associated with several hemoglobinopathies, including hemoglobin SS (sickle cell disease), hemoglobin SC, and sickle thalassemia. The reported prevalence of osteonecrosis in these populations has been 4% to 20%.[15,16]

Dysbaric osteonecrosis is largely of historic interest and now occurs quite rarely. It has been associated with working environments using compressed air (caisson disease) and with deep sea diving with poorly controlled decompression. Occupational Safety and Health Administration standards mandating atmospheric pressures of less than 17 psi and safe decompression schedules for divers have made dysbaric osteonecrosis relatively uncommon.[9]

Pathophysiology

Contemporary studies of the pathophysiology of osteonecrosis have focused on the vulnerable microcirculation of the femoral head and the ischemic consequences of microvascular occlusion. The microcirculation of the femoral head is vulnerable to occlusion both from intravascular thrombi and from extravascular compression. A 1.6-fold reduction in femoral head blood flow reduces local PO_2 by one third.[17] Osteocyte necrosis occurs after 2 to 3 hours of ischemia, although histologic signs of osteocyte death are apparent only after 24 to 72 hours. Adipocyte necrosis and necrosis of hematopoietic marrow occur before osteocyte necrosis. A unifying concept of the pathophysiology of osteonecrosis has recently been presented[18] (Fig. 1). This concept emphasizes the central role of vascular occlusion and ischemia leading to both marrow-cell and osteocyte necrosis. Vascular occlusion may occur through mechanical interruption from fractures or dislocations, intravascular occlusion from thrombi or lipid emboli, or extravascular compression associated with intraosseous hypertension. Unusual causes of direct osteocyte death may be high-dose radiation or chemotherapy.

The most likely common pathophysiologic event in nontraumatic osteonecrosis is intravascular coagulation and microcirculatory thrombosis. Indeed, thrombotic and fat emboli have been found in both arterioles and venules in specimens of osteonecrotic tissue and have been associated with osteocyte necrosis in some animal models, if not with full-blown human osteonecrosis.

Thrombotic occlusion of the microcirculation in the femoral head has been associated with hypercoagulability caused by hereditary thrombophilia, impaired fibrinolysis, antiphospholipid antibodies, or hyperlipidemia. Three thrombophilic mutations occur with some frequency (Table 1).

Factor V_{Leiden} results from an arginine-to-glutamine substitution in the factor-V peptide chain because of a CGA→CAA mutation. This substitution occurs at the point of cleavage of factor V, by its regulatory protein (protein C), making factor V more resistant to inactivation.[19] This is measured clinically as resistance to activated protein C (RAP-C). Elevations in plasminogen activator inhibitor and decreases in tissue plasminogen activator (tPA) result in impaired fibrinolysis and poorly regulated clotting, leading to hypercoagulability. The presence of lipoprotein-associated antigen Lp(a) has also been associated with impaired fibrinolysis. Lp(a) has sequence homology with plasminogen and competes for tPA but does not result in a fibrinolytic product. Finally, the presence of circulating antiphospholipid antibodies is associated with hypercoagulability. These antibodies include anticardiolipin antibodies and lupus anticoagulants. They react against a β-2 glycoprotein in endothelial cell membranes and promote the activation of soluble clotting factors.

Hypercoagulability associated with any one of these conditions may represent an underlying predisposition for microvascular thrombosis and osteonecrosis.[20] However, thrombosis is a complex event,

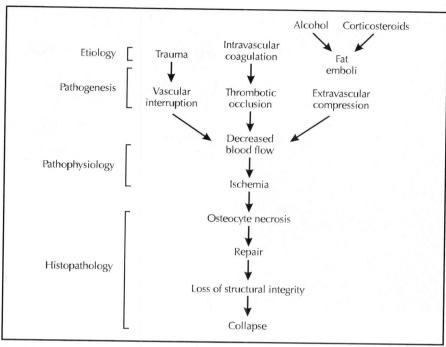

Fig. 1 A concept of pathogenesis of osteonecrosis that unifies several hypotheses. Many etiologies may contribute to the pathogenic mechanisms of mechanical interruption, thrombotic occlusion, or extravascular compression. These mechanisms all may decrease blood flow, leading to ischemia and subsequently to osteocyte necrosis. The presence of necrotic bone induces a repair process in which bone resorption exceeds production, leading to a loss of structural integrity of the subchondral trabeculae and eventually to subchondral collapse. (Reproduced with permission from Aaron RK: Osteonecrosis: Etiology, pathophysiology and diagnosis, in Callaghan JJ, Rosenberg AG, Rubash HE (eds): *The Adult Hip.* Philadelphia, PA, Lippincott-Raven, 1998, p 457.)

Table 1
Prevalence of Thrombophilic Mutations

Mutation	General Population	Patients With Thrombosis
Factor V_{Leiden}	3% to 5%	20%
Prothrombin G20210A	1% to 3%	5% to 10%
Hyperhomocysteinemia	5% to 10%	25%

and more than one risk factor may be needed to produce clinical manifestations. Genetic predisposition may require one or several epigenetic factors to result in clinical disease syndromes. Certain environmental or acquired risk factors have been specifically associated with osteonecrosis, including hyperlipidemia and fat embolism, hypersensitivity and endotoxin reactions, and conditions associated with thromboplastin release. Local hyperlipidemia and intravascular lipid deposits have been noted in patients with corticosteroid or alcohol intake. Heritable and acquired risk factors for hypercoagulability have been identified in many patients with osteonecrosis, suggesting that, of a variety of etiologic associations, intravascular coagulation with microcirculatory occlusion is, indeed, the most

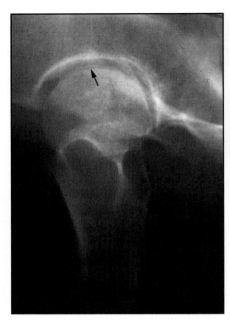

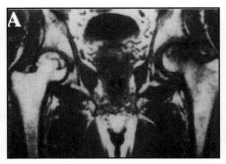

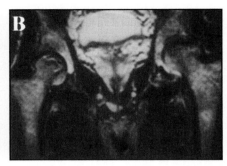

Fig. 3 A, T1-weighted MRI scan demonstrating a small osteonecrotic lesion of the right hip, and a large lesion and loss of signal intensity beyond the lesion of the left hip. **B,** T2-weighted MRI scan demonstrating the double-line sign on the right hip, with the outer dark line representing the sclerotic rim and the inner, high-intensity signal line representing hypervascularity of the repair zone. (Reproduced from Hoffman S, Kramer J, Plenk H, Kneeland JB: Imaging of osteonecrosis, in Urbaniak JR, Jones JP (eds): *Osteonecrosis: Etiology, Diagnosis and Treatment*. Rosemont, IL, American Academy of Orthopaedic Surgeons, 1997, p 218.)

Fig. 2 A lateral radiograph of the hip demonstrating the crescent sign (*arrow*).

likely final common pathophysiologic pathway for nontraumatic osteonecrosis.

Clearly defining the pathophysiology of osteonecrosis would enhance our ability to treat this problem. The development of osteonecrosis is not caused by a single precipitating event; it is a multifactorial process. In a study of the vascular anatomy of 99 hips undergoing vascularized fibular grafting for osteonecrosis of the femoral head, 93 (94%) had abnormal vascular patterns. In contrast, in a control group only 31% had abnormal vascular patterns. Absence or hypoplasia of the superior capsular artery was the most common abnormality.[21] These findings suggest that there is also a population of patients at risk for osteonecrosis as a result of anomalies of the macrovascular circulation of the femoral head.

Diagnosis

A prompt diagnosis of osteonecrosis allows early treatment, which may result in a better outcome. As with any diagnosis, the history is critical. A high index of suspicion is essential, especially if the

patient has one of the atraumatic conditions that are associated with osteonecrosis. An associated risk factor should be sought out during the initial evaluation. The most common presenting symptom is a deep pain in the groin. The findings on physical examination can be unremarkable or can include pain on internal rotation of the hip, a decreased range of motion, an antalgic gait, and clicking in the hip when the necrotic fragment has collapsed. Pain with internal rotation of the hip and a limited range of hip motion are often signs that the femoral head has already collapsed.

Radiographic studies are essential for a definitive diagnosis of the disease.[22-25] Plain radiography should still be the first step in the diagnostic evaluation. Adequate AP and frog-leg lateral radiographs are essential. Radiographic changes in the femoral head usually occur many months after the onset of the disease and include cysts, sclerosis, or a crescent sign. The crescent sign results from subchondral collapse of the necrotic segment (Fig. 2). Technetium Tc 99m bone scans were previously used for high-risk patients who had a negative radiographic examination. However, recent studies have shown that bone scans have limited value and are often misleading because they are false-

negative in 25% to 45% of cases that have been confirmed by MRI or histologic evaluation.[25-28] MRI has become the standard for diagnosing osteonecrosis. It is 99% sensitive and specific. A single-density line on the T1-weighted image demarcates the normal ischemic bone interface, and a double-density line on the T2-weighted image represents the hypervascular granulation tissue (Fig. 3). CT scans and plain tomograms can identify collapse of the femoral head. However, they are seldom used because of the high cost and the amount of radiation exposure.[28,29] Functional evaluation of bone, which involves direct measurements of marrow pressure, venography, and biopsy,[30] is not widely used at present because of its invasive nature and the high accuracy of MRI.

The most important differential diagnosis to consider for patients with suspected osteonecrosis is transient osteoporosis of the hip[31-37] (Fig. 4). Transient osteoporosis of the hip is a self-limiting condition that is usually seen in women in the third trimester of pregnancy and in men in the fifth and sixth decades of life. MRI of these patients shows edema into the femoral neck and metaphysis, which is not common with osteonecrosis. Osteonecrosis has been reported in 2% to 5% of

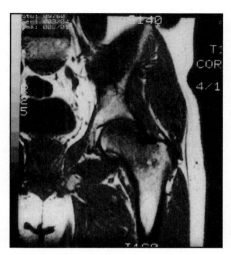

Fig. 4 T1-weighted MRI scan with low-intensity signal representing bone marrow edema in the femoral head, neck, and metaphysis consistent with transient osteopenia of bone.

Table 2
Radiographic Classifications of Osteonecrosis of the Femoral Head

Classification System	Criteria
Ficat and Arlet classification system[30,39]	
Stage I	Normal
Stage II	Sclerotic or cystic lesions
Stage III	Subchondral collapse
Stage IV	Osteoarthritis with decreased articular collapse
University of Pennsylvania system of classification and staging[41]	
Stage 0	Normal or nondiagnostic radiograph, bone scan, and MRI
Stage I	Normal radiograph; abnormal bone scan and/or MRI
A	Mild (< 15% of head affected)
B	Moderate (15% to 30% of head affected)
C	Severe (> 30% of head affected)
Stage II	Lucent and sclerotic changes in femoral head
A	Mild (< 15% of head affected)
B	Moderate (15% to 30% of head affected)
C	Severe (> 30% of head affected)
Stage III	Subchondral collapse (crescent sign) without flattening
A	Mild (< 15% of articular surface)
B	Moderate (15% to 30% of articular surface)
C	Severe (> 30% of articular surface)
Stage IV	Flattening of femoral head
A	Mild (< 15% of surface and < 2-mm depression)
B	Moderate (15% to 30% of surface or 2- to 4-mm depression)
C	Severe (> 30% of surface or > 4-mm depression)
Stage V	Joint narrowing and/or acetabular changes
A	Mild
B	Moderate
C	Severe
Stage VI	Advanced degenerative changes

patients who initially had transient osteoporosis of the hip. Such patients often have severe pain in the groin and an antalgic gait. They are instructed to use crutches while the condition resolves, which often takes 6 months. In addition, one should be cautious about instituting aggressive treatment of patients who have changes consistent with early osteonecrosis on MRI. In one study, more than 95% of such cases did not progress.[38]

Classification and Staging

The goal of any classification system is to provide guidelines for treatment and prognosis. A number of different classification systems have been developed to evaluate patients with osteonecrosis, but there is no standard unified classification system for determining the extent and location of the necrotic area in the femoral head and the involvement of the acetabulum. These are the critical elements in developing an appropriate treatment plan.

Ficat and Arlet originally developed a four-stage classification system based on radiographic changes and the functional exploration of bone, which included intraosseous venography and measurement of bone marrow pressure.[30,39] A number of different classification systems have been developed, including that of Marcus and associates,[40] the University of Pennsylvania system of classification and staging,[41] that of the Association Research Circulation Osseous,[42] and that of the Japanese Investigation Committee on Osteonecrosis.[43] The development of the University of Pennsylvania system is a major advancement because it includes findings of MRI (Table 2). In addition, in this system the extent of the involvement of the femoral head is classified as A (< 15%), B (15% to 30%), or C (> 30%).

Treatment
Core Decompression
Core decompression of the hip currently is the most common procedure used to treat the early stages of osteonecrosis of the femoral head. However, despite the fact that this procedure has been employed for approximately 3 decades and there are numerous reports analyzing its efficacy, there is no general consensus regarding either the indications for this procedure or the techniques that optimize results.

Originally, core decompression was used by Ficat and Arlet to obtain histologic specimens to confirm that patients actually had osteonecrosis of the femoral head.[30] Intraosseous venography was performed to confirm an abnormal pattern of blood flow within the femoral head, and bone marrow pressure was also found to be elevated in these patients. Ficat and Arlet then started to use core decompression as a therapeutic, rather than just as a diagnostic, procedure. Because decompression of the femoral head allowed the intraosseous pressure to return to normal, it was referred to as a core decompression. The goal of a core decompression was to decompress the femoral head and thereby reduce the intraosseous pressure in the femoral head, restore normal vascular flow, and subsequently alleviate the pain in the hip.

Does core decompression change the natural history of osteonecrosis of the hip? This question is difficult to answer because the true natural history of osteonecrosis remains unknown. Furthermore, despite numerous studies, the true success rate of core decompression is difficult to determine because of differences among studies with regard to selection of patients (ie, differences in patient diagnoses), classification systems, surgical procedures, postoperative management, and evaluation of clinical outcome.[44]

Osteonecrosis is associated with a number of medical conditions, and because earlier investigators did not have MRI available to analyze the extent and location of the osteonecrotic lesion, it is often difficult to compare the results of different series. This is one explanation for the substantial differences in success rates reported in various studies. In addition, core decompression is a generic term, and the procedure itself is often accompanied by supplemental procedures. For example, core decompression can be performed alone or combined with nonvascularized grafts (allograft bone or demineralized bone matrix), vascularized bone grafts (fibula or iliac crest), electrical stimulation, or electromagnetic fields.[45-52]

We are aware of only a few randomized trials in which the efficacy of core decompression was assessed. Stulberg and associates[53] compared core decompression alone with conservative treatment in a prospective, randomized study of 55 hips. On the basis of Harris hip scores, surgical treatment was successful in approximately 70% of hips with Ficat

stage I, II, or III osteonecrosis. In contrast, nonsurgical treatment was successful for 20% of hips with Ficat stage I disease, 0% with stage II, and 10% with stage III. The authors concluded that core decompression was more effective than nonsurgical management of early osteonecrosis.

Koo and associates[54] performed a randomized trial comparing core decompression with nonsurgical management in 37 hips. Those authors noted radiographic signs of progression in 72% of the hips treated with core decompression, and 72% of those hips eventually required a total hip arthroplasty (THA). Of the patients treated nonsurgically, 79% had radiographic signs of progression and 68% eventually required a THA. In contrast to the study by Stulberg and associates,[53] Koo and associates[54] concluded that there was no important improvement of outcome when osteonecrosis was treated with core decompression.

Recently, there have been a number of extensive literature reviews assessing the clinical results of core decompression. Smith and associates[55] reviewed 12 articles published between 1979 and 1991 that included a total of 702 hips with an average duration of follow-up of 38 months. Using the University of Pennsylvania staging system, they reported a successful result in 78% of the Ficat stage I hips, 62% of the stage II hips, and 41% of the stage III hips. In another comprehensive literature review, Mont and associates[56] assessed 42 studies in which a total of 1,206 hips had been treated with core decompression and 819 with various nonsurgical means. Of the hips treated prior to collapse, 71% had a good result after core decompression and 35% had a good result after nonsurgical management. Overall, a satisfactory clinical result was reported in 64% of the hips in the 24 studies of core decompression and in only 23% of those in the 21 studies of nonsurgical management.

There have been several fairly large retrospective reviews assessing the results

of core decompression performed with various techniques.[55-58] In all of these studies, the authors found that the results of core decompression were substantially worse when there had been collapse of the femoral head preoperatively. Smith and associates[55] retrospectively evaluated 114 hips and noted a substantial decrease in the rate of satisfactory results when a crescent sign had been present. The success rate for Ficat stage I hips was 81%, but the rates for hips with a crescent sign or definitive collapse were 20% and 0%, respectively. In a retrospective review of 128 hips, Fairbank and associates[57] also reported a poor rate of success (27%; 14 of 52 hips) for patients with collapse of the femoral head. Using the University of Pennsylvania system of classification and staging, Steinberg[58] retrospectively assessed 297 hips in 205 patients who had undergone core decompression combined with placement of a loose cancellous graft in the core tract and had been followed for a minimum of 2 years. The author concluded that the stage and site of the lesion clearly influence the results of core decompression. THA was required in 22% of the stage I and II hips with a small area of involvement (stages IA and IIA). In contrast, 39% of the stage I hips and 40% of the stage II hips with involvement of ≥ 15% of the head (stages IB, IIB, and IIC) eventually required a THA.

Surgical Technique There are a number of different surgical techniques for core decompression. Some surgeons prefer a single core tract, whereas others make multiple core holes. There is general agreement that these procedures should be done with fluoroscopic guidance in two planes. The patients are usually placed on a fracture table. A guidewire should be placed into the area of osteonecrosis. It is critical that the starting hole for the core decompression be made just proximal to the level of the lesser trochanter to avoid the development of stress fractures in the femur. A biopsy specimen should be obtained whenever possible to provide definitive confirmation of the diagnosis. Protective weight bearing with crutches is recommended for a minimum of 6 weeks after the surgical procedure.

Some surgeons have recommended combining core decompression with nonvascularized or vascularized grafts to enhance bone formation in the femoral head and to prevent fracture through the proximal part of the femur. Grafting of the femoral head with demineralized bone matrix is an attractive option because it may enhance the healing potential of the femoral head but it does not change the anatomy of the femoral neck if a THA is necessary. However, we are not aware of any randomized trials comparing core decompression alone with core decompression combined with use of demineralized bone matrix. There is also interest in using growth factors that can enhance either the patient's osteogenic potential (bone morphogenetic protein) or the patient's angiogenic potential (fibroblast growth factor or vascular endothelial growth factor). Hopefully, the efficacy of these growth factors will be evaluated in future randomized, controlled trials.

Core decompression seems to be more effective than symptomatic treatment. In order to optimize the results of core decompression, the osteonecrosis must be diagnosed and treated early. The prognosis is better when the hip is treated before collapse, when the lesion is smaller, and when there is a sclerotic rim.[59] In addition, patients who continue to take steroids seem to have a worse prognosis.[58]

Free Vascularized Fibular Grafts
The use of vascularized bone grafts to treat osteonecrosis of the femoral head was developed to prevent collapse of the femoral head and to enhance vascularization of the bone in this region.[47-50,60] The rationale for management of osteonecrosis of the femoral head with a free vascu-

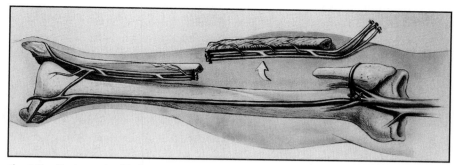

Fig. 5 The fibular graft with the peroneal vessels is harvested from the ipsilateral calf for insertion into the core in the femoral neck and head.

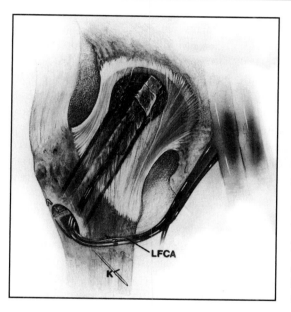

Fig. 6 Cancellous bone harvested from the greater trochanteric area is inserted into the cavity formed by removal of the necrotic bone. The fibular graft is inserted into the core tract and stabilized with a 0.62-mm Kirschner wire (K). The peroneal veins and artery are anastomosed to the ascending branches of the lateral femoral circumflex artery (LFCA) and vein.

larized fibular graft is based on five principles: (1) decompression of the femoral head, (2) removal of the necrotic bone, (3) replacement with fresh autogenous cancellous bone, (4) support of the subchondral bone with a viable strong bone strut, and (5) revascularization and osteogenesis of the femoral head.

Full details of the surgical procedure have been provided previously,[50] so we will discuss only the highlights of the technique. With the patient in a lateral decubitus position, two teams operate simultaneously; one performs the hip exposure, and the other harvests the ipsilateral fibula (Fig. 5). The proximal part of the femur is exposed through an inter-

val between the gluteus medius and the tensor fasciae latae muscles. With use of fluoroscopy, a core (16 to 19 mm) is made just distal to the vastus ridge and precisely into the necrotic area of the femoral head. Most of the necrotic bone is removed and is replaced with autogenous fresh cancellous bone from the greater trochanteric area. The sufficiency of the packing of the cavity with the cancellous bone is assessed with water-soluble contrast medium and fluoroscopy. The fibula with its peroneal artery and two veins is inserted into the core to within 3 to 5 mm of the subchondral area and is stabilized with a 0.62-mm Kirschner wire (Fig. 6). With use of microvascular surgical techniques, the ascending branches of the lateral femoral circumflex artery and vein are anastomosed to the peroneal vessels of the fibula. At the conclusion of the repair, retrograde flow must be visible from the exposed endosteum of the fibula.

The average hospital stay is less than 4 days. Patients use crutches and do not bear weight on the treated side for 6 weeks and graduate to partial weight bearing in 3 to 6 months, depending on the stage and size of the lesion.

Successful results with this technique have been reported at a number of centers.[48,50,60] In 1995, Urbaniak and associates[50] reported on 103 patients with osteonecrosis of the femoral head treated with a free vascularized fibular graft. After a median duration of follow-up of 7 years (range, 4.5 to 12.2 years), 31 of the 103 hips had required conversion to a THA. Patients with preoperative collapse of the femoral head had a worse prognosis. In an update of their experience, Urbaniak and Harvey[61] analyzed 646 consecutive grafts in patients followed for 1 to 16 years. The expected 10-year survivorship was 82%.

Urbaniak reviewed the results in 1,523 hips treated with a free vascularized fibular graft for osteonecrosis between 1979 and October 1, 2000 (unpublished data). Again, the best results were obtained in the patients who had had no collapse of the subchondral bone or articular cartilage preoperatively. Unfortunately, 1,021 of the hips (67%) had joint space narrowing or advanced degenerative changes. Of the hips that had not had preoperative subchondral or articular collapse, 91% had a successful result (no subsequent surgery) after 6 months to 22 years of follow-up. However, if collapse had been present, the success rate was 85%, and if there had also been joint-space narrowing, it was 73%. Of course, it was projected that failure rates would increase with time.

The results of core decompression have been compared with those of free vascularized fibular grafts in two studies. Kane and associates[62] reported a prospective study of 39 hips treated with core decompression or a free vascularized fibular graft and followed for 2 to 5 years. The core decompression was successful (no subsequent surgery) in 8 of 19 hips (42%), whereas treatment with the free vascularized fibular graft was successful in 16 of 20 hips (80%). Scully and associates[63] reported a retrospective matched-group comparison of patients treated with a free vascularized fibular graft or core decompression. When evaluating patients with Ficat stage III osteonecrosis (articular collapse), they found an 81% 50-month rate of survival of the femoral head (405 of 500 hips) in the group treated with the free vascularized fibular graft compared with a 21% rate (10 of 47 hips) in the group treated with core decompression. Unfortunately, there have been no large randomized, controlled trials comparing the efficacy of these treatment modalities, to our knowledge.

Although free vascularized fibular grafts have proven to be successful, there are some potential disadvantages to such an extensive surgical procedure. First, complications associated with the harvesting of the fibula have been noted. In a review of the cases of 198 patients (247 free vascularized fibular grafts), Vail and Urbaniak[64] reported a 19% rate of complications, including motor weakness, subjective discomfort in the ankle and other sites in the leg, and sensory abnormalities in the lower limb. The prevalence of pain in the ankle and the lower limb increased with time and was 11.5% at 5 years after the operation. In addition, the rate of fracture of the proximal part of the femur after use of a free vascularized fibular graft in the hip was noted to be 2.5% (18 of 707) in one large series.[65] The investigators recommended that the patient not bear weight and use crutches during the early postoperative period. Second, the placement of vascularized graft alters the bone stock in the femoral

neck and calcar region and may make a THA more difficult to perform. It has not been established whether this procedure has a negative effect on the longevity of a total hip prosthesis.

If the use of free vascularized fibular grafts provides a long-term solution with respect to preserving the femoral head, then the benefits of the procedure clearly outweigh the risks. The relative indications for the procedure in patients with osteonecrosis continue to evolve. At this time, it is generally reserved for symptomatic patients. It is a reasonable option for patients younger than 50 years without collapse of the femoral head. The procedure is more controversial in patients with collapse of the femoral head, and whether it is used should be determined by the diagnosis, the age of the patient, and the extent of progression of the disease. Other treatment options should be considered for patients older than 40 years with extensive involvement of the femoral head and evidence of femoral head collapse. However, some advocates of the procedure consider a vascularized fibular graft a treatment option to avoid performing an arthroplasty in patients younger than 20 years with even 2 or 3 mm of collapse and acetabular involvement.[50]

Osteotomies

Various types of osteotomies have been reported for the treatment of osteonecrosis of the femoral head.[66-81] One rationale for performing an osteotomy is based on the biomechanical effect of removing the necrotic or collapsing segment of the femoral head from the principal weight-bearing area of the hip joint. This area is replaced with a segment of articular cartilage of the femoral head that is supported by healthy, viable bone. Some authors have attributed the efficacy of osteotomies to the reduction of venous hypertension and the subsequent decrease in intramedullary pressure that occur after such procedures.[82]

Osteotomies are not widely accepted as a standard method of treatment of osteonecrosis of the femoral head because the outcomes have been variable and it is difficult to convert failed cases to a total hip replacement.[66-68,70,77,78,81] It is difficult to compare the results of different reports because the series have varied with regard to the patients' associated risk factors, the methods of radiographic staging, the indications for the procedure, and the methods of osteotomy.

Two main types of osteotomies have been utilized: transtrochanteric rotational osteotomies and intertrochanteric varus or valgus osteotomies (usually combined with flexion or extension). To our knowledge, transtrochanteric rotational osteotomies were first reported by Wagner and Zeiler[81] in the 1960s. They performed a double osteotomy with a maximum of 180° of rotation of the necrotic segment. In a cohort of 71 patients who had a total of 83 rotational osteotomies and were followed for 10 years, the best results were obtained in patients who had had minimal osteoarthritic changes and a small radiographic combined necrotic angle preoperatively. (Kerboul and associates[68] described the combined necrotic angle as an estimation of lesion size. It is calculated by combining the arc of surface involvement by the osteonecrotic lesion on AP radiographs with that on lateral radiographs. Small combined necrotic angles are ≤ 150°, medium angles are between 151° and 200°, and large angles are > 200°.)

To our knowledge, the best results with transtrochanteric rotational osteotomies were achieved by Sugioka and associates[72,80] in Japan, who reported that 229 of 295 hips (78%) had a successful outcome at a mean of 11 years (range, 3 to 16 years) postoperatively. Other Japanese surgeons[71,79] have also reported favorable results with this technically difficult procedure. Masuda and associates[79] reported a good result in 36 of 52 hips (69%) that were followed for a mean of 5 years (range, 1 to 10 years). Sugano and associates[71] had a similar success rate at 6 years, with a satisfactory result in 23 of 41 hips (56%). However, these success rates in Japan have not been reproduced in the United States.[73,75,76] In one representative report, the procedure failed in 15 of 18 hips that had been followed for a mean of 5 years.[75]

The less technically demanding varus and valgus osteotomies have been used commonly in Europe with variable success rates. In 1965, Merle D'Aubigné and associates[83] reported good to excellent pain reduction in 59 of 75 hips (79%) with Ficat stage II or III disease that had been followed for 1 to 6 years. In a follow-up report from the same institution, 28 of 47 hips (60%) were pain free at a mean of 5 years.[68] In a report by Maistrelli and associates,[78] 75 of 106 hips (71%) in 98 patients had a successful clinical result at 2 years postoperatively. At a mean of 8 years (range, 4 to 15 years), 61 of the 106 hips (58%) had a good or excellent result and only 24 (23%) needed a total hip replacement or an arthrodesis. Mont and associates[69] reported a good or excellent Harris hip score[84] in 28 of 37 hips (76%) at a mean of 11.5 years after treatment with varus osteotomy combined with flexion or extension.

In a number of different series, the size of the osteonecrotic lesion was determined to be a critical factor in the rate of success of the osteotomy.[70,77,81,85] Kerboul and associates[68] stressed the importance of preoperative radiographic evaluation of hips to determine if it is possible to move the necrotic area away from the point of maximum pressure with the acetabulum, which is easier if the lesion is small. For example, a varus osteotomy is appropriate only if a 20° arc of the lateral aspect of the femoral head is free of necrosis. Otherwise, some other type of osteotomy should be considered. Patients with a combined necrotic angle of less than 200° who are younger than 45 years have a better prognosis.[68] In a study by Scher and Jakim,[70] valgus osteotomy combined with bone grafting was successful in 36 of 45 young patients (80%) who were not taking corticosteroids. This finding is in concordance with the results in the report by Mont and associates,[69] in which patients receiving corticosteroids had a lower rate of clinical success. The osteotomy was clinically successful (a Harris hip score of > 80 points) in only 11 of 17 hips (65%) in the corticosteroid group, whereas it was successful in 17 of 20 hips (85%) in patients who had not received corticosteroids (Fig. 7).

A major concern about using an osteotomy as an interim procedure is that it may be difficult to convert the osteotomized hip to a THA if necessary. Benke and associates[86] reported that the long-term results of 105 THAs in 93 patients were not affected by previous osteotomies. However, the rate of intraoperative complications was 17% (18 of 105). The problems encountered included difficulty in removing the screws or plate and in reaming or broaching the femur. Broken screws were encountered, and some patients had a fracture of the shaft, calcar, or greater trochanter. These technical difficulties appear to be manageable as long as the surgeon has prepared for them preoperatively and intraoperatively.

On the basis of the results of these different studies, the criteria for the selection of patients for osteotomy include: (1) age younger than 45 years and a painful hip; (2) an early postcollapse or late precollapse status of the hip, with no narrowing of the joint space or acetabular involvement; (3) a small to medium lesion (a combined necrotic angle of ≤ 200°); and (4) no chronic use of high doses of corticosteroids.

Nonvascularized Bone Grafting

Nonvascularized bone grafting has numerous theoretical advantages for the treatment of precollapse and early post-

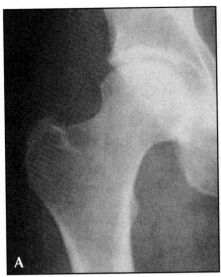 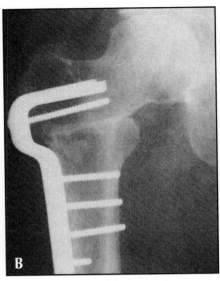 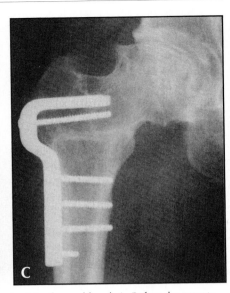

Fig. 7 AP radiographs of the right hip of a 30-year-old woman who had Ficat stage III osteonecrosis of the femoral head. **A,** Before the osteotomy, there was minimal evidence of collapse of the femoral head. **B,** Two months after the corrective osteotomy with insertion of a blade-plate. **C,** Eleven years postoperatively; despite some evidence of additional collapse, the patient had done well, with a Harris hip score of 92 points. (Reproduced with permission from Mont MA, Fairbank AC, Krackow KA, Hungerford DS: Corrective osteotomy for osteonecrosis of the femoral head: The results of a long-term follow-up study. *J Bone Joint Surg Am* 1996;78:1035.)

collapse osteonecrosis of the femoral head when the articular cartilage is relatively undamaged.[87-98] The procedure provides decompression of the osteonecrotic lesion, removal of the necrotic bone, and structural support and scaffolding for repair and remodeling of subchondral bone. Currently, three distinct approaches can be used to introduce bone graft into the femoral head; the cortical strut graft can be introduced through (1) a core tract, (2) a window in the femoral neck (a lightbulb procedure), or (3) a trapdoor that is made through the articular cartilage in the femoral head.

Cortical strut grafting, a procedure popularized by Phemister,[99] Boettcher and associates,[90] and Bonfiglio and associates,[91,92] is not commonly used today. This technique involves the removal of an 8- to 10-mm–diameter cylindrical core of bone from the femoral head and neck. This core tract is then filled with cortical strut grafts harvested from the ilium, fibula, or tibia. Postoperatively, protected weight bearing is used for 3 to 6 months.

A wide range of success rates has been reported with cortical strut-grafting techniques. Boettcher and associates[90] reported clinical and radiographic success in 27 of 38 hips (71%) 6 years after the use of tibial strut grafts. However, in a long-term evaluation by Smith and associates[97] that included the original 38 patients evaluated by Boettcher and associates, 40 of 56 hips (71%) had a poor clinical result after a mean duration of follow-up of 14 years (range, 4 to 27 years). In a short-term follow-up study (range, 2 to 4 years), Marcus and associates[100] found a satisfactory clinical result in 7 of 11 hips treated with the Phemister technique of bone grafting. However, Dunn and Grow[93] reported only four good results in 23 patients so treated. Buckley and associates[88] reported their results with a similar procedure involving core decompression combined with tibial autogenous grafts (three hips), fibular autogenous grafts (seven hips), or fibular allografts (10 hips). They reported an excellent clinical result, after a mean

duration of follow-up of 8 years (range, 2 to 19 years), in 18 of 20 hips (90%) that had Ficat stage I or II disease.

Another method of introducing bone graft is through a window in the femoral neck. An anterior hip arthrotomy is performed through a lateral or anterolateral approach. A cortical window is removed from the inferior aspect of the femoral neck, and the necrotic bone is excavated from within the femoral head. To our knowledge, Ganz and Büchler[101] were the first to use this procedure combined with an osteotomy, filling the defect of the femoral head with cancellous bone graft. This procedure was modified by Japanese investigators, who used autogenous cortical iliac strut grafts.[94,102] Itoman and Yamamoto[94] reported a good or excellent clinical result in 23 of 38 Ficat stage II or III hips (61%) at an average of 9 years (range, 2 to 15 years) postoperatively. Scher and Jakim[70] further modified this procedure by combining a valgus osteotomy with the autogenous cortical iliac strut graft. They reported a good or

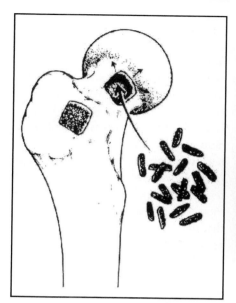

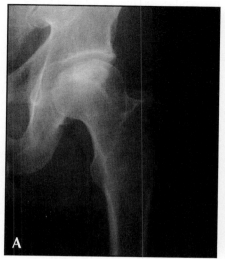

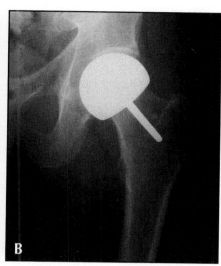

Fig. 9 A, Preoperative AP radiograph of the left hip joint showing collapse of the femoral head with an intact joint space. **B,** AP radiograph of the same hip joint 3 years after limited femoral resurfacing.

Fig. 8 Schematic diagram demonstrating the cortical window at the femoral head-neck junction. The defect within the femoral head can be filled with autogenous bone graft or various bone graft substitutes. (Reproduced with permission from Rosenwasser MP, Garino JP, Kiernan HA, Michelsen CB: Long term followup of thorough debridement and cancellous bone grafting of the femoral head for avascular necrosis. *Clin Orthop* 1994;306:21.)

excellent result in 36 of 45 hips (80%) at a mean of 5 years (range, 3 to 11 years).

The term lightbulb procedure was introduced by Rosenwasser and associates.[89] In this procedure, the cortical window is lifted from the femoral head-neck junction (Fig. 8). Cancellous bone graft from the iliac crest is used to fill the defect in the femoral head after complete evacuation of the necrotic bone. In their series, 13 of 15 hips were asymptomatic at a mean of 12 years (range, 10 to 15 years).

Another approach to bone grafting of the femoral head is through a trapdoor that is made through the articular cartilage of the femoral head. Intraoperatively, the femoral head is dislocated and the collapsed segment is exposed. An approximately 2-cm[2] flap is elevated from the chondral surface with use of scalpels and osteotomes. The necrotic bone is then removed from the femoral head with curets and burrs until viable bone is reached. This void can then be filled with various types of autogenous grafts or bone-graft extenders. This procedure was first delineated in detail by Meyers and associates.[103,104] The void in the femoral head was packed with cancellous bone graft. At a mean of 3 years (range, 1 to 9 years), a good to excellent clinical result was reported in eight of nine Ficat stage III hips. Ko and associates[105] modified this technique by adding a containment osteotomy and reported a good to excellent result in 8 of 10 hips at a mean of 4.5 years. Mont and associates[95] subsequently described filling the void in the femoral head with a combination of cortical struts and cancellous bone. At a mean of 56 months (range, 30 to 60 months), 20 of 24 Ficat stage III hips (83%) had a good or excellent clinical result, whereas only two of six Ficat stage IV hips were considered to have a successful result.

There is no consensus regarding the indications for nonvascularized bone-grafting. Proponents of these procedures recommend them for hips with less than 2 mm of femoral head depression or those in which a core decompression has failed and there is no acetabular involvement. Some investigators have reported good results in patients with a collapsed femoral head, but only small numbers of patients have been studied.[89,95,103-105] The procedures that use either a window in the femoral neck or elevation of a flap of cartilage require extensive surgical dissection, and these techniques need to be assessed in randomized trials with larger numbers of patients in order to determine their true efficacy. However, in the future, the indications for and efficacy of nonvascularized bone grafting may increase with the addition of growth factors and cytokines and the use of various bone-graft substitutes.

Limited Femoral Resurfacing Arthroplasty

Limited femoral resurfacing or hemiresurfacing arthroplasty is a viable option in young patients with either an extensive precollapse lesion or a postcollapse lesion without acetabular involvement (Fig. 9). This procedure offers several advantages:

(1) the damaged cartilage on the femoral head is removed, (2) femoral head and neck bone stock is preserved, and (3) revision to a subsequent THA is not complicated.[106] When there is moderate to severe involvement of the femoral head, a THA may be the only alternative. Because osteonecrosis is a disease that commonly affects patients in the third, fourth, or fifth decade of life (average age, 36 years), if femoral head resurfacing can consistently delay the necessity for a THA, it is a viable treatment option.

The principle of limited femoral resurfacing originated from the Smith-Petersen mold arthroplasty[107] and other designs reported by Aufranc, Luck, and Thomine.[108] Langlais and associates[109] reviewed the results of 86 adjusted cup arthroplasties of different designs and reported 85% good to excellent results at a mean of 6.5 years. These particular cup prostheses were press-fit to the reamed femoral head. However, this procedure fell out of favor as a result of the advances in THA that increased longevity and durability.

Townley[110] designed a total articular resurfacing arthroplasty (TARA, DePuy, Warsaw, IN) to resurface the articulating surface of the femoral head with a metal component while resurfacing the articulating surface of the acetabulum with a thin plastic shell inserted with cement. Because of the high failure rates on the acetabular side, this prosthesis is no longer used.[111-116] However, use of the femoral cap without the acetabular resurfacing eliminates failure secondary to polyethylene wear or loosening of the acetabular component. Krackow and associates[117] reported a good to excellent result of limited femoral resurfacing in 16 of 19 Ficat stage III hips (84%) at a mean of 3 years (range, 2 to 6 years). Scott and associates[118] reported a good to excellent result in 22 of 25 hips (88%) that had been followed for a mean of 37 months (range, 25 to 60). Hungerford and associates[119] followed 33 hips from the prior

two studies and reported a good to excellent result in 91% and 61% at 5 years and 10.5 years, respectively. In a report by Nelson and associates,[120] a cemented titanium-alloy shell was used in 21 hips, and 86% (18) had a good to excellent result at a mean of 6.2 years. Finally, Beaule and associates[121] reported on a series of 37 hips followed for a mean of 6.5 years (range, 2 to 18 years); a good to excellent result was found in 79% and 62% at 5 and 10 years, respectively. Beaule and associates[121] concluded that a longer duration of preoperative symptoms was associated with more degenerative changes of the acetabulum and that these patients required revision to a THA sooner.

One concern about the use of limited femoral resurfacing as an interim treatment is the possible difficulty of conversion to a THA. Revision of the TARA device to a THA was difficult because of the osteolysis caused by the particulate debris generated by wear of the polyethylene acetabular component. However, with the use of a femoral head component as a hemiresurfacing device, osteolysis is no longer an issue. The surgical procedure of converting a hemiresurfacing arthroplasty to a THA is similar in difficulty to a primary THA.[119,122] In one study, 13 of 33 limited femoral resurfacing devices (39%) were converted to a THA at a mean of 60 months (range, 36 to 136 months).[119] These 13 THAs were all successful clinically (a Harris hip score of at least 80 points) at a mean of 30 months (range, 24 to 72 months). Ash and associates[122] reported on 58 hips in which a cup arthroplasty was converted to a THA with cement. A satisfactory clinical result was found in 92% and 74% of the hips at 10 and 20 years, respectively, and there were no cases of femoral loosening.

Further study is required to determine the specific indications for femoral head resurfacing. There is general agreement that patients do better if this procedure is performed prior to the develop-

ment of substantial degeneration of the acetabular cartilage. Potential candidates for limited resurfacing of the femoral head include (1) young patients with no or minimal degeneration of the acetabular cartilage presenting with either a crescent sign or collapse of the femoral head and (2) young patients without femoral head collapse but with extensive osteonecrotic involvement of the femoral head (a combined necrotic angle of > 200° or femoral head involvement of > 50%). However, patients need to be cautioned that the degree of pain relief following a femoral head resurfacing procedure (Fig. 9, B) is not as consistent as that following a THA and that patients 50 years of age or older may be better off with a THA.

Total Hip Arthroplasty

Of the many different operations that are available to treat osteonecrosis of the femoral head, THA is the single treatment with the highest likelihood of providing excellent early pain relief and a good functional outcome. These advantages of THA must be balanced against the fact that it sacrifices more host bone and narrows future surgical options more than do other treatment procedures.

There is a wide range of opinions concerning the indications for THA in the treatment of osteonecrosis of the femoral head. Nevertheless, a consensus has emerged about some circumstances in which THA is clearly indicated and some in which it is not. The main indications for THA are (1) osteonecrosis of the femoral head and associated advanced secondary degenerative arthritis with severe damage of the femoral head articular cartilage and loss of acetabular cartilage,[123] and (2) an older or low-demand patient with extensive involvement or collapse of the femoral head as well as sufficient symptoms to justify THA. For both of these patient groups, THA is the most reliable method for providing pain relief and prompt functional return with a single operation. The main groups in whom THA is contraindicated are (1) young patients with early-stage osteonecrosis of the femoral head for whom treatment options that save the femoral head are available, and (2) patients at excessively high risk for complications of THA (for example, those with severe ongoing alcohol abuse who might be at excessive risk for dislocation of a total hip prosthesis). A relatively large number of patients, particularly those in middle age with variable amounts of femoral head involvement and femoral head collapse, fall into a gray zone in which THA is one of several reasonable treatment options, including resurfacing hemiarthroplasty.

THA has predictably provided excellent pain relief and functional improvement for patients with osteonecrosis of the femoral head, just as it has for patients with other diagnoses, such as osteoarthritis or inflammatory arthritis. Several authors have demonstrated that THA provides more complete and reliable pain relief than does hemiarthroplasty for patients with osteonecrosis of the femoral head.[124,125] Ito and associates[124] evaluated 48 hips at a mean of 11.4 years after bipolar hemiarthroplasty performed for osteonecrosis of the femoral head and reported groin pain in 42% of patients. Cabanela[125] reported that the results of bipolar arthroplasty were poorer than those of THA in patients with osteonecrosis of the femoral head. The less predictable results of hemiarthroplasty in comparison with those of THA may be related to pain that occurs when only one side of the joint is resurfaced (particularly in young, active patients) and may also be explained by the finding that the acetabular articular cartilage of many patients with osteonecrosis of the femoral head is histologically abnormal even before radiographs demonstrate loss of joint space.[126] Thus, the acetabular cartilage is predisposed to degenerative change when only the femoral head is replaced or resurfaced. The amount of acetabular cartilage abnormality correlates with the degree of femoral head collapse.[127]

The most controversial issue with regard to the results of THA for the treatment of osteonecrosis is the durability of the prosthesis relative to that in patients with osteoarthritis. One body of literature suggests that total hip prostheses in patients with osteonecrosis of the femoral head are less durable than those in the general patient population,[128] while another body of literature suggests that osteonecrosis of the femoral head itself is not a risk factor for failure of THA.[129,130] Ritter and Meding[129] found no significant difference between the long-term complication rate after 64 THAs performed for osteonecrosis and after 65 THAs performed for osteoarthritis. Xenakis and associates[130] compared 29 THAs performed for osteonecrosis with 29 performed for osteoarthritis. At a mean follow-up of between 7 and 8 years, there was no significant difference in the failure rates of the two groups, which were also equivalent with regard to postoperative pain, function, and improvement in hip scores. In contrast, in an evaluation of the variables associated with implant durability in a large group of THAs with cement, Sarmiento and associates[131] concluded that the diagnosis of osteonecrosis had a negative impact. Saito and associates[132] compared 29 THAs performed for osteonecrosis with 63 performed for osteoarthritis and found a higher failure rate in the patients with osteonecrosis. However, the group with osteonecrosis had a different gender distribution and mean weight than the patients with osteoarthritis. Finally, Ortiguera and associates[133] compared 178 patients with osteonecrosis with a group with osteoarthritis matched by age, sex, surgeon, and implant (all cemented Charnley total hip prostheses). At a mean follow-up of 17.8 years, there was no significant difference between groups with regard to the durability of the total hip prosthesis in patients older than 50 years. However, in the group of 35 patients who were younger than 50 years, those with osteonecrosis had a significantly greater risk of mechanical failure than did the matched osteoarthritis cohort ($P < 0.05$).[133]

The underlying diagnosis associated with osteonecrosis of the femoral head appears to have an impact on implant durability. Chiu and associates[134] compared 36 cementless THAs performed for osteonecrosis with 36 performed for osteoarthritis. Of the patients with osteonecrosis, those who used corticosteroids or abused alcohol had worse prosthetic durability than did the group with osteoarthritis, but there was no difference in prosthetic durability between the patients with posttraumatic or idiopathic osteonecrosis and those with osteoarthritis. Brinker and associates[135] reported on 90 young patients (mean age, 39.9 years) treated with THA for osteonecrosis. Patients who were younger than 35 years at the time of the THA had a high failure rate, and the results varied by underlying diagnosis. Patients with systemic lupus erythematosus or an organ transplant had worse results than did those with idiopathic osteonecrosis of the femoral head. The effect of osteonecrosis of the femoral head on the longevity of total hip prostheses remains unresolved because it has proven difficult to disentangle the variables involved. Most patient cohorts with osteonecrosis may have a high percentage of individuals with demographic factors and underlying diagnoses that also put them at higher risk for mechanical failure of the arthroplasty. In addition, many of these patients are young and active or may have poor bone quality secondary to chronic corticosteroid use, alcohol abuse, or sickle cell disease.[136-138] Whether something about osteonecrosis of the femoral head itself leads to changes in the bone around the hip joint and poorer implant durability remains uncertain. However, it is likely that at least some of the reported problems with the durability of total hip prostheses in patients with osteonecrosis can be explained by patient demographics and the underlying diagnoses leading to osteonecrosis rather than by the osteonecrosis itself.

The reported results of THA, with and without cement, for patients with osteonecrosis of the femoral head vary with the success of the specific implants used in each series and with the demographic features of the patients in each cohort. Despite the difficulty of comparing different series, several generalizations can be made. On the acetabular side, the greatest problem with cemented sockets has been loosening, and the greatest problems with uncemented sockets have been polyethylene wear and periprosthetic osteolysis.[139-141] On the femoral side, components cemented with early techniques have had a high failure rate in patients with osteonecrosis in most reports. However, a number of studies have demonstrated improved results with modern cementation methods.[142-144] Garino and Steinberg[142] reported on 123 cemented and hybrid THAs performed with second-generation cement techniques in patients with osteonecrosis. At 2 to 10 years, the overall revision rate was only 4%. Kantor and associates[143] reviewed the results of 24 THAs performed for osteonecrosis with second-generation femoral cementing techniques; at a mean of 7.7 years, three had been revised for loosening, and the 10-year survivorship was 85.7%. The authors concluded that second-generation cementing techniques improved results but the failure rate was still high.

A number of reports on uncemented femoral components have demonstrated good implant fixation and durability. Fye and associates[145] reported a 94% rate of good or excellent clinical results and a 98% 11-year rate of survival of selected uncemented femoral stems in a large series of THAs performed in young patients with osteonecrosis. In a study of 29 patients with osteonecrosis treated with an uncemented stem, Xenakis and associates[130] found only one femoral failure at a mean of 7.1 years postoperatively. Piston and associates[140] reported on 35 THAs performed with a porous-coated uncemented stem in patients with osteonecrosis; at a mean of 7.5 years (range, 5 to 10 years), 94% of the stems demonstrated bone ingrowth and only one had been revised. D'Antonio and associates[146] found no stem failures, after a minimum of 5 years, in 53 hips treated with a hydroxyapatite-coated uncemented femoral stem for osteonecrosis. Good results with the use of uncemented stems in patients with osteonecrosis of the femoral head mostly have been achieved with implant designs that also have had a high success rate in the general hip arthroplasty population.

Patients with osteonecrosis of the femoral head, in general and in certain subgroups, may be at increased risk for specific complications of THA. Patients being managed with immunusuppression (such as long-term corticosteroid therapy or posttransplant regimens) may be at increased risk for infection. There is some evidence that patients with osteonecrosis of the femoral head may be at higher risk for postoperative dislocation.[134] This risk may be higher because specific subgroups (such as alcohol abusers) are at risk for dislocation or because patients with osteonecrosis of the femoral head frequently have less capsular hypertrophy than patients with osteoarthritis and therefore may have less optimal soft-tissue restraints against dislocation.

Specific technical issues are important to consider when THA is performed for patients with osteonecrosis of the femoral head. Patients with risk factors for dislocation such as alcohol abuse may be considered candidates for specific measures to reduce the risk of dislocation, such as an anterolateral surgical approach or methods of enhanced posterior soft-tissue repair with the posterior approach. Implant choice is based on the preference and experience of the surgeon, but the individual patient's circumstances also should be kept in mind. For example, a young, active, healthy patient with good bone might be considered a good candidate for an uncemented implant and an alternative bearing surface, whereas an older, sicker patient with poor bone stock might be better treated with hybrid or cement fixation. When THA is performed in patients with osteonecrosis of the femoral head but without advanced secondary arthritis, the acetabular bone may not be as hard or sclerotic as the bone in most osteoarthritic hips. When implanting a socket without cement, the surgeon should be aware that this weaker acetabular bone may be at greater risk for fracture. The femoral anatomy may have been altered by a previous osteotomy, core decompression, or bone graft. Previous bone grafts in the femoral neck and head can leave behind hard sclerotic bone that is difficult to shape with rasps or broaches and can force instruments and implants into malposition (Fig. 10). Fehrle and associates[147] found that previous tibial cortical grafts led to suboptimal implant position in the coronal plane in 10 of 13 hips. Milling techniques and high-speed burrs can help to remove the sclerotic bone safely, and intraoperative radiographs are recommended for checking of broach alignment.

There is a good likelihood that THA will provide excellent pain relief and function for patients with osteonecrosis of the femoral head. The durability of total hip prostheses in cohorts with osteonecrosis of the femoral head may be poorer than the durability in the general population, in part because of patient demographics and reduced bone quality in some patient subgroups. Good surgical technique and implant choice may minimize the negative impact of osteonecrosis of the femoral head on implant durability. Osteonecrosis of the femoral head is associated with a disparate group of diagnoses and affects patients with very different levels of activity and bone quality.

Individualizing surgical technique and implant choice accordingly may help to optimize results and to minimize complications of THA in these patients.

Potential Treatment Algorithm

Because osteonecrosis presents with a wide spectrum of disease, a number of different treatment modalities are appropriate depending on the age and diagnosis of the patient, the extent and location of the osteonecrosis, and whether the femoral head has collapsed. The primary goals of treatment should be to relieve pain, to maintain a congruent hip joint, and to delay the need for a THA for as long as possible. When this disease is diagnosed in a younger patient, it may be advisable to perform the most conservative surgical procedure possible with the knowledge that a future intervention may be necessary.

There are a number of findings on plain radiographs and MRI scans that clearly should influence the choice of treatment. First, it is essential to determine whether the femoral head has collapsed. A good indication of collapse is the crescent sign, which can be seen on radiographic examination, especially the frog-leg lateral view. The crescent sign represents subchondral collapse or fracture. In general, once the femoral head has collapsed, the success of procedures such as core decompression or vascularized fibular grafting decreases substantially. The second factor is the size and location (extent of involvement of the weight-bearing surface) of the lesion. Studies have shown that both the size and the location of the lesion are crucial in determining both clinical and radiographic outcomes.[148,149] Size and location can be determined on plain radiographs or MRI scans.[148] Clearly, if there is extensive involvement of the femoral head (> 30%) and almost complete involvement of the weight-bearing surface, then the success rate of procedures that save the femoral head will be decreased, and

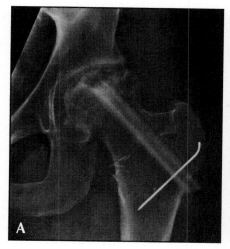
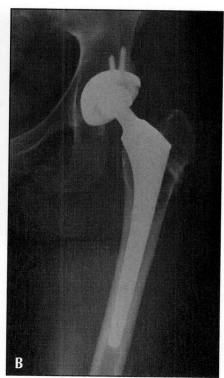

Fig. 10 A, AP radiograph of a failed vascularized fibular graft used for treatment of osteonecrosis of the femoral head. **B,** AP radiograph made after conversion to a cementless THA. A power burr and broaches were used to facilitate shaping of the proximal part of the femur.

Table 3
Treatment Algorithm According to the University of Pennsylvania System of Classification and Staging[41]

Radiographic Stage	Symptoms	Procedure
I and II	Asymptomatic	Observation, pharmacologic treatment, possible core decompression ± bone grafting
IA, IB, IC, IIA, IIB, and IIC	Symptomatic	Core decompression ± bone grafting, vascularized graft
IC, IIC, IIIA, IIIB, IIIC, and IVA	Symptomatic	Bone grafting (vascularized or nonvascularized), osteotomy, limited femoral head resurfacing, THA
IVB and IVC	Symptomatic	Limited femoral head resurfacing, THA
V and VI	Symptomatic	THA

this must be discussed with the patient. The third factor is the amount of depression of the femoral head. Treatment of patients who have femoral head depression is somewhat controversial. Some surgeons attempt bone grafting procedures if the collapse is less than 2 mm, whereas others believe that some type of arthroplasty should be performed because of the inconsistent results and limited data available on the efficacy of

bone grafting in these patients. There is general agreement that patients with less than 2 mm of femoral head depression should have an arthroplasty. The final factor in the choice of treatment of osteonecrosis of the femoral head is acetabular involvement. If the acetabular cartilage is markedly involved, THA is the only appropriate surgical treatment.

An intraoperative assessment of the femoral head and/or acetabular cartilage is necessary if one is considering performing a bone grafting procedure that involves elevation of the cartilage, a window in the femoral neck, or a limited femoral head resurfacing. The intraoperative examination is essential to confirm findings seen on radiographs or MRI scans. For example, preoperatively, one might plan a bone grafting procedure of the femoral head, but if the femoral head cartilage is noted to be damaged and the acetabular cartilage is seen to be pristine at the time of the operation, a limited femoral resurfacing would be appropriate. However, if the femoral head and acetabular cartilage appear healthy and undamaged, the bone grafting procedure is a reasonable option. If degeneration of the acetabular cartilage is noted on intraoperative examination, then a THA should be performed. Some authors have recommended hip arthroscopy to assess the cartilage prior to performing a vascularized fibular graft procedure, but further study of the efficacy of this diagnostic step is necessary.[150]

On the basis of the aforementioned treatment criteria, we developed an algorithm that uses the University of Pennsylvania radiographic classification of the disease. These are just general guidelines. A treatment program must be individualized for each patient (Table 3).

Summary

Osteonecrosis remains a difficult condition to treat because of a lack of understanding of the etiology of the disease and because it often affects young patients during the prime of their lives. The multitude of treatment modalities being used confirms both a lack of consensus and the difficulty in successfully treating these patients. The availability of growth factors that will promote bone formation and angiogenesis may revolutionize treatment of this condition. Hopefully, research efforts to enhance our understanding of the pathophysiology of this disease will enable us to improve our ability to treat patients with osteonecrosis of the hip in the future.

References

1. Mont MA, Hungerford DS: Non-traumatic avascular necrosis of the femoral head. *J Bone Joint Surg Am* 1995;77:459-474.

2. Cruess RL: Steroid-induced osteonecrosis. *J Roy Coll Surg Edinb* 1981;26:69-77.

3. Roeder LF Jr, DeLee JC: Femoral head fractures associated with posterior hip dislocation. *Clin Orthop* 1980;147:121-130.

4. Upadhyay SS, Moulton A, Srikrishnamurthy K: An analysis of the late effects of traumatic posterior dislocation of the hip without fractures. *J Bone Joint Surg Br* 1983;65:150-152.

5. Brav EA: Traumatic dislocation of the hip: Army experience and results over a twelve-year period. *J Bone Joint Surg Am* 1962;44:1115-1134.

6. Barnes R, Brown JT, Garden RS, Nicoll EA: Subcapital fractures of the femur: A prospective review. *J Bone Joint Surg Br* 1976;58:2-24.

7. Garden RS: Malreduction and avascular necrosis in subcapital fractures of the femur. *J Bone Joint Surg Br* 1971;53:183-197.

8. Jacobs B: Epidemiology of traumatic and nontraumatic osteonecrosis. *Clin Orthop* 1978;130:51-67.

9. Felson DT, Anderson JJ: A cross-study evaluation of association between steroid dose and bolus steroids and avascular necrosis of bone. *Lancet* 1987;1:902-906.

10. Jones JP Jr: Etiology and pathogenesis of osteonecrosis. *Semin Arthroplasty* 1991;2:160-168.

11. Vakil N, Sparberg M: Steroid-related osteonecrosis in inflammatory bowel disease. *Gastroenterology* 1989;96:62-67.

12. Zizic TM, Marcoux C, Hungerford DS, Dansereau JV, Stevens MB: Corticosteroid therapy associated with ischemic necrosis of bone in systemic lupus erythematosus. *Am J Med* 1985;79:596-604.

13. Matsuo K, Hirohata T, Sugioka Y, Ikeda M, Fukuda A: Influence of alcohol intake, cigarette smoking, and occupational status on idiopathic osteonecrosis of the femoral head. *Clin Orthop* 1988;234:115-123.

14. Ono K, Sugioka Y: Epidemiology and risk factors in avascular osteonecrosis of the femoral head, in Schoutens A, Arlet J, Gardeniers JWM, Hughs SPF (eds): *Bone Circulation and Vascularization in Normal and Pathological Conditions.* New York, NY, Plenum Press, 1993, pp 243-248.

15. Tanaka KD, Clifford GO, Axelrod AR: Sickle cell anemia (homozygous S) with aseptic necrosis of the femoral head. *Blood* 1956;11:998-1008.

16. Barton CJ, Cockshott WP: Bone changes in hemoglobin SC disease. *AJR Am J Roentgenol* 1962;88:523-532.

17. Kiaer T, Pedersen NW, Kristensen KD, Starklint H: Intra-osseous pressure and oxygen tension in avascular necrosis and osteoarthritis of the hip. *J Bone Joint Surg Br* 1990;72:1023-1030.

18. Aaron RK: Osteonecrosis: Etiology, pathophysiology, and diagnosis, in Callaghan JJ, Rosenberg AG, Rubash HE (eds): *The Adult Hip.* Philadelphia, PA, Lippincott-Raven, 1998, pp 451-466.

19. Rosendaal FR, Koster T, Vandenbroucke JP, Reitsma PH: High risk of thrombosis in patients homozygous for factor V Leiden (activated protein C resistance). *Blood* 1995;85:1504-1508.

20. Aaron RK, Ciombor DM: Coagulopathies and osteonecrosis. *Curr Opin Orthop* 2001;12:370-383.

21. Wheeless CR, Lins RE, Knelson MH, Urbaniak JR: Digital subtraction angiography in patients with osteonecrosis of the femoral head, in Urbaniak JR, Jones JP Jr (eds): *Osteonecrosis: Etiology, Diagnosis, and Treatment.* Rosemont, IL, American Academy of Orthopaedic Surgeons, 1997, pp 241-245.

22. Norman A, Bullough P: The radiolucent crescent line: An early diagnostic sign of avascular necrosis of the femoral head. *Bull Hosp Joint Dis* 1963;24:99-104.

23. Steinberg ME, Steinberg DR: Avascular necrosis of the femoral head, in Steinberg ME (ed): *The Hip and Its Disorders.* Philadelphia, PA, WB Saunders, 1991, pp 623-647.

24. Totty WG, Murphy WA, Ganz WI, Kumar B, Daum WJ, Siegel BA: Magnetic resonance imaging of the normal and ischemic femoral head. *AJR Am J Roentgenol* 1984;143:1273-1280.

25. Beltran J, Herman LJ, Burk JM, et al: Femoral head avascular necrosis: MR imaging with clinical-pathologic and radionuclide correlation. *Radiology* 1988;166:215-220.

26. Jiang CC, Shih TT: Epiphyseal scar of the femoral head: Risk factor of osteonecrosis. *Radiology* 1994;191:409-412.

27. Markisz JA, Knowles RJ, Altchek DW, Schneider R, Whalen JP, Cahill PT: Segmental patterns of avascular necrosis of the femoral head: Early detection with MR imaging. *Radiology* 1987;162:717-720.

28. Mitchell DG, Rao VM, Dalinka MK, et al: Femoral head avascular necrosis: Correlation of MR imaging, radiographic staging, radionuclide imaging, and clinical findings. *Radiology* 1987;162:709-715.

29. Mitchell MD, Kundel HL, Steinberg ME, Kressel HY, Alavi A, Axel L: Avascular necrosis of the hip: Comparison of MR, CT, and scintigraphy. *AJR Am J Roentgenol.* 1986;147:67-71.

30. Functional investigation of bone under normal conditions, in Ficat RP, Arlet J, Hungerford DS (ed): *Ischemia and Necrosis of Bone.* Baltimore, MD, Williams and Wilkins, 1980, pp 29-52.

31. Bramlett KW, Killian JT, Nasca RJ, Daniel WW: Transient osteoporosis. *Clin Orthop* 1987;222:197-202.

32. Kaplan SS, Stegman CJ: Transient osteoporosis of the hip: A case report and review of the literature. *J Bone Joint Surg Am* 1985; 67:490-493.

33. Potter H, Moran M, Schneider R, Bansal M, Sherman C, Markisz J: Magnetic resonance imaging in diagnosis of transient osteoporosis of the hip. *Clin Orthop* 1992;280:223-229.

34. Takatori Y, Kokubo T, Ninomiya S, Nakamura T, Okutsu I, Kamogawa M: Transient osteoporosis of the hip: Magnetic resonance imaging. *Clin Orthop* 1991;271:190-194.

35. Turner DA, Templeton AC, Selzer PM, Rosenberg AG, Petasnick JP: Femoral capital osteonecrosis: MR findings of diffuse marrow abnormalities without focal lesions. *Radiology* 1989;171:135-140.

36. Unger E, Moldofsky P, Gatenby R, Hartz W, Broder G: Diagnosis of osteomyelitis by MR imaging. *AJR Am J Roentgenol* 1988;150:605-610.

37. Guerra JJ, Steinberg ME: Distinguishing transient osteoporosis from avascular necrosis of the hip. *J Bone Joint Surg Am* 1995;77:616-624.

38. Kopecky KK, Braunstein EM, Brandt KD, et al: Apparent avascular necrosis of the hip: Appearance and spontaneous resolution of MR findings in renal allograft recipients. *Radiology* 1991;179:523-527.

39. Ficat RP: Idiopathic bone necrosis of the femoral head: Early diagnosis and treatment. *J Bone Joint Surg Br* 1985;67:3-9.

40. Marcus ND, Enneking WF, Massam RA: The silent hip in idiopathic aseptic necrosis: Treatment by bone-grafting. *J Bone Joint Surg Am* 1973;55:1351-1366.

41. Steinberg ME, Hayken GD, Steinberg DR: A quantitative system for staging avascular necrosis. *J Bone Joint Surg Br* 1995;77:34-41.

42. ARCO (Association Research Circulation Osseous): Committee on Terminology and Classification. *ARCO News* 1992;4:41-46.

43. Ohzono K, Saito M, Takaoka K, et al: Natural history of nontraumatic avascular necrosis of the femoral head. *J Bone Joint Surg Br* 1991;73:68-72.

44. Mont MA, Jones LC, Sotereanos DG, Amstutz HC, Hungerford DS: Understanding and treating osteonecrosis of the femoral head. *Instr Course Lect* 2000;49:169-185.

45. Smith KR, Bonfiglio M, Montgomery WJ: Non-traumatic necrosis of the femoral head treated with tibial bone-grafting: A follow-up note. *J Bone Joint Surg Am* 1980;62:845-847.

46. Aaron RK, Ciombor DM, Lord CF: Core decompression augmented with human decalcified bone matrix graft for osteonecrosis of the femoral head, in Urbaniak JR, Jones JP (eds): *Osteonecrosis: Etiology, Diagnosis, and Treatment.* Rosemont, IL, American Academy of Orthopaedic Surgeons, 1997, pp 301-307.

47. Meyers MH: The treatment of osteonecrosis of the hip with fresh osteochondral allografts and with the muscle pedicle graft technique. *Clin Orthop* 1978;130:202-209.

48. Yoo MC, Chung DW, Hahn CS: Free vascularized fibula grafting for the treatment of osteonecrosis of the femoral head. *Clin Orthop* 1992;277:128-138.

49. Iwata H, Torii S, Hasegawa Y, et al: Indications and results of vascularized pedicle iliac bone graft in avascular necrosis of the femoral head. *Clin Orthop* 1993;295:281-288.

50. Urbaniak JR, Coogan PG, Gunneson EB, Nunley JA: Treatment of osteonecrosis of the femoral head with free vascularized fibular grafting: A long-term follow-up study of one hundred and three hips. *J Bone Joint Surg Am* 1995;77:681-694.

51. Steinberg ME, Larcom PG, Stafford BB, et al: Treatment of osteonecrosis of the femoral head by core decompression, bone grafting, and electrical stimulation, in Urbaniak JR, Jones JP Jr (eds): *Osteonecrosis: Etiology, Diagnosis, and Treatment.* Rosemont, IL, American Academy of Orthopaedic Surgeons, 1997, pp 293-299.

52. Aaron RK, Lennox D, Bunce GE, Ebert T: The conservative treatment of osteonecrosis of the femoral head: A comparison of core decompression and pulsing electromagnetic fields. *Clin Orthop* 1989;249:209-218.

53. Stulberg BN, Davis AW, Bauer TW, Levine M, Easley K: Osteonecrosis of the femoral head: A prospective randomized treatment protocol. *Clin Orthop* 1991;268:140-151.

54. Koo KH, Kim R, Ko GH, Song HR, Jeong ST, Cho SH: Preventing collapse in early osteonecrosis of the femoral head: A randomised clinical trial of core decompression. *J Bone Joint Surg Br* 1995;77:870-874.

55. Smith SW, Fehring TK, Griffin WL, Beaver WB: Core decompression of the osteonecrotic femoral head. *J Bone Joint Surg Am* 1995;77:674-680.

56. Mont MA, Carbone JJ, Fairbank AC: Core decompression versus nonoperative management for osteonecrosis of the hip. *Clin Orthop* 1996;324:169-178.

57. Fairbank AC, Bhatia D, Jinnah RH, Hungerford DS: Long-term results of core decompression for ischaemic necrosis of the femoral head. *J Bone Joint Surg Br* 1995;77:42-49.

58. Steinberg ME: Core decompression. *Semin Arthroplasty* 1998;9:213-220.

59. Bozic KJ, Zurakowski D, Thornhill TS: Survivorship analysis of hips treated with core decompression for nontraumatic osteonecrosis of the femoral head. *J Bone Joint Surg Am* 1999;81:200-209.

60. Sotereanos DG, Plakseychuk AY, Rubash HE: Free vascularized fibula grafting for the treatment of osteonecrosis of the femoral head. *Clin Orthop* 1997;344:243-256.

61. Urbaniak JR, Harvey EJ: Revascularization of the femoral head in osteonecrosis. *J Am Acad Orthop Surg* 1998;6:44-54.

62. Kane SM, Ward WA, Jordan LC, Guilford WB, Hanley EN Jr: Vascularized fibular grafting compared with core decompression in the treatment of femoral head osteonecrosis. *Orthopedics* 1996;19:869-872.

63. Scully SP, Aaron RK, Urbaniak JR: Survival analysis of hips treated with core decompression or vascularized fibular grafting because of avascular necrosis. *J Bone Joint Surg Am* 1998;80:1270-1275.

64. Vail TP, Urbaniak JR: Donor-site morbidity with use of vascularized autogenous fibular grafts. *J Bone Joint Surg Am* 1996;78:204-211.

65. Aluisio FV, Urbaniak JR: Proximal femur fractures after free vascularized fibular grafting to the hip. *Clin Orthop* 1998;356:192-201.

66. Mont MA, Hungerford DS: Non-traumatic avascular necrosis of the femoral head. *J Bone Joint Surg Am* 1995;77:459-474.

67. Gottschalk F: Indications and results of intertrochanteric osteotomy in osteonecrosis of the femoral head. *Clin Orthop* 1989;249:219-222.

68. Kerboul M, Thomine J, Postel M, Merle d'Aubigné R: The conservative surgical treatment of idiopathic aseptic necrosis of the femoral head. *J Bone Joint Surg Br* 1974;56:291-296.

69. Mont MA, Fairbank AC, Krackow KA, Hungerford DS: Corrective osteotomy for osteonecrosis of the femoral head. *J Bone Joint Surg Am* 1996;78:1032-1038.

70. Scher MA, Jakim I: Intertrochanteric osteotomy and autogenous bone-grafting for avascular necrosis of the femoral head. *J Bone Joint Surg Am* 1993;75:1119-1133.

71. Sugano N, Takaoka K, Ohzono K, Matsui M, Saito M, Saito S: Rotational osteotomy for non-traumatic avascular necrosis of the femoral head. *J Bone Joint Surg Br* 1992;74:734-739.

72. Sugioka Y, Hotokebuchi T, Tsutsui H: Transtrochanteric anterior rotational osteotomy for idiopathic and steroid-induced necrosis of the femoral head: Indications and long-term results. *Clin Orthop* 1992;277:111-120.

73. Tooke SM, Amstutz HC, Hedley AK: Results of transtrochanteric rotational osteotomy for femoral head osteonecrosis. *Clin Orthop* 1987;224:150-157.

74. Willert HG, Buchhorn G, Zichner L: Results of flexion osteotomy on segmental femoral head necrosis in adults, in Weil UH (ed): *Progress in Orthopaedic Surgery: Segmental Idiopathic Necrosis of the Femoral Head.* Berlin, Germany, Springer-Verlag, 1981, vol 5, pp 63-80.

75. Dean MT, Cabanela ME: Transtrochanteric anterior rotational osteotomy for avascular necrosis of the femoral head: Long-term results. *J Bone Joint Surg Br* 1993;75:597-601.

76. Eyb R, Kotz R: The transtrochanteric anterior rotational osteotomy of Sugioka: Early and late results in idiopathic aseptic femoral head necrosis. *Arch Orthop Trauma Surg* 1987;106:161-167.

77. Jacobs MA, Hungerford DS, Krackow KA: Intertrochanteric osteotomy for avascular necrosis of the femoral head. *J Bone Joint Surg Br* 1989;71:200-204.

78. Maistrelli G, Fusco U, Avai A, Bombelli R: Osteonecrosis of the hip treated by intertrochanteric osteotomy: A four- to 15-year follow-up. *J Bone Joint Surg Br* 1988;70:761-766.

79. Masuda T, Matsuno T, Hasegawa I, Kanno T, Ichioka Y, Kaneda K: Results of transtrochanteric rotational osteotomy for nontraumatic osteonecrosis of the femoral head. *Clin Orthop* 1988;228:69-74.

80. Sugioka Y, Katsuki I, Hotokebuchi T: Transtrochanteric rotational osteotomy of the femoral head for the treatment of osteonecrosis: Follow-up statistics. *Clin Orthop* 1982;169:115-126.

81. Wagner H, Zeiler G: Idiopathic necrosis of the femoral head: Results of intertrochanteric

osteotomy and joint resurfacing, in Weil UH (ed): *Progress in Orthopaedic Surgery: Segmental Idiopathic Necrosis of the Femoral Head.* Berlin, Germany, Springer-Verlag, 1981, vol 5, pp 87-116.

82. Arnoldi CC, Lemperg R, Linderholm H: Immediate effect of osteotomy on the intramedullary pressure in the femoral head and neck in patients with degenerative osteoarthritis. *Acta Orthop Scand* 1971;42:454-455.

83. Merle D'Aubigne R, Postel M, Mazabraud A, Massias P, Gueguen J, France P: Idiopathic necrosis of the femoral head in adults. *J Bone Joint Surg Br* 1965;47:612-633.

84. Harris WH: Traumatic arthritis of the hip after dislocation and acetabular fractures: Treatment by mold arthroplasty: An end-result study using a new method of result evaluation. *J Bone Joint Surg Am* 1969;51:737-755.

85. Saito S, Ohzono K, Ono K: Joint-preserving operations for idiopathic avascular necrosis of the femoral head: Results of core decompression, grafting and osteotomy. *J Bone Joint Surg Br* 1988;70:78-84.

86. Benke GJ, Baker AS, Dounis E: Total hip replacement after upper femoral osteotomy: A clinical review. *J Bone Joint Surg Br* 1982;64:570-571.

87. Wang GJ, Sweet DE, Reger SI, Thompson RC. Fat-cell changes as a mechanism of avascular necrosis of the femoral head in cortisone-treated rabbits. *J Bone Joint Surg Am* 1977;59:729-735.

88. Buckley PD, Gearen PF, Petty RW: Structural bone-grafting for early atraumatic avascular necrosis of the femoral head. *J Bone Joint Surg Am* 1991;73:1357-1364.

89. Rosenwasser MP, Garino JP, Kiernan HA, Michelsen CB. Long term followup of thorough debridement and cancellous bone grafting of the femoral head for avascular necrosis. *Clin Orthop* 1994;306:17-27.

90. Boettcher WG, Bonfiglio M, Smith K: Non-traumatic necrosis of the femoral head: Part II. Experiences in treatment. *J Bone Joint Surg Am* 1970;52:322-329.

91. Bonfiglio M, Bardenstein MB: Treatment by bone-grafting of aseptic necrosis of the femoral head and non-union of the femoral neck (Phemister technique). *J Bone Joint Surg Am* 1958;40:1329-1346.

92. Bonfiglio M, Voke EM: Aseptic necrosis of the femoral head and non-union of the femoral neck: Effect of treatment by drilling and bone-grafting (Phemister technique). *J Bone Joint Surg Am* 1968;50:48-66.

93. Dunn AW, Grow T: Aseptic necrosis of the femoral head: Treatment with bone grafts of doubtful value. *Clin Orthop* 1977;122:249-254.

94. Itoman M, Yamamoto M: Pathogenesis and treatment of idiopathic aseptic necrosis of the femoral head. *Clin Immunol* 1989;21:713-725.

95. Mont MA, Einhorn TA, Sponseller PD, Hungerford DS: The trapdoor procedure using autogenous cortical and cancellous bone grafts for osteonecrosis of the femoral head. *J Bone Joint Surg Br* 1998;80:56-62.

96. Phemister DB: Treatment of the necrotic head of the femur in adults. *J Bone Joint Surg Am* 1949;31:55-66.

97. Smith KR, Bonfiglio M, Montgomery WJ: Nontraumatic necrosis of the femoral head treated with tibial bone-grafting: A follow-up note. *J Bone Joint Surg Am* 1980;62:845-847.

98. Springfield DS, Enneking WJ: Surgery for aseptic necrosis of the femoral head. *Clin Orthop* 1978;130:175-185.

99. Phemister DB: Treatment of the necrotic head of the femur in adults. *J Bone Joint Surg Am* 1949;31:55-66.

100. Marcus ND, Enneking WF, Massam RA: The silent hip in idiopathic aseptic necrosis: Treatment by bone-grafting. *J Bone Joint Surg Am* 1973;55:1351-1366.

101. Ganz R, Büchler U: Overview of attempts to revitalize the dead head in aseptic necrosis of the femoral head: Osteotomy and revascularization, in Hungerford DS (ed): *The Hip: Proceedings of the Eleventh Open Scientific Meeting of The Hip Society.* St. Louis, MO, CV Mosby, 1983, pp 296-305.

102. Yamamoto M, Itoman M, Sagamoto N, Morita M: Strut bone graft for aseptic necrosis of the femoral head: Theory and surgical technique. *Orthop Surg* 1983;34:902-908.

103. Meyers MH, Jones RE, Bucholz RW, Wenger DR: Fresh autogenous grafts and osteochondral allografts for the treatment of segmental collapse in osteonecrosis of the hip. *Clin Orthop* 1983;174:107-112.

104. Meyers MH, Convery FR: Grafting procedures in osteonecrosis of the hip. *Semin Arthroplasty* 1991;2:189-197.

105. Ko JY, Meyers MH, Wenger DR: "Trapdoor" procedure for osteonecrosis with segmental collapse of the femoral head in teenagers. *J Pediatr Orthop* 1995;15:7-15.

106. Rubash HE, Sinha RK, Shanbhag AS, Kim SY: Pathogenesis of bone loss after total hip arthroplasty. *Orthop Clin North Am* 1998;29:173-186.

107. Smith-Petersen MN: The classic: Evolution of mold arthroplasty of the hip joint. *Clin Orthop* 1978;134:5-11.

108. Amstutz HC, Grigoris P, Dorey FJ: Evolution and future of surface replacement of the hip. *J Orthop Sci* 1998;3:169-186.

109. Langlais F, Barthas J, Postel M: Adjusted cups for idiopathic necrosis: Radiological results. *Rev Chir Orthop Reparatrice Appar Mot* 1979;65:151-155.

110. Townley CO: Hemi and total articular replacement arthroplasty of the hip with the fixed femoral cup. *Orthop Clin North Am* 1982;13:869-894.

111. Amstutz HC, Dorey F, O'Carroll PF: THARIES resurfacing arthroplasty: Evolution and longterm results. *Clin Orthop* 1986;213:92-114.

112. Bierbaum BE, Sweet R: Complications of resurfacing arthroplasty. *Orthop Clin North Am* 1982;13:761-775.

113. Drinker H, Murray WR: The universal proximal femoral endoprosthesis: A short-term comparison with conventional hemiarthroplasty. *J Bone Joint Surg Am* 1979;61:1167-1174.

114. Head WC: Total articular resurfacing arthroplasty: Analysis of component failure in sixty seven hips. *J Bone Joint Surg Am* 1984;66:28-34.

115. Jolley MN, Salvati EA, Brown GC: Early results and complications of surface replacement of the hip. *J Bone Joint Surg Am* 1982; 64:366-377.

116. Kim WC, Grogan T, Amstutz HC, Dorey F: Survivorship comparison of THARIES and conventional hip arthroplasty in patients younger than 40 years old. *Clin Orthop* 1987;214:269-277.

117. Krackow KA, Mont MA, Maar DC: Limited femoral endoprosthesis for avascular necrosis of the femoral head. *Orthop Rev* 1993;22:457-463.

118. Scott RD, Urse JS, Schmidt R, Bierbaum BE: Use of TARA hemiarthroplasty in advanced osteonecrosis. *J Arthroplasty* 1987;2:225-232.

119. Hungerford MW, Mont MA, Scott R, Fiore C, Hungerford DS, Krackow KA: Surface replacement hemiarthroplasty for the treatment of osteonecrosis of the femoral head. *J Bone Joint Surg Am* 1998;80:1656-1664.

120. Nelson CL, Walz BH, Gruenwald JM: Resurfacing of only the femoral head for osteonecrosis. Long-term follow-up study. *J Arthroplasty* 1997;12:736-740.

121. Beaule PE, Schmalzried TP, Campbell P, Dorey F, Amstutz HC: Duration of symptoms and outcome of hemiresurfacing for hip osteonecrosis. *Clin Orthop* 2001;385:104-117.

122. Ash SA, Callaghan JJ, Johnston RC: Revision total hip arthroplasty with cement after cup arthroplasty: Long-term follow-up. *J Bone Joint Surg Am* 1996;78:87-93.

123. Lavernia CJ, Sierra RJ, Grieco FR: Osteonecrosis of the femoral head. *J Am Acad Orthop Surg* 1999;7:250-261.

124. Ito H, Matsuno T, Kaneda K: Bipolar hemiarthroplasty for osteonecrosis of the femoral head: A 7- to 18-year followup. *Clin Orthop* 2000;374:201-211.

125. Cabanela ME: Bipolar versus total hip arthroplasty for avascular necrosis of the femoral head: A comparison. *Clin Orthop* 1990;261:59-62.

126. Steinberg ME, Corces A, Fallon M: Acetabular involvement in osteonecrosis of the femoral head. *J Bone Joint Surg Am* 1999;81:60-65.

127. Im GI, Kim DY, Shin JH, Cho WH, Lee CJ: Degeneration of the acetabular cartilage in osteonecrosis of the femoral head: Histopathologic examination of 15 hips. *Acta Orthop Scand* 2000;71:28-30.

128. Salvati EA, Cornell CN: Long-term follow-up of total hip replacement in patients with avascular necrosis. *Instr Course Lect* 1988;37:67-73.

129. Ritter MA, Meding JB: A comparison of osteonecrosis and osteoarthritis patients following total hip arthroplasty: A long-term follow-up study. *Clin Orthop* 1986;206:139-146.

130. Xenakis TA, Beris AE, Malizos KK, Koukoubis T, Gelalis J, Soucacos PN: Total hip arthroplasty for avascular necrosis and degenerative

osteoarthritis of the hip. *Clin Orthop* 1997;341:62-68.

131. Sarmiento A, Ebramzadeh E, Gogan WJ, McKellop HA: Total hip arthroplasty with cement: A long-term radiographic analysis in patients who are older than fifty and younger than fifty years. *J Bone Joint Surg Am* 1990;72:1470-1476.

132. Saito S, Saito M, Nishina T, Ohzono K, Ono K: Long-term results of total hip arthroplasty for osteonecrosis of the femoral head: A comparison with osteoarthritis. *Clin Orthop* 1989;244:198-207.

133. Ortiguera CJ, Pulliam IT, Cabanela ME: Total hip arthroplasty for osteonecrosis: Matched pair analysis of 188 hips with long-term followup. *J Arthroplasty* 1999;14:21-28.

134. Chiu KH, Shen WY, Ko CK, Chan KM: Osteonecrosis of the femoral head treated with cementless total hip arthroplasty: A comparison with other diagnoses. *J Arthroplasty* 1997;12:683-688.

135. Brinker MR, Rosenberg AG, Kull L, Galante JO: Primary total hip arthroplasty using noncemented porous-coated femoral components in patients with osteonecrosis of the femoral head. *J Arthroplasty* 1994;9:457-468.

136. Clarke HJ, Jinnah RH, Brooker AF, Michaelson JD: Total replacement of the hip for avascular necrosis in sickle cell disease. *J Bone Joint Surg Br* 1989;71:465-470.

137. Hanker GJ, Amstutz HC: Osteonecrosis of the hip in the sickle-cell diseases: Treatment and complications. *J Bone Joint Surg Am* 1988;70:499-506.

138. Moran MC: Osteonecrosis of the hip in sickle cell hemoglobinopathy. *Am J Orthop* 1995;24:18-24.

139. Phillips FM, Pottenger LA, Finn HA, Vandermolen J: Cementless total hip arthroplasty in patients with steroid-induced avascular necrosis of the hip: A 62-month follow-up study. *Clin Orthop* 1994;303:147-154.

140. Piston RW, Engh CA, De Carvalho PI, Suthers K: Osteonecrosis of the femoral head treated with total hip arthroplasty without cement. *J Bone Joint Surg Am* 1994;76:202-214.

141. Stulberg BN, Singer R, Goldner J, Stulberg J: Uncemented total hip arthroplasty in osteonecrosis: A 2- to 10-year evaluation. *Clin Orthop* 1997;334:116-123.

142. Garino JP, Steinberg ME: Total hip arthroplasty in patients with avascular necrosis of the femoral head: A 2- to 10-year follow-up. *Clin Orthop* 1997;334:108-115.

143. Kantor SG, Huo MH, Huk OL, Salvati EA: Cemented total hip arthroplasty in patients with osteonecrosis: A 6-year minimum follow-up study of second-generation cement techniques. *J Arthroplasty* 1996;11:267-271.

144. Ritter MA, Helphinstine J, Keating EM, Faris PM, Meding JB: Total hip arthroplasty in

patients with osteonecrosis: The effect of cement techniques. *Clin Orthop* 1997;338:94-99.

145. Fye MA, Huo MH, Zatorski LE, Keggi KJ: Total hip arthroplasty performed without cement in patients with femoral head osteonecrosis who are less than 50 years old. *J Arthroplasty* 1998;13:876-881.

146. D'Antonio JA, Capello WN, Manley MT, Feinberg J: Hydroxyapatite coated implants: Total hip arthroplasty in the young patient and patients with avascular necrosis. *Clin Orthop* 1997;344:124-138.

147. Fehrle MJ, Callaghan JJ, Clark CR, Peterson KK: Uncemented total hip arthroplasty in patients with aseptic necrosis of the femoral head and previous bone grafting. *J Arthroplasty* 1993;8:1-6.

148. Steinberg ME, Bands RE, Parry S, Hoffman E, Chan T, Hartman KM: Does lesion size affect the outcome in avascular necrosis? *Clin Orthop* 1999;367:262-271.

149. Mont MA, Jones LC, Pacheco I, Hungerford DS: Radiographic predictors of outcome of core decompression for hips with osteonecrosis stage III. *Clin Orthop* 1998;354:159-168.

150. Sekiya JK, Ruch DS, Hunter DM, et al: The role of arthroscopy in the diagnosis and staging of osteonecrosis, in: Urbaniak JR, Jones JP Jr (eds): *Osteonecrosis: Etiology, Diagnosis, and Treatment.* Rosemont, IL, American Academy of Orthopaedic Surgeons, 1997, pp 253-260.

Osteoporotic Femoral Neck Fractures: Management and Current Controversies

Michael J. Gardner, MD
Dean G. Lorich, MD
Joseph M. Lane, MD

Abstract

Osteoporosis is a pervasive disease among the growing elderly population. Femoral neck fractures are often a direct result of osteoporosis and are challenging to treat. Surgical interventions seek to return the patient to preinjury function as quickly as possible, but many obstacles exist. Disruption of the blood supply occurs regardless of the fracture pattern, and in the active elderly population, reduction and fixation should be done as soon as possible to minimize healing problems. Closed reduction with percutaneous cannulated screw instrumentation is currently the fixation method of choice, but even with meticulous technique, moderate complication rates persist. Newer devices and biologic bone augmentation cement show promise in decreasing postoperative fracture collapse. Patients in whom a stable reduction cannot be achieved or who have a limited life expectancy should undergo arthroplasty. Unipolar and bipolar arthroplasty have both been effective in restoring function and have been the standard of care in these patients. Recent evidence suggests that active elderly patients who have acetabular disease or severely displaced fractures may benefit most from primary total hip arthroplasty.

Fractures of the femoral neck and osteoporosis are epidemic diseases that occur in elderly patients. As the population continues to age, so does the rate of hip fracture and incidence of osteoporosis. More than 28 million Americans are affected, and this number is predicted to rise substantially over the next 20 years.[1] Osteoporosis leads to bone fragility and is directly linked to risk of hip fracture. Approximately 250,000 hip fractures occur annually in the United States, and 87% occur in people older than age 65 years, and 75% occur in women.[2,3]

Femoral neck fractures in the patient with osteoporosis pose a formidable challenge to the orthopaedic surgeon. Most of these patients have significant medical comorbidities, and many have a declining mental status. It is agreed that surgical intervention leads to superior outcomes, but deciding between closed reduction with percutaneous fixation or arthroplasty can be difficult. Treatment strategies must be altered in patients with severe radiographic osteopenia. Fixation techniques rely on hardware purchase in the femoral neck and head and is often inade-

quate in the osteoporotic hip.

Anatomy

Articular cartilage invests the entire femoral head and extends distally onto the neck of the femur. The synovial membrane and capsule of the hip joint envelop the entire femoral head and anterior neck, but only the proximal aspect of the posterior neck. The anatomy of the femoral head has implications in treatment decisions, as posteriorly displaced or angulated fractures are more likely to rupture the posterior capsule and relieve intra-articular pressure.

Osseous Anatomy

The angle of the femoral neck in the coronal plane in relation to the femoral shaft is approximately 128°, ranging from 122° to 134° in 95% of both men and women.[4] The angle of the neck in the axial plane is in approximately 10° of anteversion, but may range from 3° to 17°.[4] Posterolaterally on the femoral neck is the calcar femorale, a thickened plate of bone that extends superiorly and blends with the greater trochanter posteriorly. This transfers the majority of force to the femur during weight bearing, and its integrity after a femoral neck fracture plays a large part in favorable outcome following internal fixation.[5]

Vascular Anatomy

Blood supply to the femoral head is a crucial factor when evaluating fracture pattern, surgical timing, and choosing the method of treatment. Three arterial sources contribute to the femoral head. The artery of the ligamentum teres arises from the obturator artery and supplies a small area at the apex of the head. Intramedullary arteries penetrate the proximal head, but also contribute little to the overall blood supply. The major arterial source arises from the medial femoral circumflex artery, which encircles the superior neck posteriorly, and the lateral femoral circumflex, which lies anterior to the femoral neck. Both arise from the profunda femoris artery. These two branches form an intracapsular and extracapsular anastomotic ring,[6] which are connected by ascending cervical arteries, and which subsequently give off the lateral epiphyseal arteries (usually between two and six.) This arterial system pierces the capsule superolaterally to supply the majority of the head.[7-9]

When the femoral neck is fractured, some disruption of the blood supply invariably occurs. If the slightest bit of displacement occurs, the intraosseous vessels are initially damaged, and up to 60% of the blood supply may be compromised.[5,10,11] The level of the neck fracture also results in variable amounts of devascularization. Following a subcapital fracture, the ascending cervical arteries are frequently disrupted; however, when a basicervical fracture occurs, these arteries are more likely to be spared.[12]

Aside from direct vascular shear injuries, impediment of blood flow can increase intracapsular pressure and lead to osteonecrosis of the femoral head. The pressure threshold for impediment of perfusion has been reported between 40 and 80 mm Hg.[13-15] Woodhouse[13] found necrosis to be inevitable when this pressure threshold was maintained for 12 hours in a canine model. In a minimally displaced fracture, capsular rupture is infrequent and hematoma accumulation is likely. In two studies,[16,17] increased pressures were found in 64% of 25 femoral neck fractures, 70% of which returned to normal levels after aspiration. Despite this, there is no consensus that aspiration is beneficial. Other authors have reported average intra-articular pressures to be 18 mm Hg and 29 mm Hg.[18,19] Maruenda and associates[20] found no correlation between intracapsular pressure and patient outcomes. Although there is some evidence that capsular hematoma may reach critical levels, it currently remains unclear whether evacuation of the hematoma protects against osteonecrosis. Gill and associates[21] reported on 63 patients who underwent intraoperative drilling of the femoral head. Bleeding was correlated to union with 100% sensitivity and specificity.

Classification

Multiple classification systems exist for femoral neck fractures. The Garden classification[22,23] is the most widely recognized in the literature, using the amount of displacement to grade fracture patterns. Type I fractures are incomplete and may be valgus impacted. Type II fractures are complete fractures but are nondisplaced. Type III fractures are complete, but retain some bony contact between the proximal and distal fragment. Type IV fractures are completely displaced without cortical contact. These may be rotated in any plane, and often the trabeculae of the acetabulum and femoral head are aligned, as the soft tissues provide the only stabilizing force. In practice, most fractures are classified as nondisplaced (Garden I and II) or displaced (Garden III and IV), which have a much higher rate of nonunion and osteonecrosis when treated with internal fixation. Fractures are also frequently described by their location: subcapital, transcervical, or basilar. The former two are usually intracapsular, whereas basilar fractures may or may not occur within the capsule.

The Pauwels classification quantifies the angle of the fracture plane as viewed on the AP radiograph.[24,25] Type I fractures are between 30° and 50° from the horizontal, and tend to compress with weight bearing. Type II fractures are between 50° and 70°. Type III fractures are greater than 70°, and weight bearing causes a high shear force and tends to displace the fracture.

Diagnosis

Fractures of the femoral neck have a bimodal distribution, with a small peak among young adults involved in high-energy trauma, but most fractures occur in the elderly following a fall while standing or walking. After nondisplaced fractures, the patient may still be able to ambulate. Other pertinent elements of the history include past medical history, medications, and review of symptoms, paying particular attention to any signs indicating a possible myocardial or cerebrovascular event. Physical examination often reveals slight shortening and external rotation of the affected leg, although usually less so than with intertrochanteric fractures. Point tenderness is present over the groin, and any hip motion will perform or produce pain. Gentle axial force to the heel often causes pain, and the patient is unable to straight leg raise. Close inspection of the soft tissues and a thorough neurovascular examination are essential.

Imaging

A standard radiographic series includes an AP view of the pelvis and AP and lateral views of the hip and will show an obvious deformity in most femoral neck fractures. It is important to obtain a cross-table lateral view as opposed to a frog-leg view to minimize pain and risk of fracture displacement. An adequate lateral radiograph will show the presence or absence of crucial posterior comminution.[26,27] If initial studies are not diagnostic, repeating the AP hip radiograph with the leg in 15° of internal rotation may be helpful, to view the femoral neck en face.

Plain radiographs have been reported to be negative in femoral neck fractures in 6% to 8% of patients.[28,29] Delay in diagnosis of a fracture delays surgery and increases morbidity.[26,27,30,31] When radiographs are negative and clinical suspicion persists, bone scanning may be useful[29,32,33] and has been reported to have its highest sensitivity and specificity at least 3 days after fracture.[34,35] MRI is more sensitive and specific than bone scan,[36-40] particularly in the acute period, and is often the test of choice to rule out occult femoral neck fractures. Diagnosing occult fractures is particularly important when treating an elderly population with a high incidence of osteoporosis, in whom stress fractures of the femoral neck are more common.[41]

Surgical Treatment

Patients in whom a femoral neck fracture is diagnosed are ideally managed surgically, with a goal of prompt return to preoperative levels of function. Nonsurgical treatment of femoral neck fractures leads to unacceptably high complication rates,[42,43] with incidence of nonunion as high as 40%,[44] and is of historical interest only. Whenever possible, surgical intervention is preferred to provide stable fixation and allow immediate full weight bearing.

Currently, two categories of patients exist for whom nonsurgical treatment may be warranted. In patients who are medically unstable, surgery should be delayed. Following a myocardial infarction, the patient's cardiovascular status should be optimized before surgery. Surgery should be postponed in patients who are coagulopathic or therapeutically anticoagulated who cannot safely be reversed for at least 72 hours.[3] In patients who are severely demented or nonambulators, no function will be regained following surgical stabilization, and conservative treatment may be indicated. However, these patients are not treated with traction and bed rest as in the past; rather, they are mobilized after acute pain is controlled to prevent decubiti, pneumonia, and thrombophlebitis.

The age-old controversy in managing femoral neck fractures, for which there is still no consensus, is in deciding between arthroplasty and fixation. The preoperative functional status and physiologic age of the patient are the key elements in making a decision.[45] In a study of 836 hip fractures, Richmond and associates[46] found that patient age of 85 years or older was not associated with increased mortality; preoperative medical comorbidities were the significant factor. Some authors believe that all patients, regardless of age, fracture pattern, or time to surgery should be treated with internal fixation.[25,47] Proponents of this approach claim that a healed neck with the native femoral head is always superior to arthroplasty. Though healing complications following fixation of displaced fractures range from 16% to 40%,[47-50] only a fraction of these are symptomatic and require additional surgery for late head collapse secondary to nonunion or osteonecrosis.[23,47,51] Stromqvist and associates[47] reviewed 215 femoral neck fractures treated with internal fixation. At 2-year follow-up, 83% of the survivors had retained their native femoral head. It is generally agreed that patients younger than 65 years of age should undergo emergent internal fixation following anatomic reduction to minimize risk of osteonecrosis and allow the patient to retain the native femoral head. Patients who are physiologically older than 75 or 80 years old, or minimal community ambulators with or without severe dementia, should be considered for prosthetic replacement. Traditionally, this has included unipolar or bipolar hemiarthroplasty,[52-55] but with improved technology and materials in arthroplasty, total hip replacement may provide superior results.[56-60]

A gray area exists around the appropriate management of the "young elderly," patients between 65 and 75 years old. There have been many reports comparing internal fixation versus arthroplasty, but few have been prospectively controlled. In a meta-analysis, Lu-Yao and associates[50] found only four suitable studies. They reported a 20% to 36% revision rate within 2 years following internal fixation, though not all studies used parallel cannulated screws. Hemiarthroplasty yielded a 6% to 18% revision surgery rate, with earlier mobility and better functional results at 1 year. There was no difference in mortality at 1 year. Despite

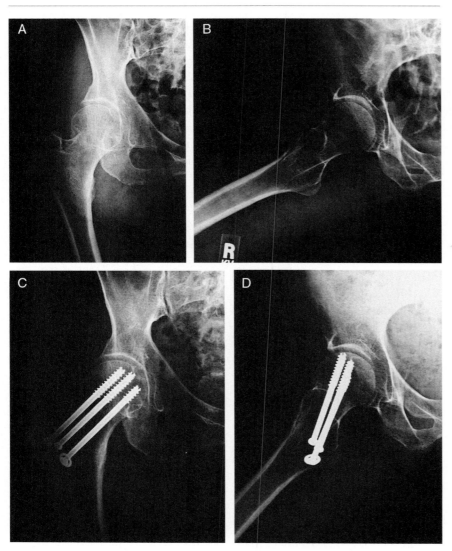

Figure 1 A and **B,** Radiographs showing Garden II femoral neck fracture in an 81-year-old woman. **C** and **D,** Three months after fixation, the fracture has healed in its initial stable position.

tion of femoral neck fractures. The current gold standard implant is three 7.3-mm partially threaded cannulated screws, inserted percutaneously through stab incisions[45,61,66] (Figure 1). Asnis and Wanek-Sgaglione[48] examined 141 fractures, 65% of which were displaced. With an average follow-up of 8 years, they reported no wound complications, a 96% healing rate, and an osteonecrosis rate of 22%.

An adequately stable reduction increases perfusion to the femoral head,[5,12,67] and the reduction achieved is far more important than implant selection or insertion technique.[27,68-73] Although some damage to the vascular supply inevitably occurs immediately following a femoral neck fracture, anatomic reduction decreases incidence of osteonecrosis and nonunion, giving way to a mechanically optimal environment for healing.[68-70,73,74] Various closed reduction techniques have been described with minor differences. The essential components include gentle traction with the hip in abduction and slight extension, followed by internal rotation and adduction to slightly beyond neutral. It is important to take care to achieve the optimal reduction on the first attempt, as subsequent reductions can further damage the remaining tenuous blood supply.[75] It is generally agreed that varus alignment places the fracture site in a mechanically disadvantageous position, and any residual varus is unacceptable.[68,69] Garden described a system of measuring the angle between the proximal and distal trabeculae, which normally measures 160°.[76] He reported 155° to 180° in both the AP and lateral views to be satisfactory. Lindequist and Tornkvist[77] used similar measurements and stated that displacement of 2 mm or less, with less than 10° of angulation, was acceptable. If a satisfactory reduction

these results, many other authors have reported increased wound complication, more frequent medical complications, prosthetic loosening, and dislocation rates up to 11% with hemiarthroplasty.[49,61-64] Most of the literature in the last few decades regarding superior outcomes is frequently methodologically flawed and inconclusive, and decisions must be based individually on preoperative function, bone quality, and comorbidities.[5] With the increasing awareness and improved medical treatment of osteoporosis,[65] coupled with the increasing numbers of active elderly patients and longer life expectancy, many patients in this age group are better candidates for fixation techniques. Closed reduction and percutaneous fixation can be attempted in these patients.

Internal Fixation
Dozens of devices have been developed over the past 70 years for fixa-

is achieved, pinning may proceed (Figure 2). Ideally, three screws should be placed in an inverted triangle configuration,[45,61,66,78] with the screws spread apart to abut cortical bone. The most crucial aspect of screw placement is obtaining cortical support along the posteromedial calcar.[77,79,80] Two screws should be placed inferiorly and posteriorly within 3 mm of the cortex to prevent postoperative varus deformity[48,77-79] (Figure 3). Entry point of the screws should begin no lower than the superior border of the lesser trochanter to prevent a stress riser and possible subtrochanteric fracture.

If the fracture remains unreduced, particularly in the lateral fluoroscopic view in the presence of posterior comminution, a decision must be made whether to proceed or convert to arthroplasty. This decision must be based on the physiologic age and functional demands of the patient. A prosthetic replacement should be performed in a patient who is older than age 75 years or who is sedentary with other medical health issues and has a displaced fracture. However, severe dementia has correlated with a high mortality rate following hemiarthroplasty,[81] and pinning in situ should be performed. For younger, more active elderly patients, open reduction and percutaneous pinning is the treatment of choice. A lateral Watson-Jones approach with an anterior capsulotomy affords excellent visualization while avoiding damage to the crucial posterior blood supply to the head.

In patients with a basicervical fracture, there is ample bone for purchase in the proximal fragment. The rotational moment behaves similarly to an intertrochanteric fracture[45,82-84] and may be treated with a sliding hip screw or intramedullary device such as a Trochanteric Fixation Nail

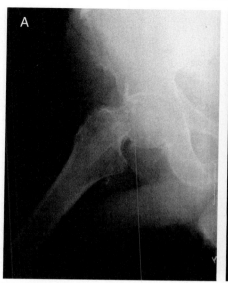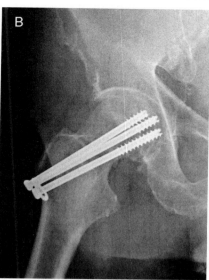

Figure 2 A, Radiograph showing Garden III fracture with varus angulation. **B,** Following reduction on a fracture table, the deformity is corrected and pinning is performed.

(TFN; Synthes USA, Paoli, PA). For Pauwels type III fractures with a steep fracture angle, biomechanical studies have shown superior results using a dynamic condylar screw or crossed screw fixation with purchase in the calcar,[85] or a sliding hip screw.[86] Consideration must be given to the potential rotation of the head and neck about its axis with insertion of the lag screw or spiral blade, and a supplemental provisional or permanent device can be used to prevent this.[82] It is also critical to avoid superolateral placement of the head fixation device to avoid damage to the main blood supply to the femoral head.[87,88]

Primary Arthroplasty
In a patient with low functional demands or whose medical condition prohibits early fixation to salvage the femoral head, primary arthroplasty is indicated. In a recent study of 90 hip fractures treated with internal fixation, Tidermark and associates[89] reported that patients with displaced fractures had a higher nonunion rate,

and patients whose fractures healed well had a significant decrease in quality of life. This adds more support to performing primary arthroplasty in patients with Garden IV fractures. Bipolar prostheses were designed with stems similar to those used in total hip arthroplasty, but with two bearing surfaces. This theoretically increases the arc range and protects the cement-bone and cement-prosthesis interface from loosening forces and leads to less acetabular erosion than unipolar stems.[52-54,90] However, increased range of motion afforded by a bipolar prosthesis is rarely noticed by the patient, and one of the articulations may lock in place soon after implantation. Cornell and associates[55] and others[91,92] have found no difference in outcomes between bipolar and unipolar hemiarthroplasty and advocated use of the less expensive unipolar prosthesis. Other authors have reported significant failures with bipolar prostheses, including early failure caused by the addition of a poly-

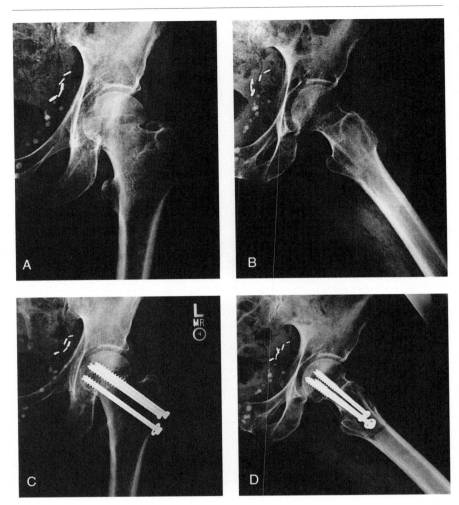

Figure 3 A and **B,** Valgus impacted femoral neck fracture. After cannulated screw fixation, the fracture remains stable. **C** and **D,** Radiographs show screw apposition to the inferior and posterior cortices along the calcar femorale.

ethylene bearing surface.[93,94] In addition, although dislocation rates may be lower after bipolar hemiarthroplasty,[92] open reduction is frequently required to reduce a dislocated bipolar head.[5,95] Modern stems do allow conversion to total arthroplasty without stem removal, with little diminution in function.[96]

Recent prospectively randomized studies may begin to swing the pendulum back to favoring primary hemiarthroplasty or total hip arthroplasty in the younger, active elderly patient. Parker and associates[97] randomized 455 patients older than age

70 years with displaced femoral neck fractures to receive either internal fixation or hemiarthroplasty. Internal fixation led to shorter surgical times and less blood loss, but 90 patients required 111 additional procedures, compared with 15 procedures in 12 patients following hemiarthroplasty. In another prospective study, Rogmark and associates[98] treated 409 patients older than age 70 years with either fixation or hemiarthroplasty following Garden III or Garden IV femoral neck fracture. At 5 years, the hemiarthroplasty group had a failure rate of 10%, compared with 46% in

the fixation group, and had less pain and better ambulation. Both of these studies recommend hemiarthroplasty in patients older than age 70 years, except when the hip is too unstable to tolerate the more invasive procedure. Keating and associates[57] prospectively evaluated 301 displaced neck fractures and reported that fixation led to an eightfold greater risk for revision than the hemiarthroplasty group and a fivefold greater risk than the total arthroplasty group. Both arthroplasty groups had better functional outcomes when compared with the internal fixation patients. Abboud and associates[58] followed 60 patients for at least 32 months and reported that outcomes following total hip arthroplasty were the same following hip fracture or osteoarthritis. Modern reports of poor function in patients following total hip replacement have been scant. Greenough and Jones[99] reported an anticipated 49% revision rate in their series of 37 patients and recommended against total hip arthroplasty for femoral neck fractures.

Total hip arthroplasty for femoral neck fractures has been historically notorious for high dislocation rates. However, many of these studies used techniques and prostheses that are now antiquated, and more recent studies show better results.[57-60,100] Indications for total hip arthroplasty have traditionally included preexisting moderate to severe acetabular disease in elderly patients.[100-102] Perioperative morbidity, particularly dislocation, has been reported to be slightly higher than with hemiarthroplasty, but total hip arthroplasty leads to better long-term function and pain relief.[56,59,60,102] Reports comparing total hip arthroplasty and hemiarthroplasty must be interpreted with caution, however, because randomization is often difficult and younger, healthier patients receive total hip arthroplasty.[98] Elderly patients who have sustained a displaced femoral neck fracture and have good mental status, minimal medical comorbidities, and who are relatively active appear to be the best candidates for primary hip replacement.[56,59,98,102]

Surgical Timing

A delay from admission to the hospital to surgical intervention is sometimes critical for different reasons, depending on the patient. In patients younger than 65 years old or who are active and relatively healthy, a femoral neck fracture is a true surgical emergency. Delaying surgery decreases the chance of survival of the femoral head.[103,104] For patients whose functional, medical, or mental status precludes internal fixation, arthroplasty should be planned on an urgent basis. Surgical intervention sooner than 24 hours after hospital admission may be detrimental to the patient with comorbidities, as the patient will benefit from preoperative hydration and medical evaluation.[75] However, healthier patients without significant medical problems benefit from surgery within the first 48 hours after hospital admission.[31,105,106] Zuckerman and associates[107] showed that a delay longer than after 48 hours approximately doubles the 1-year mortality risk. Elderly patients should first be assessed for preinjury function and mental status to decide for or against internal fixation. If prosthetic replacement is chosen, surgery should be expedited once all easily correctable medical conditions are stabilized. In younger active elderly patients with medical comorbidities, the timing of surgery must be individualized, weighing the benefits of early fixation to preserve the head against medical intervention.

Considerations in Osteoporosis

Osteoporosis is the most common metabolic bone disorder, which currently affects 28 million Americans (20 million are women), and is increasing as the population ages.[1,108] It is a painless disease that leads to a decrease in bone mass and increased fragility. Both cortical and cancellous bone are affected, and metabolic disturbances may lead to impaired healing.[2,109,110] Hip fracture incidence is clearly linked to osteoporosis and is one of the most debilitating consequences. Twenty percent of Caucasian women older than age 50 years have osteoporosis, and lifetime risk of a hip fracture is 17%.[108]

Low femoral bone density is the most correlative with risk for hip fracture.[111,112] The most common technique for measuring bone density is dual energy x-ray absorptiometry (DEXA). Other methods of bone density measurements exist. Quantitative CT scanning measures metabolic bone activity, but is associated with significantly greater radiation exposure, and is currently less accurate than DEXA.[108] Peripheral ultrasound evaluates quality of the calcaneus bone and is more useful as an initial screening tool than for following patients undergoing treatment. Correlations between peripheral measurements and the hip have been low.[113] Clinically, obtaining these studies in the setting of an acute femoral neck fracture is impractical. Obtaining good-quality plain radiographs and evaluating the presence or absence of groups of trabeculae in the femoral neck and head may give a general idea of the osteopenia. The Singh Index, first described in 1970,[114] grades osteopenia based on the trabecular pattern of an AP radiograph of the hip. Grades from 1 to 6 are given, with 1 being the most severe. Though this system has not been shown to correlate well with regard to specific grades,[115,116] familiarity with these patterns will give a rough estimate of the degree of osteopenia, and may predict poor outcome.

Femoral Neck Fixation in Osteoporotic Bone

Treating osteoporotic hip fractures requires special attention and different treatment algorithms because of the abnormal mechanical bone properties and extensive comminution commonly present. Due to the aging population and high prevalence of osteoporosis, the development of alternate fixation techniques is essential. General surgical principles of early stable fixation for immediate restoration of function apply in patients with osteoporotic hip fractures. Second to reduction position, bone quality is the most important factor to maintaining rigid internal fixation. Microarchitectural changes in porotic bone are characterized by a thinner cortex with an increased cancellous to cortical bone ratio.[117,118] Trabeculae lose their cross-connectivity, a major component in overall strength of the bone.[119] The most common mode of failure following fixation is bone cutout rather than implant failure, and it has been found that patients with lower trabecular bone mass have a higher rate of fixation failure.[120-122] When the surrounding cancellous bone is inadequate to anchor the screw threads with the force of weight bearing, the interface at the edge of the implant fails, leading to toggle of the screw and motion at the fractured neck. Approaches to this problem have centered around increasing stability of the entire system and have involved

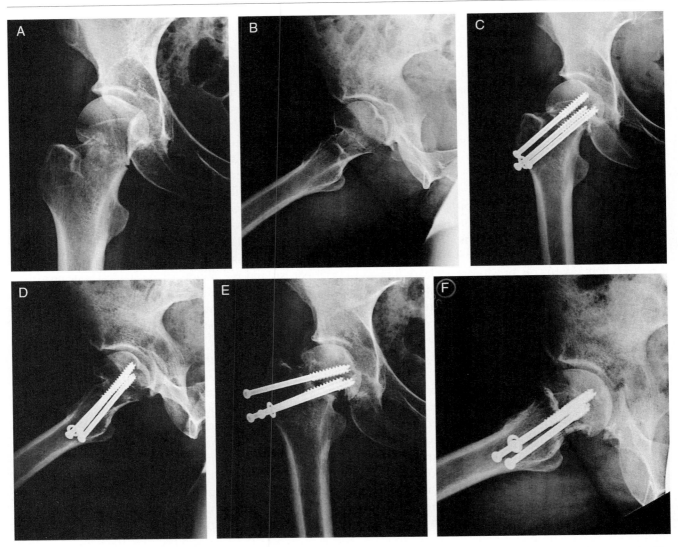

Figure 4 Radiographs of a 62-year-old woman with a femoral neck fracture, angled in valgus (**A**) and displaced posteriorly (**B**). **C** and **D,** Initial fixation caused impaction initially, but appeared adequate. By 6 months postoperatively, the head had impacted further and the hardware backed out (**E** and **F**), causing the patient significant discomfort.

redesigning implants and fixation, augmentation.[123] Ideally, at the time of fixation, a stable construct would distribute force throughout the cancellous bone and shift most of the load bearing from the implant to the bone.

The current gold standard for fixation of subcapital and transcervical femoral neck fractures is three parallel, partially threaded cancellous cannulated screws[48,61,66] One of the advantages of using parallel partially threaded screws is that axial sliding allows impaction of the neck fragments into stable position. This effectively gradually shifts the load-bearing from the implants to the bone. Unfortunately, it is difficult to control the degree of impaction, and overimpaction with screw backout is not uncommon (Figures 4 and 5). Although prominent hardware may necessitate a second procedure and proximal migration of the distal fragment may lead to impingement at extremes of motion, this is usually well tolerated in the elderly patient.[123] Nevertheless, hardware pullout and loss of fixation remains a significant problem in osteoporotic bone. A new "cement screw" has been designed to increase fixation in cancellous bone and has potential use in the femoral head.[124,125] This screw is cannulated and has holes radially along its axis in the threaded portion of the screw. After insertion of the screw over a Kirschner wire, the wire is removed, and cement is injected through the screw head. Cement then flows from the side holes and interdigitates in the trabeculae.[124] Because the holes are located only among the threads of the screw, cement does not accrue in the distal fragment, and axial impaction may still occur.

Artificial materials have been studied extensively to augment internal fixation. The traditional method of screw augmentation has been with polymethylmethacrylate. After insertion of the Kirschner wires into the femoral neck, the wires are over-drilled. The cement is injected, and the screw is partially inserted. Once the cement has hardened, insertion is completed.[126-128] Although polymethylmethacrylate has been shown to significantly improve screw anchorage in porotic bone,[126,129,130] its toxicity, nonresorbability, and exothermic reaction have precluded its widespread use.[123,125] More recently, a calcium phosphate cement has been developed to gain purchase of screw threads in trabecular bone of the femoral head.[128,131-133] This cement is nonexothermic and has the advantages of providing sufficient stability to allow early weight bearing and load transfer to host bone in the short-term, and is resorbed and replaced by host bone in the long-term.[128,132] Early clinical results are encouraging.[132]

It would seem clear that with the potential fixation difficulties, patients with osteopenia should undergo hemiarthroplasty. Although hemiarthroplasty may be more reliable than fixation, the patient must be able to tolerate a longer surgery with more blood loss. Hemiarthroplasty may lead to better short-term results, but techniques that allow for predictable healing in osteoporotic femoral neck fractures are preferable to arthroplasty. If prosthetic replacement is

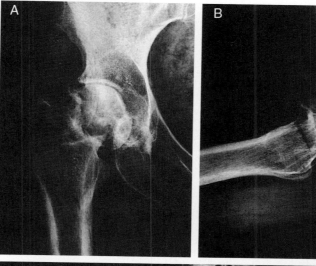
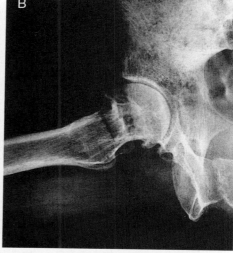
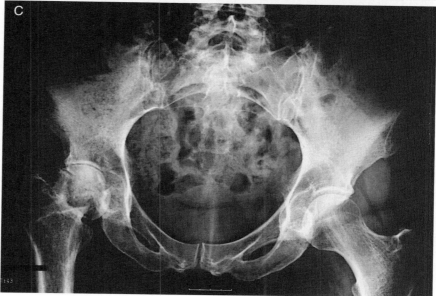

Figure 5 A through **C**, Additional postoperative radiographs of the patient described in Figure 4. By 9 months postoperatively the fracture still had not fully healed, and the neck was significantly shortened. Removal of the screws alleviated local irritation, but the patient continued to complain to intermittent impingement symptoms.

selected, total hip arthroplasty may still be an option in the active elderly patient with a displaced osteoporotic fracture and acetabular pathology. In this case, acetabular cement fixation may be considered.[45]

Because fixation of osteoporotic fractures is fraught with difficulties, fracture prevention is of paramount importance. All postmenopausal women and elderly men should undergo a risk factor assessment and DEXA scanning. Patients with osteoporosis should receive physiologic calcium and an antiresorptive agent, either estrogen or a bisphosphonate. In addition, exercise programs including balance, strengthening, and moderate impact activities should be initiated. Tai chi has been shown to be effective in decreasing the risk of falls.[134]

Summary

Improved general medical prevention and treatment have increased life expectancy. As the population ages, so does the incidence of osteoporosis. Fractures of the femoral neck are directly correlated to osteoporosis, and as this epidemic evolves, development of novel treatment methods has become increasingly important. The two categories of management options include internal fixation and arthroplasty. Hemiarthroplasty is a time-tested alternative, but when the clinical situation allows, fixation of the native femoral head is preferable. Obtaining stable fixation in osteoporotic bone is a formidable challenge, and presently no solution is universally accepted for this unsolved fracture. The current treatment of choice for fixation is parallel cannulated screws inserted percutaneously. Ongoing research in implant design and newly developed biologic augmentation cement is likely to change future treatment methods.

References

1. National Osteoporosis Foundation: *1996 and 2015 Osteoporosis Prevalence Figures: State-by-State Report.* Washington, DC, National Osteoporosis Foundation, 1997.

2. Brunelli MP, Einhorn TA: Medical management of osteoporosis: Fracture prevention. *Clin Orthop* 1998;348:15-21.

3. Koval KJ, Zuckerman JD: Hip fractures: I. Overview and evaluation and treatment of femoral-neck fractures. *J Am Acad Orthop Surg* 1994;2:141-149.

4. Reikeras O, Hoiseth A, Reigstad A, Fonstelien E: Femoral neck angles: A specimen study with special regard to bilateral differences. *Acta Orthop Scand* 1982;53:775-779.

5. Swiontkowski MF: Intracapsular fractures of the hip. *J Bone Joint Surg Am* 1994;76:129-138.

6. Chung SM: The arterial supply of the developing proximal end of the human femur. *J Bone Joint Surg Am* 1976;58:961-970.

7. Sevitt S, Thompson RG: The distribution and anastomoses of arteries supplying the head and neck of the femur. *J Bone Joint Surg Br* 1965;47:560-573.

8. Trueta J, Harrison MHM: The normal vascular anatomy of the femoral head in adult man. *J Bone Joint Surg Br* 1953;35:442-461.

9. Crock HV: An atlas of the arterial supply of the head and neck of the femur in man. *Clin Orthop* 1980;152:17-27.

10. Arnoldi CC, Lemperg RK: Fracture of the femoral neck: II. Relative importance of primary vascular damage and surgical procedure for the development of necrosis of the femoral head. *Clin Orthop* 1977;129:217-222.

11. Arnoldi CC, Linderholm H: Fracture of the femoral neck: I. Vascular disturbances in different types of fractures, assessed by measurements of intraosseous pressures. *Clin Orthop* 1972;84:116-127.

12. Claffey TJ: Avascular necrosis of the femoral head: An anatomical study. *J Bone Joint Surg Br* 1960;42:802-809.

13. Woodhouse CF: Dynamic influences of vascular occlusion affecting the development of avascular necrosis of the femoral head. *Clin Orthop* 1964;32:119-129.

14. Swiontkowski MF, Tepic S, Perren SM, Moor R, Ganz R, Rahn BA: Laser Doppler flowmetry for bone blood flow measurement: Correlation with microsphere estimates and evaluation of the effect of intracapsular pressure on femoral head blood flow. *J Orthop Res* 1986;4:362-371.

15. Calandruccio RA, Anderson WE III: Post-fracture avascular necrosis of the femoral head: Correlation of experimental and clinical studies. *Clin Orthop* 1980;152:49-84.

16. Wingstrand H, Stromqvist B, Egund N, Gustafson T, Nilsson LT, Thorngren KG: Hemarthrosis in undisplaced cervical fractures: Tamponade may cause reversible femoral head ischemia. *Acta Orthop Scand* 1986;57:305-308.

17. Stromqvist B, Nilsson LT, Egund N, Thorngren KG, Wingstrand H: Intracapsular pressures in undisplaced fractures of the femoral neck. *J Bone Joint Surg Br* 1988;70:192-194.

18. Drake JK, Meyers MH: Intracapsular pressure and hemarthrosis following femoral neck fracture. *Clin Orthop* 1984;182:172-176.

19. Soto-Hall R, Johnson R, Johnson LH: Abstract: Alterations in the intra-articular pressure in transcervical fractures of the hip. *J Bone Joint Surg Am* 1963;45:662.

20. Maruenda JI, Barrios C, Gomar-Sancho F: Intracapsular hip pressure after femoral neck fracture. *Clin Orthop* 1997;340:172-180.

21. Gill TJ, Sledge JB, Ekkernkamp A, Ganz R: Intraoperative assessment of femoral head vascularity after femoral neck fracture. *J Orthop Trauma* 1998;12:474-478.

22. Garden RS: Reduction and fixation of subcapital fractures of the femur. *Orthop Clin North Am* 1974;5:683-712.

23. Barnes R, Brown JT, Garden RS, Nicoll EA: Subcapital fractures of the femur: A prospective review. *J Bone Joint Surg Br* 1976;58:2-24.

24. Pauwels F (ed): *Der Schenkelhalsbruch, ein Mechanisches Problem: Grundlagen des Heilungsvorganges, Prognose und Kausale Therapie.* Stuttgart, Germany, Ferdinand Enke Verlag, 1935.

25. Chapman MW: Fractures of the hip and proximal femur, in Chapman MW (ed): *Chapman's Orthopaedic Surgery*, ed 3. Philadelphia, PA, Lippincott Williams and Wilkins, 2001, pp 617-670.

26. Scheck M: The significance of posterior comminution in femoral neck fractures. *Clin Orthop* 1980;152:138-142.

27. Frangakis EK: Intracapsular fractures of the neck of the femur: Factors influencing nonunion and ischaemic necrosis. *J Bone Joint Surg Br* 1966;48:17-30.

28. Lewis SL, Rees JI, Thomas GV, Williams LA: Pitfalls of bone scintigraphy in suspected hip fractures. *Br J Radiol* 1991;64:403-408.

29. Fairclough J, Colhoun E, Johnston D, Williams LA: Bone scanning for suspected hip fractures: A prospective study in elderly patients. *J Bone Joint Surg Br* 1987;69:251-253.

30. Hoenig H, Rubenstein LV, Sloane R, Horner R, Kahn K: What is the role of timing in the surgical and rehabilitative care of community-dwelling older persons with acute hip fracture? *Arch Intern Med* 1997;157:513-520.

31. Hamlet WP, Lieberman JR, Freedman EL, Dorey FJ, Fletcher A, Johnson EE: Influence of health status and the timing

of surgery on mortality in hip fracture patients. *Am J Orthop* 1997;26:621-627.

32. Geslien GE, Thrall JH, Espinosa JL, Older RA: Early detection of stress fractures using 99mTc-polyphosphate. *Radiology* 1976;121:683-687.

33. Batillas J, Vasilas A, Pizzi WF, Gokcebay T: Bone scanning in the detection of occult fractures. *J Trauma* 1981;21:564-569.

34. Prather JL, Nusynowitz ML, Snowdy HA, Hughes AD, McCartney WH, Bagg RJ: Scintigraphic findings in stress fractures. *J Bone Joint Surg Am* 1977;59:869-874.

35. Matin P: The appearance of bone scans following fractures, including immediate and long-term studies. *J Nucl Med* 1979;20:1227-1231.

36. Lee JK, Yao L: Stress fractures: MR imaging. *Radiology* 1988;169:217-220.

37. Lang P, Genant HK, Jergesen HE, Murray WR: Imaging of the hip joint: Computed tomography versus magnetic resonance imaging. *Clin Orthop* 1992;274:135-153.

38. Deutsch AL, Mink JH, Waxman AD: Occult fractures of the proximal femur: MR imaging. *Radiology* 1989;170:113-116.

39. Glickstein MF, Burk DL Jr, Schiebler ML, et al: Avascular necrosis versus other diseases of the hip: Sensitivity of MR imaging. *Radiology* 1988;169:213-215.

40. Evans PD, Wilson C, Lyons K: Comparison of MRI with bone scanning for suspected hip fracture in elderly patients. *J Bone Joint Surg Br* 1994;76:158-159.

41. Lucas TS, Einhorn TA: Osteoporosis: The role of the orthopaedist. *J Am Acad Orthop Surg* 1993;1:48-56.

42. Bentley G: Treatment of nondisplaced fractures of the femoral neck. *Clin Orthop* 1980;152:93-101.

43. Holmberg S, Kalen R, Thorngren KG: Treatment and outcome of femoral neck fractures: An analysis of 2418 patients admitted from their own homes. *Clin Orthop* 1987;218:42-52.

44. Tanaka J, Seki N, Tokimura F, Hayashi Y: Conservative treatment of Garden stage I femoral neck fracture in elderly patients. *Arch Orthop Trauma Surg* 2002;122:24-28.

45. Baumgaertner MR, Higgins TF: Femoral neck fractures, in Bucholz RW, Heckman JD (eds): *Rockwood and Green's Fractures in Adults*, ed 5. Philadelphia, PA, Lippincott Williams and Wilkins, 2001, vol 2, pp 1579-1634.

46. Richmond J, Aharonoff GB, Zuckerman JD, Koval KJ: Mortality risk after hip fracture. *J Orthop Trauma* 2003;17:53-56.

47. Stromqvist B, Hansson LI, Nilsson LT, Thorngren KG: Hook-pin fixation in femoral neck fractures: A two-year follow-up study of 300 cases. *Clin Orthop* 1987;218:58-62.

48. Asnis SE, Wanek-Sgaglione L: Intracapsular fractures of the femoral neck: Results of cannulated screw fixation. *J Bone Joint Surg Am* 1994;76:1793-1803.

49. Soreide O, Molster A, Raugstad TS: Internal fixation versus primary prosthetic replacement in acute femoral neck fractures: A prospective, randomized clinical study. *Br J Surg* 1979;66:56-60.

50. Lu-Yao GL, Keller RB, Littenberg B, Wennberg JE: Outcomes after displaced fractures of the femoral neck: A meta-analysis of one hundred and six published reports. *J Bone Joint Surg Am* 1994;76:15-25.

51. Parker MJ: Internal fixation or arthroplasty for displaced subcapital fractures in the elderly? *Injury* 1992;23:521-524.

52. Devas M, Hinves B: Prevention of acetabular erosion after hemiarthroplasty for fractured neck of femur. *J Bone Joint Surg Br* 1983;65:548-551.

53. Lausten GS, Vedel P, Nielsen PM: Fractures of the femoral neck treated with a bipolar endoprosthesis. *Clin Orthop* 1987;218:63-67.

54. Giliberty RP: Hemiarthroplasty of the hip using a low-friction bipolar endoprosthesis. *Clin Orthop* 1983;175:86-92.

55. Cornell CN, Levine D, O'Doherty J, Lyden J: Unipolar versus bipolar hemiarthroplasty for the treatment of femoral neck fractures in the elderly. *Clin Orthop* 1998;348:67-71.

56. Taine WH, Armour PC: Primary total hip replacement for displaced subcapital fractures of the femur. *J Bone Joint Surg Br* 1985;67:214-217.

57. Keating JF, Masson M, Scott N, Forbes J, Grant A: Abstract: Randomized trial of reduction and fixation versus bipolar hemiarthroplasty versus total hip arthroplasty for displaced subcapital fractures in the fit older patient. *70th Annual Meeting Proceedings*. Rosemont, IL, American Academy of Orthopaedic Surgeons, 2003, p 96.

58. Abboud JA, Patel RV, Nazarian DG, Booth RE: Abstract: A comparison of

outcomes following total hip arthroplasty for femoral neck fractures versus osteoarthritis. *70th Annual Meeting Proceedings*. Rosemont, IL, American Academy of Orthopaedic Surgeons, 2003, p 101.

59. Lee BP, Berry DJ, Harmsen WS, Sim FH: Total hip arthroplasty for the treatment of an acute fracture of the femoral neck: Long-term results. *J Bone Joint Surg Am* 1998;80:70-75.

60. Gebhard JS, Amstutz HC, Zinar DM, Dorey FJ: A comparison of total hip arthroplasty and hemiarthroplasty for treatment of acute fracture of the femoral neck. *Clin Orthop* 1992;282:123-131.

61. Bray TJ: Femoral neck fracture fixation: Clinical decision making. *Clin Orthop* 1997;339:20-31.

62. Jarnlo GB, Thorngren KG: Background factors to hip fractures. *Clin Orthop* 1993;287:41-49.

63. Kenzora JE, Magaziner J, Hudson J, et al: Outcome after hemiarthroplasty for femoral neck fractures in the elderly. *Clin Orthop* 1998;348:51-58.

64. Beckenbaugh RD, Tressler HA, Johnson EW Jr: Results after hemiarthroplasty of the hip using a cemented femoral prosthesis: A review of 109 cases with an average follow-up of 36 months. *Mayo Clin Proc* 1977;52:349-353.

65. Gardner MJ, Flik KR, Mooar P, Lane JM: Improvement in the undertreatment of osteoporosis following hip fracture. *J Bone Joint Surg Am* 2002;84:1342-1348.

66. Husby T, Alho A, Ronningen H: Stability of femoral neck osteosynthesis: Comparison of fixation methods in cadavers. *Acta Orthop Scand* 1989;60:299-302.

67. Stromqvist B: Femoral head vitality after intracapsular hip fracture: 490 cases studied by intravital tetracycline labeling and Tc-MDP radionuclide imaging. *Acta Orthop Scand Suppl* 1983;200:1-71.

68. Weinrobe M, Stankewich CJ, Mueller B, Tencer AF: Predicting the mechanical outcome of femoral neck fractures fixed with cancellous screws: An in vivo study. *J Orthop Trauma* 1998;12:27-37.

69. Chua D, Jaglal SB, Schatzker J: Predictors of early failure of fixation in the treatment of displaced subcapital hip fractures. *J Orthop Trauma* 1998;12:230-234.

70. Garden RS: Malreduction and avascular necrosis in subcapital fractures of the femur. *J Bone Joint Surg Br* 1971;53:183-197.

71. Keller CS, Laros GS: Indications for open reduction of femoral neck fractures. *Clin Orthop* 1980;152:131-137.

72. Parker MJ, Porter KM, Eastwood DM, Schembi Wismayer M, Bernard AA: Intracapsular fractures of the neck of femur: Parallel or crossed garden screws? *J Bone Joint Surg Br* 1991;73:826-827.

73. Alberts KA, Jervaeus J: Factors predisposing to healing complications after internal fixation of femoral neck fracture: A stepwise logistic regression analysis. *Clin Orthop* 1990;257:129-133.

74. Smyth EH, Shah VM: The significance of good reduction and fixation in displaced subcapital fractures of the femur. *Injury* 1974;5:197-209.

75. Kenzora JE, McCarthy RE, Lowell JD, Sledge CB: Hip fracture mortality: Relation to age, treatment, preoperative illness, time of surgery, and complications. *Clin Orthop* 1984;186:45-56.

76. Garden RS: Low-angle fixation in fractures of the femoral neck. *J Bone Joint Surg Br* 1961;43:647-663.

77. Lindequist S, Tornkvist H: Quality of reduction and cortical screw support in femoral neck fractures: An analysis of 72 fractures with a new computerized measuring method. *J Orthop Trauma* 1995;9:215-221.

78. Booth KC, Donaldson TK, Dai QG: Femoral neck fracture fixation: A biomechanical study of two cannulated screw placement techniques. *Orthopedics* 1998;21:1173-1176.

79. Lindequist S: Cortical screw support in femoral neck fractures: A radiographic analysis of 87 fractures with a new mensuration technique. *Acta Orthop Scand* 1993;64:289-293.

80. Lindequist S, Wredmark T, Eriksson SA, Samnegard E: Screw positions in femoral neck fractures: Comparison of two different screw positions in cadavers. *Acta Orthop Scand* 1993;64:67-70.

81. van Dortmont LM, Douw CM, van Breukelen AM, et al: Outcome after hemi-arthroplasty for displaced intracapsular femoral neck fracture related to mental state. *Injury* 2000;31:327-331.

82. Deneka DA, Simonian PT, Stankewich CJ, Eckert D, Chapman JR, Tencer AF: Biomechanical comparison of internal fixation techniques for the treatment of unstable basicervical femoral neck fractures. *J Orthop Trauma* 1997;11:337-343.

83. Blair B, Koval KJ, Kummer F, Zuckerman JD: Basicervical fractures of the proximal femur: A biomechanical study of 3 internal fixation techniques. *Clin Orthop* 1994;306:256-263.

84. Ort PJ, LaMont J: Treatment of femoral neck fractures with a sliding compression screw and two Knowles pins. *Clin Orthop* 1984;190:158-162.

85. Sirkin M, Grossman MG, Renard RL, et al: Abstract: A biomechanical analysis of fixation constructs in high angle femoral neck fractures. Proceedings of the Annual Orthopaedic Trauma Association Meeting. Rosemont, IL, 1999.

86. Baitner AC, Maurer SG, Hickey DG, et al: Vertical shear fractures of the femoral neck: A biomechanical study. *Clin Orthop* 1999;367:300-305.

87. Nilsson LT, Johansson A, Stromqvist B: Factors predicting healing complications in femoral neck fractures: 138 patients followed for 2 years. *Acta Orthop Scand* 1993;64:175-177.

88. Brodetti A: The blood supply of the femoral neck and head in relation to the damaging effects of nails and screws. *J Bone Joint Surg Br* 1960;42:794-801.

89. Tidermark J, Zethraeus N, Svensson O, Tornkvist H, Ponzer S: Quality of life related to fracture displacement among elderly patients with femoral neck fractures treated with internal fixation. *J Orthop Trauma* 2002;16:34-38.

90. Coates RL, Armour P: Treatment of subcapital femoral fractures by primary total hip replacement. *Injury* 1979;11:132-135.

91. Wathne RA, Koval KJ, Aharonoff GB, Zuckerman JD, Jones DA: Modular unipolar versus bipolar prosthesis: A prospective evaluation of functional outcome after femoral neck fracture. *J Orthop Trauma* 1995;9:298-302.

92. Ong BC, Maurer SG, Aharonoff GB, Zuckerman JD, Koval KJ: Unipolar versus bipolar hemiarthroplasty: Functional outcome after femoral neck fracture at a minimum of thirty-six months of follow-up. *J Orthop Trauma* 2002;16:317-322.

93. Coleman SH, Bansal M, Cornell CN, Sculco TP: Failure of bipolar hemiarthroplasty: A retrospective review of 31 consecutive bipolar prostheses converted to total hip arthroplasty. *Am J Orthop* 2001;30:313-319.

94. Eiskjaer S, Ostgard SE: Survivorship analysis of hemiarthroplasties. *Clin Orthop* 1993;286:206-211.

95. Drinker H, Murray WR: The universal proximal femoral endoprosthesis: A short-term comparison with conventional hemiarthroplasty. *J Bone Joint Surg Am* 1979;61:1167-1174.

96. Skinner P, Riley D, Ellery J, Beaumont A, Coumine R, Shafighian B: Displaced subcapital fractures of the femur: A prospective randomized comparison of internal fixation, hemiarthroplasty and total hip replacement. *Injury* 1989;20:291-293.

97. Parker MJ, Khan RJ, Crawford J, Pryor GA: Hemiarthroplasty versus internal fixation for displaced intracapsular hip fractures in the elderly: A randomised trial of 455 patients. *J Bone Joint Surg Br* 2002;84:1150-1155.

98. Rogmark C, Carlsson A, Johnell O, Sernbo I: A prospective randomised trial of internal fixation versus arthroplasty for displaced fractures of the neck of the femur: Functional outcome for 450 patients at two years. *J Bone Joint Surg Br* 2002;84:183-188.

99. Greenough CG, Jones JR: Primary total hip replacement for displaced subcapital fracture of the femur. *J Bone Joint Surg Br* 1988;70:639-643.

100. Papandrea RF, Froimson MI: Total hip arthroplasty after acute displaced femoral neck fractures. *Am J Orthop* 1996;25:85-88.

101. Kyle RF, Cabanela ME, Russell TA, et al: Fractures of the proximal part of the femur. *Instr Course Lect* 1995;44:227-253.

102. Dorr LD, Glousman R, Hoy AL, Vanis R, Chandler R: Treatment of femoral neck fractures with total hip replacement versus cemented and noncemented hemiarthroplasty. *J Arthroplasty* 1986;1:21-28.

103. Manninger J, Kazar G, Fekete G, et al: Significance of urgent (within 6h) internal fixation in the management of fractures of the neck of the femur. *Injury* 1989;20:101-105.

104. Swiontkowski MF, Winquist RA, Hansen ST Jr: Fractures of the femoral neck in patients between the ages of twelve and forty-nine years. *J Bone Joint Surg Am* 1984;66:837-846.

105. Rogers FB, Shackford SR, Keller MS: Early fixation reduces morbidity and mortality in elderly patients with hip fractures from low-impact falls. *J Trauma* 1995;39:261-265.

106. Parker MJ, Pryor GA: The timing of surgery for proximal femoral fractures. *J Bone Joint Surg Br* 1992;74:203-205.

107. Zuckerman JD, Skovron ML, Koval KJ, Aharonoff G, Frankel VH: Postoperative complications and mortality associated with operative delay in older patients who have a fracture of the hip. *J Bone Joint Surg Am* 1995;77:1551-1556.

108. Lane JM, Nydick M: Osteoporosis: Current modes of prevention and treatment. *J Am Acad Orthop Surg* 1999;7:19-31.

109. Lane JM, Cornell CN, Healey JH: Osteoporosis: The structural and reparative consequences for the skeleton. *Instr Course Lect* 1987;36:71-83.

110. Einhorn TA, Bonnarens F, Burstein AH: The contributions of dietary protein and mineral to the healing of experimental fractures: A biomechanical study. *J Bone Joint Surg Am* 1986;68:1389-1395.

111. Seeger LL: Bone density determination. *Spine* 1997;22(suppl 24):49S-57S.

112. Greenspan SL, Myers ER, Maitland LA, Resnick NM, Hayes WC: Fall severity and bone mineral density as risk factors for hip fracture in ambulatory elderly. *JAMA* 1994;271:128-133.

113. Lane JM, Russell L, Khan SN: *Osteoporosis. Clin Orthop* 2000;372:139-150.

114. Singh M, Nagrath AR, Maini PS: Changes in trabecular pattern of the upper end of the femur as an index of osteoporosis. *J Bone Joint Surg Am* 1970;52:457-467.

115. Masud T, Jawed S, Doyle DV, Spector TD: A population study of the screening potential of assessment of trabecular pattern of the femoral neck (Singh index): The Chingford Study. *Br J Radiol* 1995;68:389-393.

116. Koot VC, Kesselaer SM, Clevers GJ, de Hooge P, Weits T, van der Werken C: Evaluation of the Singh index for measuring osteoporosis. *J Bone Joint Surg Br* 1996;78:831-834.

117. Bloom RA, Laws JW: Humeral cortical thickness as an index of osteoporosis in women. *Br J Radiol* 1970;43:522-527.

118. An YH, Burgoyne CR, Crum MS, Glaser JA: Current methods and trends in fixation in osteoporotic bone, in An YH (ed): *Internal Fixation in Osteoporotic Bone.* New York, NY, Thieme, 2002.

119. Bailey AJ, Sims TJ, Ebbesen EN, Mansell JP, Thomsen JS, Mosekilde L: Age-related changes in the biochemical properties of human cancellous bone collagen: Relationship to bone strength. *Calcif Tissue Int* 1999;65:203-210.

120. Halpin PJ, Nelson CL: A system of classification of femoral neck fractures with special reference to choice of treatment. *Clin Orthop* 1980;152:44-48.

121. Van Audekercke R, Martens M, Mulier JC, Stuyck J: Experimental study on internal fixation of femoral neck fractures. *Clin Orthop* 1979;141:203-212.

122. Cornell CN: Management of fractures in patients with osteoporosis. *Orthop Clin North Am* 1990;21:125-141.

123. Hertel R, Jost B: Basic principles and techniques of internal fixation in osteoporotic bone, in An YH (ed): *Internal Fixation in Osteoporotic Bone.* New York, NY, Thieme, 2002.

124. Reynders PA, Labey LA: A cement screw for fixation in osteoporotic metaphyseal bone, in An YH (ed): *Internal Fixation in Osteoporotic Bone.* New York, NY, Thieme, 2002.

125. McKoy BE, An YH: An injectable cementing screw for fixation in osteoporotic bone. *J Biomed Mater Res* 2000;53:216-220.

126. Cameron HU, Jacob R, Macnab I, Pilliar RM: Use of polymethylmethacrylate to enhance screw fixation in bone. *J Bone Joint Surg Am* 1975;57:655-656.

127. Motzkin NE, Chao EY, An KN, Wikenheiser MA, Lewallen DG: Pull-out strength of screws from polymethylmethacrylate cement. *J Bone Joint Surg Br* 1994;76:320-323.

128. Cornell CN: Internal fixation of osteoporotic long bone, in An YH (ed): *Internal Fixation in Osteoporotic Bone.* New York, NY, Thieme, 2002.

129. Benum P: The use of bone cement as an adjunct to internal fixation of supracondylar fractures of osteoporotic femurs. *Acta Orthop Scand* 1977;48:52-56.

130. Schatzker J, Ha'eri GB, Chapman M: Methylmethacrylate as an adjunct in the internal fixation of intertrochanteric fractures of the femur. *J Trauma* 1978;18:732-735.

131. Larsson S, Mattsson P, Bauer TW: Resorbable bone cement for augmentation of internally fixed hip fractures. *Ann Chir Gynaecol* 1999;88:205-213.

132. Goodman SB, Bauer TW, Carter D, et al: Norian SRS cement augmentation in hip fracture treatment: Laboratory and initial clinical results. *Clin Orthop* 1998;348:42-50.

133. Stankewich CJ, Swiontkowski MF, Tencer AF, Yetkinler DN, Poser RD: Augmentation of femoral neck fracture fixation with an injectable calcium-phosphate bone mineral cement. *J Orthop Res* 1996;14:786-793.

134. Wolf SL, Barnhart HX, Ellison GL, Coogler CE: The effect of Tai Chi Quan and computerized balance training on postural stability in older subjects: Atlanta FICSIT Group: Frailty and Injuries: Cooperative Studies on Intervention Techniques. *Phys Ther* 1997;77:371-384.

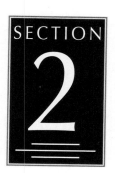

SECTION

2

New Directions in Hip Replacement

New Directions in Hip Replacement

Total hip arthroplasty (THA) is widely recognized as a clinically successful and cost-effective procedure for patients with debilitating hip disease. Surgical techniques and implant technologies have evolved over the past 4 decades, allowing more patients with diverse clinical and demographic characteristics to benefit from THA. Implant survivorship beyond 10 to 15 years is not uncommon, with most patients reporting substantial improvements in pain, function, and quality of life. However, many problems remain unsolved, particularly bearing surface wear, soft-tissue balancing, and perioperative pain management. The articles in this section explore new directions for addressing each of these current limitations in THA.

Harry McKellop, who is one of the leading experts on bearing surface wear, thoroughly outlines the current problems with THA bearing surfaces and describes how new technologies have impacted them. One of the primary limitations of traditional metal-on-polyethylene bearings has been particle-induced osteolysis. Newer bearing technologies, including metal-on-metal, ceramic-on-ceramic, ceramic-on-polyethylene, and enhanced highly cross-linked polyethylenes have shown great promise in the laboratory in terms of reducing bearing surface wear. However, each of these combinations has associated risks, including metal ion toxicity and hypersensitivity, ceramic fracture, and a reduction in material properties associated with highly cross-linked polyethylene bearings. Furthermore, as Dr. McKellop points out, the clinical performance of these new technologies to date has been comparable to that of conventional metal-on-polyethylene hips, calling into question whether the laboratory-proven benefits of reduced wear will translate into improvements in clinical outcomes and implant survivorship. Given the small numbers of patients and limited follow-up, only time will tell whether these technologies will prove to be worth the additional risk and associated cost.

Heisel and associates build on McKellop's article with additional details regarding the biomechanical and histologic consequences of alternative bearing surfaces. Specifically, they describe the relationship between the degree of cross-linking and reductions in wear and the material properties of highly cross-linked polyethylene bearings, the potential local effects of metal wear particles and the systemic effects of metal ion release, and the sensitivity of ceramic bearings to design, manufacturing, and implantation variables. Since this review was written in 2004, additional studies have been published that provide further insight into the clinical performance of alternative bearings in THA. Several clinical and radiographic studies have reported excellent clinical outcomes and very low wear rates with metal-on-highly cross-linked polyethylene, metal-on-metal, ceramic-on-ceramic, and ceramic-on-polyethylene bearings. However, reports describing the potential pitfalls associated with these technologies also have surfaced, including highly cross-linked polyethylene acetabular liner fractures, local effects of metal hypersensitivity (including loosening and osteolysis associated with metal-on-metal bearings), and a "squeaking" noise associated with ceramic bearings. As the authors point out, the degree of wear reduction associated with newer bearing materials may not translate into increased implant longevity. One possible explanation for this lack of correlation between laboratory success and clinical performance is that substantial reductions in wear below the osteolysis threshold (0.1 mm per year) may not provide any additional clinical benefit in terms of better long-term implant survivorship.

Sharkey and associates also comment on the challenges associated with THA in young patients with a review of the poor results associated with THA and the problems associated with bearing surface wear in this population. Although THA is more commonly accepted and performed today in young patients with hip disease, the authors emphasize the need to exercise caution and provide realistic expectations when discussing THA as a treatment alternative for this challenging group of patients.

Seyler and associates provide an excellent review of the history and current status of arthroplasty treatment options for patients with osteonecrosis. They emphasize that although THA provides excellent pain relief and good functional outcomes, it traditionally has been associated with high implant failure rates in this young, highly active patient population. Furthermore, while certain other arthroplasty procedures (eg, bipolar hemiarthroplasty) have been consistently associated with poor results and thus avoided in patients with osteonecrosis, other newer treatment options (eg, metal-on-metal hip resurfacing) have had promising early results but require longer-term follow-up. The wide variety of current surgical options for osteonecrosis of the hip is evidence of the lack of consensus regarding the appropriate treatment for this often debilitating condition.

Hing and colleagues provide an interesting overview of the indications and results of hip resurfacing, a procedure that has become increasingly popular over the past few years.

The importance of this article lies in its presentation of data collected by the authors and data reported in the Australian Hip Registry, resulting in a cogent discussion of the appropriate indications for, limitations of, and unique complications associated with hip resurfacing procedures. Their data suggest that the incidence of early revision surgery is higher with hip resurfacing than with standard THA, with femoral neck fracture the reason for most revision procedures. Early failure also occurs in women of all ages, men over the age of 65, and patients with inflammatory arthritis. Theoretical concerns regarding metal ion sensitivity, metal hypersensitivity, and osteonecrosis of the femoral head have not yet proved to be major clinical obstacles. The article is further evidence that with careful patient selection, proper training, and meticulous surgical technique, hip resurfacing can be a valuable treatment option for young, active patients with degenerative arthritis of the hip.

Charles and associates provide a useful commentary on the importance of soft-tissue balancing in THA. This subject is often overlooked by surgeons, despite its influence on functional outcomes. The benefits of restoring femoral offset, including reduced joint reactive forces, lower bearing surface wear rates, enhanced stability, and

improved abductor muscle function, were originally elucidated by Sir John Charnley in the early 1960s. However, only recently have orthopaedic surgeons and implant design engineers come to understand the biomechanical and clinical implications of failure to restore femoral offset in THA. Techniques to increase and restore femoral offset have involved both implant design factors, including decreasing the neck-shaft angle, medializing the femoral neck (eg, "high-offset" femoral components), and lateralized polyethylene acetabular liners, as well as surgical techniques, including medializing the acetabular component and advancing the trochanter. Regardless of the technique(s) used, careful preoperative templating and planning and intraoperative attention to detail are essential to restoring femoral offset. Although it is too early for definitive conclusions given limited clinical experience, intraoperative computer-assisted surgical navigation tools may prove to be beneficial for soft-tissue balancing in this context.

Finally, the article by Viscusi and colleagues provides a glimpse into a current topic of interest among arthroplasty surgeons and their patients: pain management in total joint arthroplasty (TJA). Multimodal pain management has only recently been recognized as an important factor in perioperative management of and return to function of patients undergoing TJA. Many of the benefits of minimally invasive techniques for TJA that were previously attributed to surgical technique are now widely believed to be the result of improved pain management techniques. Preoperative preemptive analgesia, improved intraoperative techniques, including hypotensive epidural techniques and longer-acting intrathecal agents, and indwelling peripheral nerve catheters have revolutionized perioperative management of TJR patients, allowing more aggressive physical therapy, shorter hospitalization, and earlier return to function. The indications for newer techniques, including intra-articular wound catheters and patient-activated transdermal analgesia patches, have yet to be defined. More experience will be needed to understand the benefits, limitations, and complications associated with these techniques. For all of these reasons, multimodal pain management will remain an area of active clinical and basic science investigation in the years to come.

The articles in this section of *Instructional Course Lectures Hip* collectively summarize the benefits and limitations of new technologies and techniques in THA. Although many of these developments have the potential to improve clinical outcomes and expand the indications for THA to allow a broader range of patients to benefit from these quality-of-life enhancing procedures, many questions remain unanswered. These problems underscore the need for well-designed investigations to critically evaluate the impact of these changes on patient outcomes. This is especially true given the overwhelming success of THA procedures using currently available techniques and implant technologies.

Kevin J. Bozic, MD, MBA
Assistant Professor in Residence
UCSF Department of Orthopaedic
    Surgery and Institute for Health
    Policy Studies
San Francisco, California

Bearing Surfaces in Total Hip Replacements: State of the Art and Future Developments

Harry A. McKellop, PhD

Mechanisms, Damage, and Modes of Wear

To understand and compare the wear performance of bearing materials, it is convenient to define some key terms relating to the tribology of artificial joints. For joint replacements, it is most meaningful to define wear as the removal of material from the bearing surfaces in the form of wear particles, because the intensity of the biologic reaction is a function of the rate of release of this debris. This definition distinguishes wear from damage, which, as it is used in the orthopaedic literature, typically refers to visible changes in the surface of the bearings (polishing, scratching, etc)[1,2] that may or may not be accompanied by actual wear (Fig. 1).

Wear is caused by fundamental mechanisms that include adhesion, abrasion, and fatigue.[3] Adhesive wear occurs if the bond strength of micro contacts, for example, between the polyethylene of the cup and the metal of the ball, exceeds the inherent strength of either material. Typically, polyethylene is pulled from the surface, forming fibrils and/or small pits. When adhesive wear occurs on a micron or submicron scale, the bearing surface still can appear highly polished to the

The author or the departments with which he is affiliated have received something of value from a commercial or other party related directly or indirectly to the subject of this chapter.

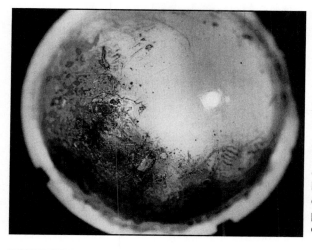

Fig. 1 Polyethylene acetabular cup worn in vivo (stained with ink to emphasize the morphology), showing highly polished area corresponding to high wear but low visible damage and damaged area (scratches, pits, and so forth) corresponding to low wear.

eye.[4-7] Nevertheless, the billions of wear particles that are released into the tissues annually[6,8] are the driving force behind progressive osteolysis.[9-13]

Abrasive wear occurs when a hard projection on one surface cuts a scratch on the opposing surface during sliding. These projections can include the edge of an existing scratch, protruding carbides, embedded third-body particles, or even original contaminants that were exposed by the wear process itself. As with adhesive wear, abrasive scratching may be visible to the eye or, if it occurs on a microscopic scale, the surfaces may appear very smooth (undamaged), even though substantial wear has occurred. This wear is analogous to sanding a piece of wood with very fine sandpaper. The wood appears progressively

smoother precisely because of the substantial amount of abrasive wear occurring. Fatigue wear is cracking, pitting, and/or delamination that is caused by cyclic stresses applied to the bearing surface. Again, this wear can occur on a micron scale, being nearly invisible to the eye, or on a millimeter scale, resulting in visible damage to the implant. Corrosion of a metal component and oxidation of a polyethylene component are not wear mechanisms per se, but they can substantially lower the wear resistance of the material.

Any number of these wear mechanisms may operate while the prosthesis is functioning in one of the following four distinct wear modes.[3,6] Mode 1 corresponds to articulation between two bearing surfaces only, which is necessary

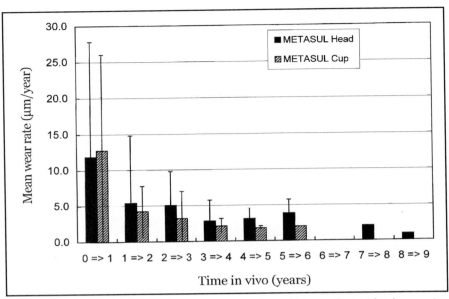

Fig. 2 Wear rate for retrieved, second-generation metal-metal hip prostheses. The decrease in wear rate after the initial wear-in phase has also been observed in hip simulator studies of metal-metal bearings. (Reproduced with permission from Rieker C, Kottig P, Schon R, Windler M, Wyss U: Clinical tribological performance of 144 metal-on-metal hip articulations, in Rieker C, Windler M, Wyss U (eds): *METASUL: A Metal-On-Metal Bearing.* Bern, Switzerland, Hans Huber, 1999, pp 83-91.)

for the prosthesis to function. Mode 2 corresponds to articulation between a bearing surface and a nonbearing surface; for example, if the femoral ball penetrates the polyethylene liner (after excessive mode 1 wear) and contacts the metal backing. Mode 3 wear corresponds to motion between two bearing surfaces, but with third-body abrasive contaminants present. Mode 4 wear corresponds to motion between two nonbearing surfaces, such as backside wear between the inside of a metal acetabular shell and the outside of the polyethylene liner or fretting of the Morse taper junction between the ball and the stem. Porous-coated prostheses that tend to shed particles are particularly susceptible to mode 3 wear, and the loaded interfaces between the components of a modular prosthesis provide additional opportunities for mode 4 wear. Furthermore, the debris produced in mode 4 may induce local osteolysis or it can migrate to the bearing

surfaces, initiating mode 3 wear. Bearing surfaces for prosthetic joints should have high wear resistance under ideal conditions (mode 1) and adverse conditions (modes 2, 3, and 4).

Metal-on-Metal Bearings

The first widely used total hip replacements featured cobalt-chromium alloy bearing against itself, primarily the McKee-Farrar (Howmedica, Limerick, Ireland) design,[14] along with the Mueller (Sulzer AG, Winterthur, Switzerland), Ring (Downs, Ltd, Mitchham, England) and others.[15-18] Because of a relatively high rate of early failure, the first-generation metal-on-metal hips were largely supplanted by the Charnley prosthesis, which featured a stainless steel ball and a polyethylene socket.[19] However, in hindsight, it has become apparent that a large percentage of the early failures of the McKee-Farrar hips comprised implants from a single supplier and involved relatively thin acetabular shells

and a small ball-cup clearance, possibly leading to distortion of the cups under physiologic loading, jamming, excessively high frictional torque, and rapid wear. Disregarding the early failures, the long-term survivorship of the early metal-on-metal designs has been comparable to that of the metal-on-polyethylene Charnley.[15,16,23,24] In particular, the steady-state wear rates have been on the order of a few micrometers per year[17,25,26] compared with the average of 100 to 200 μm of polyethylene wear per year typically reported for metal-on-polyethylene hips.[27-32]

In view of the growing awareness of the problem of extensive osteolysis caused by polyethylene wear debris, a number of second-generation metal-on-metal implants have been developed, including conventional total hips and surface replacements.[33-35] The first to be widely used clinically was the Metasul (Sulzer AG, Winterthur, Switzerland) hip,[16,36-38] which recently received United States Food and Drug Administration (FDA) approval for use in the United States. Hip simulator studies[39-42] and clinical retrievals[37,43,44] of modern metal-on-metal bearings also typically have shown steady-state wear rates on the order of a few micrometers per million cycles (with one million cycles being the equivalent of about 1 year's use in a patient of average activity[45]). It is also apparent that metal-on-metal implants have the ability to self-heal, that is, to polish-out isolated surface scratches caused by third-body particles or subluxation damage.[26,46] The overall clinical performance of second-generation metal-on-metal hips to date has been comparable to that of conventional metal-on-polyethylene hips and somewhat better than that of first-generation metal-on-metal hips.[37,47]

Clinical and laboratory wear studies have indicated that metal-on-metal implants often exhibit 10 to 20 times greater wear-in during the initial 1 to 2 years of clinical use (Fig. 2), or one to two million cycles in a hip simulator[37,39-41,43] In addition, some first-generation and second-generation metal-on-metal hips have exhibited extensive surface micropitting, possibly due to a fatigue-corrosion mechanism associated with the smaller carbides.[43,46,48] Although the high wear-in rate is a transitory phenomenon, and the presence of the micropits does not appear to be associated with a high wear rate,[43] they represent areas for potential improvement of metal-on-metal implants.

Ceramic-on-Ceramic Implants
Alumina-on-Alumina Bearings

As with metal-on-metal bearings, the earliest designs of alumina-on-alumina hip bearings often experienced unacceptably high wear rates.[49-55] The United States' experience with ceramic-on-ceramic primarily involved the Autophor/Xenophor prostheses (Osteo, Selzach, Switzerland), which were first developed and used in Europe by Mittelmeier and Heisel.[50] The clinical results with the Autophor were subject to greater problems of pain, neck-socket impingement, ceramic fracture, and component loosening than for contemporary metal-on-polyethylene designs, and ceramic-on-ceramic implants were never widely used in the United States.[52,56] The causes of high wear included poor quality ceramic (by today's standards), edge contact of the cup on the ball due to inadequate range of motion and/or vertical cup placement, and other design shortcomings. For example, hips with a lateral opening smaller than 30° or larger than 55° and/or a high neck shaft angle (larger than about 140°) were at greater risk for neck socket impingement and/or high wear as a result of increased contact stress.[57]

Fortunately, the past two decades have seen substantial improvement in prosthesis design, implantation technique, and, most importantly, the quality of the alumina.[53,57-59] Changes in the

Table 1			
Physical properties of alumina and zirconia[85]			
Property	Alumina Sintered in air	Alumina Hipped	Zirconia (Y-TZP)
Grain size (μm)	3	1.8	< 0.5
Density (g/cm³)	≥ 3.96	≥ 3.98	> 6.00
Modulus (GPa)	380	380	210
Bending strength (Mpa)	> 500	> 500	> 950
Fracture toughness (MPa m$^{1/2}$)	4	4	8

latter have included higher purity, finer grain structure, and improved sintering techniques. Hip simulator studies and clinical retrievals have indicated that the steady-state wear rate of alumina-on-alumina bearings can be as low as 1 to 2 μm/yr.[60-64]

Modern alumina-on-alumina bearings are not, however, immune to high wear.[65-67] For example, in one study severe wear and osteolysis were reported in 22% of the patients after an average of only 7.7 years follow-up.[68] Although the causes of such unusually rapid wear in alumina-on-alumina bearings are a subject of continuing study,[57,69] these results emphasize the importance of observing proper surgical technique with ceramic-on-ceramic bearings.[53,58] For example, edge-chipping of ceramic balls or cups during insertion can be avoided by careful alignment of the components prior to assembly.[67,70]

Gross fracture of a ceramic bearing component in the patient is a catastrophic failure, and the surgeon performing the revision procedure can be faced with a difficult decision. If a new ceramic ball is placed on a damaged Morse taper, there is a much greater chance of fracture of the new ball.[71,72] On the other hand, if a metal ball is used in the revision, fragments of ceramic that are left in the tissues may subsequently become trapped between the ball and cup and initiate extremely rapid wear of the metal ball and massive metallosis. From the perspective of preventing wear, the safest option is to replace the femoral stem and use a new ceramic

ball on a new taper; however, this can also be problematic if the stem is well fixed in the femur.

Fortunately, improvements in the quality of the alumina ceramic, particularly through hot isostatic pressing (Table 1), have led to a reduction in the rate of fracture to as low as one or two in 10,000 patients,[53,75,76] a risk that must be weighed against the potential benefits of very low wear and high biocompatibility of alumina-on-alumina bearings.

Ceramic-on-Ceramic Bearings Involving Zirconia

As the outside diameter of a femoral ball is reduced, for example, from 32 mm to 28 mm to 22 mm, the ball becomes progressively thinner adjacent to the Morse taper, and many surgeons are reluctant to use 22-mm diameter alumina balls. Due to its finer grain structure, yttria-stabilized zirconia ceramic (Y-TZP, where TZP refers to tetragonal zirconia polycrystals) is about 73% stronger than alumina (Table 1) and, therefore, provides a greater margin of safety, particularly with the smaller diameter balls.[77-79] For example, one survey reported only two fractures of zirconia balls out of 300,000 implanted.[80] However, at high temperatures in a wet environment, Y-TZP zirconia can undergo a phase transformation that substantially weakens the material and roughens the surface, degrading its wear properties.[81-83] Although zirconia is highly stable at physiologic temperature,[80,84] Y-TZP zirconia components should not be steam autoclaved.

To date, zirconia has been used primarily as a femoral ball articulating against an acetabular cup of polyethylene. The advisability of using Y-TZP zirconia balls against cups of alumina or zirconia is a subject of controversy. Laboratory studies using a washer-on-flat test configuration have reported severe wear of zirconia-on-zirconia and zirconia-on-alumina pairs,[85,86] possibly due to a temperature-induced degradation of the zirconia. In contrast, other investigators using a pin-on-disk machine[87] have observed very low wear of zirconia-on-alumina and zirconia-on-zirconia combinations. It seems likely that the differences in outcome of these studies were related to differences in the specimen configuration, the access of the lubricant to the bearing surfaces, and the type of lubricant used, resulting in substantial differences in the maximum temperatures generated. In particular, tests run in water gave severe wear of the zirconia, whereas tests run in serum did not. Thus, the clinical use of Y-TZP zirconia bearing against alumina or itself remains controversial, as do the optimal conditions for laboratory wear testing of ceramic-on-ceramic bearings.

Most recently, ceramics have been fabricated using a mixture of zirconia and alumina in various ratios. The resultant mixed-oxides materials appear to combine the high strength of zirconia with the thermal stability of alumina, and preliminary wear tests on a pin-on-disk machine and a hip joint simulator have indicated excellent wear resistance.[88-90] Although clinical trials have been underway in the United States for several years for alumina-on-alumina bearings, as yet, none of the ceramic-on-ceramic bearing combinations have received FDA approval.

Materials Bearing Against Polyethylene
Metal-on-Polyethylene Bearings
The metals used in conjunction with polyethylene principally have included stainless steel, cobalt-chromium alloy (in the vast majority), and titanium alloy. In some cases, the metal components have been surface hardened; for example, by nitriding or ion-implanting. In general, the wear rate of polyethylene against stainless steel has been comparable to that against cobalt-chrome alloy in laboratory tests[91,92] and in clinical use.[93-96] In contrast, although the wear rate of polyethylene against titanium alloy under clean conditions appears to be comparable to that with the other metals, the greater vulnerability of titanium alloy to abrasion by entrapped third-body particles can cause severe, runaway wear.[99-101] Hardening of the surface of the titanium alloy by techniques such as gas nitriding, solution nitriding, or ion implanting can markedly improve its resistance to abrasion by third-body particles, and good 10-year results have been reported for titanium nitride-hardened TiAlNb alloy balls used with polyethylene cups.[102] Nevertheless, if a hardened surface eventually is penetrated, severe wear of the underlying alloy still can be triggered.[101,103-105] Consequently, even hardened titanium alloys have seen limited clinical use as bearing surfaces.

The vast majority of metal-on-polyethylene bearings used in hip prostheses have involved cobalt-chrome alloy femoral balls, including cast or forged alloys, and the wear rate of this combination now forms the clinical baseline against which potentially improved bearing combinations are evaluated. As noted above, the *average* wear rate of the polyethylene against cobalt-chrome alloy is typically reported to be in the range of 0.1 to 0.2 mm/yr. However, it should be noted that this average includes those implants that have accelerated wear rates due to excessive third-body damage to the bearing surfaces, radiation-induced oxidative degradation of the polyethylene, or other causes.[30,105] Thus, the inherent wear rate of a polyethylene cup with a cobalt-chrome alloy ball under clean conditions (as are usually modeled in a hip simulator) is probably somewhat below the clinical average wear rate, possibly as low as 0.05 mm/yr.

Ion implanting and other surface hardening techniques also have been applied to cobalt-chromium alloy. Laboratory tests of hardened cobalt-chromium alloy have been reported to both markedly reduce wear and to increase wear of the opposing polyethylene,[105] and clinical results are not yet sufficient to resolve this contradiction. Whereas it seems likely that surface hardening of cobalt-chrome may improve its resistance to moderate amounts of third-body abrasion, the uncertainty of the advantage in general has limited its clinical application.

Ceramic-on-Polyethylene Bearings
Alumina and zirconia femoral balls have been used widely as bearing surfaces against polyethylene cups, and most clinical studies have shown substantially lower polyethylene wear rates than with metal balls, with the wear ratios ranging from 0.75 to as low as 0.25 with alumina balls.[53,105] A comparable advantage has been reported with zirconia against polyethylene.[106] However, in one recent radiographic study little difference was reported in the wear of polyethylene with alumina or metal balls,[96] as it was in one study of four retrieved alumina implants.[107] Unacceptably high rates of polyethylene wear, lysis, and loosening with an early type of zirconia ball were reported in another study.[82] Similarly, although the majority of the laboratory tests have indicated lower wear of polyethylene with alumina or zirconia than with metal,[105] in one hip simulator study slightly greater polyethylene wear was reported with alumina balls, but less with zirconia balls.[108]

Although the reasons for this disagreement among both clinical and laboratory studies are not clear, it may be due in part to the influence of third-body particles. That is, the greater hardness of ceramic balls renders them more resistant than metal balls to scratching by entrapped abrasive contaminants that can, in turn, accelerate the wear of the opposing polyethylene cup (wear mode 3). The differences in the relative wear rates in the various clinical studies might, therefore, reflect differences in the amount of third-body contamination, with those studies having relatively little such contamination showing comparable polyethylene wear rates for ceramic or metal balls (as in the laboratory tests run under clean conditions). Nevertheless, contamination by metal particles may be detrimental even with a ceramic ball, because the particles can adhere to the surface of the ceramic, effectively roughening it and, thereby, increasing abrasion of the polyethylene. Metal also can be transferred to the ceramic by contact against metallic components or instruments during surgery.[61] Regardless of the bearing material used, care must be taken to minimize the formation of abrasive contaminants in vivo, for example, by avoiding those porous coatings that are prone to shed particles.

Improved Polyethylenes
Historic Polyethylenes and the Effects of Gamma-Air Sterilization

The ultra-high molecular weight polyethylenes (UHMWPEs) that were used for acetabular cups implanted during the past 30 years were fabricated from raw powder (also called resin) from a variety of manufacturers. Presently, there are just two suppliers[109-111] (Table 2). The powder is converted to solid form using one of three distinct methods. In the extrusion process, the polyethylene powder is driven by a ram through a heated nozzle, fusing the flakes into a continuous bar, typically several inches in diameter. The components are machined from the bar stock. In bulk compression molding, the powder is placed in a large mold and heated under

Table 2
UHMWPE resins presently available[111]

Type	Supplier	Average Molecular Weight(10^6 g/mol)	Contains calcium stearate?
GUR 1150	Ticona*	5.5 to 6	Yes
GUR 1050	(Germany)	5.5 to 6	No
GUR 1120		3.5	Yes
GUR 1020		3.5	No
1900	Montell	4.4 to 4.9	No
1900 H	(USA)	> 4.9	No

*Ticona was formerly knows as Hoechst, and the Hoechst UHMWPEs produced in the USA prior to 1998 were GUR 4150/4050/4120/4020, with properties corresponding to the first four entries in the table, respectively

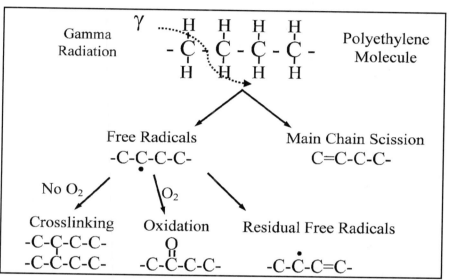

Fig. 3 Effect of radiation on the UHMWPE molecule. The radiation (gamma or electron-beam) causes chain scission and creates free radicals. In the absence of oxygen, the free radicals tend to form cross-links between adjacent molecules in the amorphous regions, improving wear resistance. Oxygen molecules present in the polyethylene, particularly near the surface, can combine with free radicals to cause chain scission, decreasing the strength, toughness, and wear resistance. Free radicals can remain trapped in the crystalline regions of the polyethylene for many years, eventually migrating to the amorphous regions and contributing to oxidative degradation. Free radicals can be neutralized very rapidly by heating above the "melt" temperature (crystalline-to-amorphous transition), or much more slowly by annealing below the melt temperature.

pressure to fuse it into a block or sheet from which the final components are machined. In net-shape molding, the powder is placed in a metal mold having the desired shape of the implant and then fused under heat and pressure, such that little or no final machining is required.

The final step in any fabrication process was sterilization. Although ethylene oxide sterilization was used initially and gas plasma more recently,[112-114] the great majority of polyethylene components implanted during the past 25 years or more were sterilized by exposure to gamma radiation, with the dose

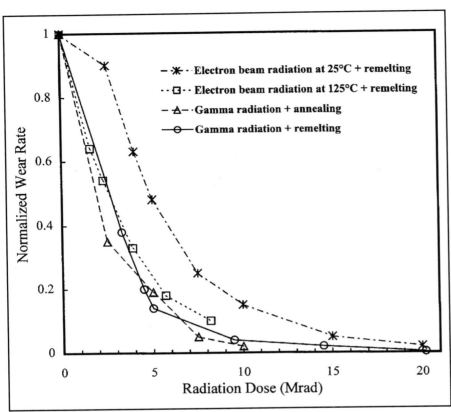

Fig. 4 Reduction in wear with increased level of cross-linking. The curves for the two gamma-radiation cross-linked polyethylenes were produced on hip joint simulators in two different laboratories.[118,119] The curves for the two electron-beam cross-linked polyethylenes were produced on a bidirectional pin-on-disk machine in a third laboratory.[120] Because two wear machines may produce different wear magnitudes for the same material due to differences in the applied load and/or the sliding distance per cycle, the original data were normalized by dividing by the wear rate for zero Mrad (no cross-linking) obtained in each test.

somewhere between 2.5 to 4 Mrads, and with the components sealed in air during irradiation and subsequent storage. Ethylene oxide and gas plasma sterilization have relatively little effect on the physical properties of polyethylene. In contrast, an extensive amount of research, particularly during the past 5 years, has shown that gamma sterilization in air, as well as extended storage in air, markedly affects the physical properties of UHMWPE components (Fig. 3). Near the surface of the component, free radicals generated by the radiation combine with oxygen that has diffused into the polymer during the period between fabrication and irradiation. Depending on how much oxygen is present, there could be immediate oxidative degradation and very little cross-linking of the surface layer. Beneath the level of diffused oxygen, free radicals generated by the radiation in the amorphous regions of the polyethylene rapidly combine to form cross-links. In contrast, free radicals generated in the crystalline regions are far less mobile but could eventually migrate to the amorphous regions and combine with any oxygen that had diffused to that level. This oxidative degradation of the polyethylene could continue for years during shelf-storage and, to a lesser extent,[115,116] during use in vivo. Oxidation leads to extensive chain-

scission, weakening and embrittling the polyethylene, directly reducing its resistance to wear, delamination, and fracture. In addition, oxidation can indirectly reduce wear resistance by reducing the level of cross-linking.[117]

While, as discussed below, gamma-induced cross-linking can markedly improve the wear resistance of UHMWPE (Fig. 4), excessive cross-linking can adversely affect other physical properties such as ultimate strength, elongation, and fracture toughness.[118-121] However, studies of retrieved implants have demonstrated that weakening of the polyethylene due to immediate and long-term oxidation could be substantially greater than that due to the moderate level of cross-linking induced by the 2.5 to 4 Mrads used for routine sterilization.[115,122-127] Consequently, the alterations in the methods for fabricating and sterilizing UHMWPE components in the past few years have been directed at minimizing oxidative degradation while simultaneously optimizing the level of cross-linking to improve wear resistance.

Alternative Sterilization Techniques

In one approach to minimizing oxidative degradation, some manufacturers now sterilize the polyethylene components without irradiation, using either ethylene oxide or gas plasma.[111] Because these methods do not generate free radicals in the polyethylene, they completely avoid the potential for immediate and long-term oxidative degradation of the mechanical properties and wear resistance. However, because ethylene oxide or gas plasma do not induce cross-linking, they do not take advantage of its potential for improving the wear resistance of the polyethylene.

Other manufacturers continue to sterilize their implants with gamma radiation, but do so with the polyethylene components sealed in some type of low-oxygen atmosphere, including vacuum,[128] inert gas,[129] or with an oxygen scavenger.[130] In addition, one manufacturer anneals the polyethylene acetabular cups after sterilization by heating them in the nitrogen packaging at 37° to 50°C (well below the melt temperature of 135°C to avoid distorting the components) for about 6 days to reduce the level of residual free radicals that were induced by the gamma radiation.[131] These approaches can markedly reduce but not necessarily eliminate the oxidation that would otherwise occur during gamma sterilization and subsequent shelf-storage,[127,132] and the remaining free radicals may induce some oxidation during long-term use in vivo. Furthermore, because the level of cross-linking is determined by the 2.5- to 4-Mrad gamma radiation dose used to sterilize the components, the improvement in wear resistance (as exhibited in laboratory wear tests) relative to non-cross-linked polyethylene ranges from about 30% to 50%, compared to the 85% or more reduction achieved with elevated cross-linking doses.

In retrospective studies of shelf-stored and/or retrieved implants, some sets of components that were fabricated from block molded or net-shape molded polyethylene, gamma-sterilized, and stored in air have undergone substantially lower levels of oxidation than similarly treated extruded-machined components. It has been suggested that the molded polyethylene was more completely fused than typical extruded material, rendering it more resistant to diffusion of oxygen and, therefore, more resistant to immediate and long-term oxidative degradation, despite the presence of free radicals.[125,133] Consequently, several suppliers have reintroduced net-shape molding of components. Specialized molding techniques include hot-isostatic pressing of the polyethylene powder in an argon atmosphere[134] and special molding protocols that can provide polyethylene with a specified crystallinity and stiffness.[111,135] How-

ever, manufacturers no longer irradiate and store the polyethylene in air; therefore the marked differences in oxidation levels that occurred between molded and extruded-machined components in the past may not occur under current techniques of manufacturing and use. Furthermore, while molded polyethylene may have superior resistance to oxidation, this fabrication technique alone does not address cross-linking of the polyethylene to improve its wear resistance.

Clinical Studies of Polyethylenes With Elevated Levels of Cross-Linking

As noted above, the moderate level of cross-linking that was present in the vast majority of UHMWPE components implanted over the past three decades was an unintentional byproduct of the 2.5 to 4 Mrads of gamma radiation used to sterilize the components. Nevertheless, intentional cross-linking has long been used to improve the wear resistance of polyethylene in industrial applications; for example, as a lining for coal chutes. In addition, polyethylene acetabular cups that were intentionally cross-linked at levels much higher than occurs with routine sterilization were used in three clinical studies over the past 25 years. Grobbelaar and associates[136,137] cross-linked finished polyethylene acetabular cups by exposing them to 10 Mrads of gamma radiation. By irradiating the cups while immersed in acetylene gas, cross-linking in the outermost 300 μm was increased substantially above what would normally occur at 10 Mrads. No postirradiation thermal processing was done to reduce the residual free radicals. In anticipation of a lower wear rate, the cross-linked polyethylene was used with 30 mm diameter femoral balls to reduce the incidence of dislocation the investigators had experienced with 22-mm diameter heads. In a 14- to 21-year follow-up based on radiographs, Grobbelaar and associates[137] reported a "lack of measurable wear" in 56 of 64

cases, and only two revisions due to osteolysis.

Oonishi and associates[138] induced very high levels of cross-linking by exposing finished cups to 100 Mrads of gamma radiation, with the cups in air. As with Grobbelaar's method, there was no thermal treatment to extinguish free radicals. In a clinical follow-up from 6 to 8 years, Oonishi and associates[139] reported steady-state wear rates of 247 and 98 μm/yr for noncross-linked polyethylene cups bearing against cobalt-chrome and alumina heads, respectively, and 76 and 72 μm/yr for 100-Mrad cross-linked polyethylene cups bearing against stainless steel and alumina heads, respectively. Subsequently, Oonishi and associates[140] reported that against cobaltchrome heads, the long-term wear rates averaged 290 and 60 μm/yr for the noncross-linked cups and cross-linked cups, respectively. While this represented about a 79% reduction with cross-linking, the average wear rate for the noncross-linked cups in the study by Oonishi and associates[140] was substantially above the range of 100 to 200 μm/yr that typically has been reported for gamma-air sterilized polyethylene cups in clinical studies.[105]

More recently, Wroblewski and associates[141] chemically cross-linked polyethylene cups using a silane process. After an initial higher rate of penetration (possibly due to greater creep), the average steady-state wear rate in 19 patients with up to 8.3 years of follow-up was only 22 μm/yr for cross-linked cups bearing against alumina ceramic heads. While this rate was well below the clinical range for gamma-air cups, as with Oonishi's study, it was not clear how much of the advantage was due to head material rather than cross-linking. Nevertheless, the results of the three clinical studies were encouraging in that, despite any reduction in strength caused by the high levels of cross-linking, and despite the lack of thermal treatment to extinguish free radicals from the gamma-cross-linked materials,[137,138] none

Table 3
Comparison among new cross-linked thermally-stabilized polyethylenes

Name and Manufacturer	FDA Approved ? (June 2000)	Radiation Type and Dose	Thermal Stabilization	Final Sterilization	Manufacturer's Rationale
Marathon™ DePuy, Inc	Yes	Gamma radiation to 5 Mrads at room temperature	Remelted at 155°C for 24 hours	Gas plasma	5 Mrads gamma cross-linking provides about 85% wear reduction (well below the threshold for lysis) while preserving other mechanical properties. Remelting eliminates free radicals and prevents oxidative degradation.
XLPE™ Smith & Nephew-Richards, Inc	Yes	Gamma radiation to 5 Mrads at room temperature	Remelted at 150°C for two hours	Ethylene oxide	5 Mrads gamma to provide wear reduction (wear data not yet available), while preserving other mechanical properties. Remelting eliminates free radicals and prevents oxidation.
Longevity™ Zimmer, Inc	Yes	Electron beam radiation to 10 Mrads at room temperature	Remelted at 150°C for about two hours	Gas plasma	10 Mrads provides about 89% wear reduction. Remelting eliminates free radicals and prevents oxidation.
Durasul™ Sulzer, Inc	Yes	Electron beam radiation to 9.5 Mrads at 125°C	Remelted at 150°C for about two hours	Ethylene oxide	9.5 Mrads provides > 95% wear reduction. E-beam cross-linking at elevated temperature provides more wear reduction than E-beam at room temperature. Remelting eliminates free radicals and prevents oxidation.
Crossfire™ Stryker-Osteonics-Howmedica, Inc	Yes	Gamma radiation to 7.5 Mrads at room temperature	Annealed at about 120°C for a proprietary duration	Gamma at 2.5 to 3.5 Mrads while packaged in nitrogen	Depending on actual sterilization dose, total gamma cross-linking dose may vary from 10 to 11 Mrads, providing about 90% wear reduction. Annealing provides a different balance of material properties than remelting. Resultant material has substantial free radicals, but oxidation is limited by sterilization and storage in nitrogen.
Aeonian™ Kyocera, Inc	Approved in Japan; not yet in US	Gamma to 3.5 Mrads at room temperature	Annealed at 110°C for 10 hours	Gamma at 2.5 to 4 Mrads while packaged in nitrogen	Depending on actual sterilization dose, total gamma cross-linking dose may vary from 6 to 7.5 Mrads. Wear data not yet available. Annealing provides a different balance of material properties than remelting. Resultant material has substantial free radicals, but oxidation is limited by sterilization and storage in nitrogen.

(The processing parameters shown in this table were compiled from various publications and information provided by the manufacturers and are subject to modification.)

of the investigators reported fractures or other mechanical failures of their cross-linked cups.

Intentionally Cross-Linked, Thermally Stabilized Polyethylenes

Over the past few years, a number of laboratory wear simulations have demonstrated that the wear rate of UHMWPE cups decreases markedly with an increasing level of radiation-induced cross-linking.[118-120] Although the baseline wear rate differed among various wear machines due to systematic differences in the load, sliding distance per cycle, and other factors, the dose-wear curve was remarkably consistent among different laboratories and with different cross-linking techniques. The greatest reduction per Mrad occurred as the dose increased from zero to about 5 Mrads, with progres-sively less improvement at higher doses and no additional benefit after 15 to 20 Mrads (Fig. 4). While this dose-wear relationship was the basis for the recent development of a variety of intentionally-cross-linked polyethylenes, the developers have arrived at very different opinions regarding the appropriate dose and other processing parameters for optimizing the clinical performance of a polyethylene implant. The fabrication and characteristics of the new, intentionally-cross-linked polyethylenes are described in the following sections, and are summarized in Table 3.

Marathon Gamma Radiation-Cross-Linked and Remelted Polyethylene

In the Marathon (DePuy, Warsaw, IN) process,[119,142-144] extruded bars of UHM-WPE are cross-linked by exposing them to 5 Mrads of gamma radiation. The bars are then heated to 155°C for 24 hours, followed by slow cooling to room temperature. When polyethylene is heated above the melt temperature, it is transformed from a partially crystalline solid to a totally amorphous solid. Because the uncombined free radicals that were generated during the gamma irradiation are trapped primarily in the crystalline regions,[145] heating above the melt temperature frees them to combine with each other, forming additional cross-links and, more importantly, minimizing the potential for long-term oxidative degradation.[119] The acetabular cup is then machined from the central portion of the cross-linked-remelted bar, thereby removing any surface-oxidized material, and is sterilized using gas plasma rather than gamma radiation to avoid increasing the level of cross-linking or reintroducing residual free radicals. In addition to reducing the wear under ideal, clean test conditions by about 85% (Fig. 4), Marathon has shown substantially less wear than noncross-linked polyethylene bearing against severely roughened femoral balls (that is, modeling third-body abrasive wear).[142] Comparable improved resistance to third-body abrasion has been demonstrated for two other cross-linked polyethylenes tested in hip simulators,[146,147] although greater wear of a cross-linked polyethylene was observed in one pin-on-plate test configuration.[148]

XLPE Gamma Radiation-Cross-Linked and Remelted Polyethylene

XLPE (Smith and Nephew Richards, Memphis, TN) is fabricated in much the same manner as Marathon, except that the final sterilization is done with ethylene oxide.[149]

Longevity Electron Beam-Cross-Linked and Remelted Polyethylene

In the Longevity (Zimmer, Warsaw, IN) process, compression molded sheets of UHMWPE are cross-linked by exposure to a 10-MeV electron beam.[150] After cross-linking, the polyethylene is heated above the melt temperature for about 2 hours to extinguish the free radicals and then

machined into cups and sterilized with gas plasma.

Durasul Electron Beam-Cross-Linked and Remelted Polyethylene

The Durasul (Sulzer, Winterthur, Switzerland) process is similar to the Longevity process, with two exceptions. The polyethylene is machined into short segments or pucks that are cross-linked from both sides with a 10-MeV electron beam to a total of 9.5 Mrads, to increase the uniformity of the cross-linking. In addition, the pucks are preheated to about 125°C while being electron-beam cross-linked because comparative tests have indicated that this procedure provides greater wear resistance (Fig. 4) and less reduction in elongation to break and toughness than electron-beam cross-linking at room temperature.[151] For either process, because the electron beam drives the cross-linking energy into the polyethylene about 2,500 times faster than with gamma radiation (that is, in seconds rather than hours), which generates substantial heating of the polyethylene. After cross-linking, the Durasul cups are remelted to remove free radicals and sterilized with ethylene oxide.[152]

Crossfire Gamma-Cross-Linked and Annealed Polyethylene

In the Crossfire (Stryker-Howmedica Osteonics, Rutherford, NJ) process,[153] extruded bars of UHMWPE are cross-linked by exposure to 7.5 Mrads of gamma radiation. The bars are then annealed (rather than melted) by heating them to just below the melt temperature for a duration that is proprietary. Cups are then machined from the bars, sealed in nitrogen, and sterilized by exposure to an additional 2.5 to 3.5 Mrads of gamma radiation (that is, to a total gamma dose of 10 to 11 Mrads). No thermal treatment to extinguish free radicals is applied after the final gamma sterilization.

The developers of the Crossfire process prefer annealing to remelting of the polyethylene on the grounds that it induces less change in material morphology and material properties than does remelting.[153] However, as noted above, melting is used in the molding or extruding processes to fuse the UHMWPE powder into a solid form. Thus, it is not clear that remelting has a deleterious effect on the properties of the polymer. In addition, because crystalline regions remain in the polyethylene unless it is heated above the melt temperature, annealing is not as effective as remelting in extinguishing the residual free radicals. Consequently, Crossfire polyethylene that was artificially aged by being heated to 80°C in air for 3 weeks underwent substantial oxidative degradation of its strength and wear resistance.[154] In contrast, artificial aging has negligible effect on radiation-cross-linked polyethylenes that have been remelted to extinguish the residual free radicals[154,155] As with other current gamma-sterilized polyethylenes, however, the manufacturer of Crossfire implants recommends that they be shelf-stored in the nitrogen-filled package, and for only a limited duration prior to implantation. In view of this, the developers argue that any oxidative degradation of Crossfire implants will be far less than historically occurred with polyethylene components that were irradiated and stored in air, or for artificially aged implants, such that the residual free radicals will have negligible effect on the clinical performance of the implants.[153] Careful clinical follow-up will be required to resolve these issues.

Aeonian Gamma-Cross-Linked and Annealed Polyethyene

Except for the use of a lower range of cross-linking dose (Table 3), the rationale and processing of Aenoian (Kyocera, San Diego, CA) parallels that for Crossfire.

Optimum Method for Cross-Linking

The optimum amount of cross-linking to use is also a subject of current debate. Because increasing the level of cross-linking causes a progressively greater reduction in some mechanical properties, such as ultimate strength, ductility, fracture toughness, and fatigue strength,[119,121,144] one extreme is to avoid cross-linking altogether (for example, by simply sterilizing with ethylene oxide or gas plasma). This avoidance is to retain the maximum values of strength, elongation, and fracture toughness, despite the fact that it results in substantially higher wear of the polyethylene.

Among those who advocate cross-linking, the particular dose used represents that manufacturer's approach to balancing reduced wear against the need to maintain other mechanical properties well above that needed for acceptable clinical performance. Those using the high levels of cross-linking (9.5 to 11 Mrads, Table 3), about 3 to 4 times the typical dose used historically to sterilize polyethylene components, maintain that these high levels are justified to obtain the additional 5% to 10% improvement in wear over that provided by a moderate dose (Fig. 4), despite the corresponding reduction in other physical properties. In contrast, advocates of a moderate cross-linking dose, such as 5 Mrads (Table 3), maintain that the corresponding reduction in wear to 85% below that of a noncrosslinked polyethylene, if realized clinically, will be sufficient to avoid an osteolytic reaction in even the most active patients, without unnecessarily reducing other physical properties.

Clearly, it is not desirable to use a dose that will result in mechanical failure of the polyethylene components. However, it is important to recall several facts when considering the likelihood of failure of a cross-linked cup in vivo: (1) the vast majority of polyethylene cups

Table 4
Overall advantages and disadvantages of current bearing choices

Bearing Combination	Potential Advantages	Potential Disadvantages
Alumina on alumina	Usually very low wear High biocompatability	Sometimes high wear Component fracture Higher cost Technique sensitive surgery
Cobalt-chrome on cobalt-chrome	Usually very low wear Can self-polish moderate surface scratches	Question of long-term local and systemic reactions to metal debris and/or ions
Hardened cobalt chrome on polyethylene	Some additional protection against third-body abrasion	Hardened layer can wear off Higher cost
Ceramic on polyethylene	Lower wear of polyethylene than with conventional metal-polyethylene Some additional protection against third-body abrasion	Component fracture Difficulty of revision (that is, if Morse taper is damaged) Higher cost
Polyethylene sterilized with ethylene oxide or gas plasma	No short- or long-term oxidation	No cross-linking so doesn't minimize polyethylene wear
Polyethylene sterilized with gamma in low-oxygen	Some cross-linking, some wear reduction	Polyethylene wear not minimized Residual free radicals (long-term oxidation?)
Cross-linked, thermally-stabilized polyethylene	Minimal polyethylene wear rate No short- or long-term oxidative degradation	Newest of low-wear bearing combinations, only early clinical results available Questions remain regarding optimum cross-linking level and optimum method for thermal stabilization (Table 3)

implanted in the past were moderately cross-linked at gamma doses ranging from 2.5 to 4 Mrads; (2) irradiation was done in air and without the benefit of postirradiation thermal treatment, such that many of these cups were subject to immediate and long-term oxidative degradation; and (3) this poststerilization oxidative degradation caused a much greater loss in strength than the moderate level of cross-linking that was induced by the gamma sterilization.[126,133] Despite their being moderately cross-linked, very few cups used in the past 20 to 30 years fractured in vivo and, when fracture did occur, it was strongly associated with oxidative degradation of the polymer.[156] It is reasonable, therefore, to predict that an acetabular cup that is moderately cross-linked and adequately stabilized against oxidative degradation will be less likely to fracture than the

gamma-air sterilized and oxidized cups that have been the clinical standard for the past three decades.

On the other hand, there is questionable justification for increasing the level of cross-linking substantially above that which is necessary to reduce the wear below the threshold for clinically significant lysis.[157] For example, in a 7-year minimum follow-up, Xenos and associates[158] and others[159] reported that, after 4 to 7.2 years, those patients without lysis averaged a total radiographic wear depth of only 0.8 mm, while patients with lysis averaged 1.2 mm. Consistent with this, Nashed and associates[160] reported no lysis in a group of patients with a hip prosthesis that averaged 0.1 mm/yr or less, 31% in a group averaging 0.13 mm/yr, 24% in a group averaging 0.17 mm/yr, and 87% in a group averaging 0.25 mm/yr. Wan and Dorr[161] found that osteolysis was more likely to be present in hips with polyethylene wear depths exceeding 0.2 mm/yr.

Together, these studies show that clinically significant osteolysis is very rare in patients with polyethylene acetabular cups wearing less than about 0.1 mm (100 μm) per year. As noted above, while the inherent wear rate of UHMWPE (absent substantial oxidative degradation) may fall in the range of 0.05 to 0.1 mm/yr in a patient with average activity, the most active patients walk three to four times the average,[45] which would be sufficient to increase the wear rate of conventional polyethylene to as much as 0.4 mm/yr, well into the range for clinical osteolysis. In contrast, the 85% reduction provided by 5 Mrads of cross-linking (Fig. 4) would reduce the wear rate in such active patients to 0.06 mm/yr or less, well below the threshold for lysis. Although increasing the dose as high as 10 Mrads provides some additional reduction in wear (Fig. 4), this also increases the risk of introducing new problems that were not encountered with the historic maximum of 4 Mrads used for routine sterilization of polyethylene components. Again, resolving these controversies will require close monitoring of the clinical performance of the new polyethylenes over the coming years.

Summary

Because the UHMWPE components fabricated by the historic process of gamma-sterilization in air are no longer marketed, a surgeon who wishes to continue performing joint replacement surgery must choose among the new polyethylenes, or he or she may choose a modern metal-metal or ceramic-ceramic bearing, each of which has its potential advantages and disadvantages (Table 4). Ultimately, it is the responsibility of the surgeon to assess the risk-benefit ratios of each of the new bearing combinations and make an informed and wise choice among them.

References

1. Rostoker W: The appearacnces of wear on poyethylene: A comparison of in vivo an in vitro wear surfaces. *J Biomed Mater Res* 1978;12:317-335.

2. Hood RW, Wright TM, Burstein AH: Retrieval analysis of total knee prostheses: A method and its application to 48 total condylar prostheses. *J Biomed Mater Res* 1983;17:829-842.

3. McKellop HA: Wear modes, mechanisms, damage, and debris: Separating cause from effect in the wear of total hip replacements, in Galante JO, Rosenberg AG, Callaghan JJ (eds): *Total Hip Revision Surgery*. New York, NY, Raven Press, 1995, pp 21-39.

4. Cooper JR, Dowson D, Fisher J: Macroscopic and microscopic wear mechanisms in ultra-high molecular weight polyethylene. *Wear* 1993;162:378-384.

5. Jasty M, Bragdon C, Jiranek W, Chandler H, Maloney W, Harris WH: Etiology of osteolysis around porous-coated cementless total hip arthroplasties. *Clin Orthop* 1994;308:111-126.

6. McKellop HA, Campbell P, Park SH, et al: The origin of submicron polyethylene wear debris in total hip arthroplasty. *Clin Orthop* 1995;311:3-20.

7. Wang A, Stark C, Dumbleton JH: Mechanistic and morphological origins of ultra-high molecular weight polyethylene wear debris in total joint replacement prostheses. *Proc Inst Mech Eng [H]* 1996;210:141-155.

8. Clarke IC, Kabo JM: Wear in total hip replacement, in Amstutz HC (ed): *Hip Arthroplasty*. New York, NY, Churchill Livingstone, 1991, pp 535-553.

9. Willert HG, Semlitsch M: Reactions of the articular capsule to wear products of artificial joint prostheses. *J Biomed Mater Res* 1977;11:157-164.

10. Goldring SR, Jasty M, Roelke MS, Rourke CM, Bringhurst FR, Harris WH: Formation of a synovial-like membrane at the bone-cement interface: Its role in bone resorption and implant loosening after total hip replacement. *Arthritis Rheum* 1986;29:836-842.

11. Howie DW, Vernon-Roberts B, Oakeshott R, Manthey B: A rat model of resorption of bone at the cement-bone interface in the presence of polyethylene wear particles. *J Bone Joint Surg Am* 1988;70:257-263.

12. Schmalzried TP, Jasty M, Harris WH: Periprosthetic bone loss in total hip arthroplasty: Polyethylene wear debris and the concept of the effective joint space. *J Bone Joint Surg Am* 1992;74:849-863.

13. Amstutz HC, Campbell P, Kossovsky N, Clarke IC: Mechanism and clinical significance of wear-debris induced osteolysis. *Clin Orthop* 1992;276:7-18.

14. McKee GK, Watson-Farrar J: Replacement of arthritic hips by the McKee-Farrar prosthesis. *J Bone Joint Surg Br* 1966;48:245-259.

15. Amstutz HC, Grigoris P: Metal on metal bearings in hip arthroplasty. *Clin Orthop* 1996;329(suppl):11-34.

16. Schmidt M, Weber H, Schon R: Cobalt chromium molybdenum metal combination for modular hip prostheses. *Clin Orthop* 1996;329(suppl):35-47.

17. Willert HG, Buchhorn GH, Gobel D, et al: Wear behavior and histopathology of classic cemented metal on metal hip endoprostheses. *Clin Orthop* 1996;329(suppl):160-186.

18. Scott ML, Lemons JE: The wear characteristics of Sivash/SRN Co-Cr-Mo THA articulating surfaces, in Jacobs JJ, Craig TL (eds): *Alternative Bearing Surfaces in Total Joint Replacement*. West Conshohocken, PA, ASTM, 1998, pp 159-172.

19. Charnley J, Cupic Z: The nine and ten year results of the low-friction arthroplasty of the hip. *Clin Orthop* 1973;95:9-25.

20. Walker PS, Salvati E, Hotzler RK: The wear on removed McKee-Farrar total hip prostheses. *J Bone Joint Surg Am* 1974;56:92-100.

21. Semlitsch M, Streicher RM, Weber H: Long-term results with meta/metal pairings in artificial hip joints, in Buchhorn G, Willert HG (eds): *Technical Principles, Design, and Safety of Joint Implants*. Seattle, WA, Hogrefe & Huber, 1994, pp 62-67.

22. Poggie RA: A review of the effects of design, contact stress, and materials on the wear of metal-on-metal hip prostheses, in Jacobs JJ, Craig TL (eds): *Alternative Bearing Surfaces in Total Joint Replacement*. West Conshohocken, PA, ASTM, 1998, pp 47-54.

23. Jacobsson S-A, Djerf K, Wahlstrom O: A comparative study between McKee-Farrar and Charnley arthroplasty with long-term follow-up periods. *J Arthroplasty* 1990;5:9-14.

24. Schmalzried TP, Szuszczewicz ES, Akizuki KH, Petersen TD, Amstutz HC: Factors correlating with long term survival of McKee-Farrar total hip prostheses. *Clin Orthop* 1996;329(suppl)48-59.

25. Kothari M, Bartel DL, Booker JF: Surface geometry of retrieved McKee-Farrar total hip replacements. *Clin Orthop* 1996;329(suppl):141-147.

26. McKellop H, Park S-H, Chiesa R, et al: In vivo wear of three types of metal on metal hip prostheses during two decades of use. *Clin Orthop* 1996;329(suppl):128-140.

27. Griffith MJ, Seidenstein MK, Williams D, Charnley J: Socket wear in Charnley low friction arthroplasty of the hip. *Clin Orthop* 1978;137:37-47.

28. Rimnac CM, Wilson PD Jr, Fuchs MD, Wright TM: Acetabular cup wear in total hip arthroplasty. *Orthop Clin North Am* 1988;19:631-636.

29. Shih CH, Lee PC, Chen JH, et al: Measurement of polyethylene wear in cementless total hip arthroplasty. *J Bone Joint Surg Br* 1997;79:361-365.

30. Schmalzried TP, Dorey FJ, McKellop H: The multifactorial nature of polyethylene wear in vivo. *J Bone Joint Surg Am* 1998;80:1234-1243.

31. Sochart DH: Relationship of acetabular wear to osteolysis and loosening in total hip arthroplasty. *Clin Orthop* 1999;363:135-150.

32. Yamaguchi M, Hashimoto Y, Akisue T, Bauer TW: Polyethylene wear vector in vivo: A three-dimensional analysis using retrieved acetabular components and radiographs. *J Orthop Res* 1999;17:695-702.

33. Wagner M, Wagner H: Preliminary results of uncemented metal on metal stemmed and resurfacing hip replacement arthroplasty. *Clin Orthop* 1996;329(suppl):78-88.

34. Schmalzried TP, Fowble VA, Ure KJ, Amstutz HC: Metal on metal surface replacement of the hip: Technique, fixation, and early results. *Clin Orthop* 1996;329(suppl):106-114.

35. McMinn D, Treacy R, Lin K, Pynsent P: Metal on metal surface replacement of the hip: Experience of the McMinn prosthesis. *Clin Orthop* 1996;329(suppl):89-98.

36. Rieker C, Windler M, Wyss U (eds): *META-SUL: A Metal-On-Metal Bearing*. Bern, Switzerland, Hans Huber, 1999.

37. Weber BG: Experience with the Metasul total hip bearing system. *Clin Orthop* 1996;329(suppl):69-77.

38. Dorr LD, Hilton KR, Wan Z, Markovich GD, Bloebaum R: Modern metal on metal articulation for total hip replacements. *Clin Orthop* 1996;333:108-117.

39. Streicher RM, Semlitsch M, Schon R, Weber H, Rieker C: Metal-on-metal articulation for artificial hip joints: Laboratory study and clinical results. *Proc Inst Mech Eng [H]* 1996;210:223-232.

40. Medley JB, Chan FW, Krygier JJ, Bobyn JD: Comparison of alloys and designs in a hip simulator study of metal on metal implants. *Clin Orthop* 1996;329(suppl):148-159.

41. Chan FW, Bobyn JD, Medley JB, Krygier JJ, Tanzer M: Wear and lubrication of metal-on-metal hip implants. *Clin Orthop* 1999;369:10-24.

42. Rieker C, Weber H, Schon R, Windler M, Wyss U: Development of the METASUL articulation, in Rieker C, Windler M, Wyss U (eds): *METASUL: A Metal-On-Metal Bearing*. Bern, Switzerland, Hans Huber, 1999, pp 15-21.

43. Rieker C, Kottig P, Schon R, Windler M, Wyss U: Clinical tribological performance of 144 metal-on-metal hip articulations, in Rieker C, Windler M, Wyss U (eds): *METASUL: A Metal-On-Metal Bearing*. Bern, Switzerland, Hans Huber, 1999, pp 83-91.

44. Campbell P, McKellop H, Alim R, et al: Metal-on-metal hip replacements: Wear performance and cellular response to wear particles, in Disegi JA, Kennedy RL, Pilliar R (eds): *Cobalt-base Alloys for Biomedical Applications*. West Conshohocken, PA, ASTM, 1999, pp 193-209.

45. Schmalzried TP, Szuszczewicz ES, Northfield MR, et al: Quantitative assessment of walking activity after total hip or knee replacement. *J Bone Joint Surg Am* 1998;80:54-59.

46. Park S-H, McKellop H, Lu B, Chan F, Chiesa R: Wear morphology of metal-metal implants: Hip simulator tests compared with clinical retrievals, in Jacobs JJ, Craig TL (eds): *Alternative Bearing Surfaces in Total Joint Replacement*. West Conshohocken, PA, ASTM, 1998, pp 129-143.

47. Dorr LD, Wan Z, Longjohn DB, Dubois B, Murken R: Total hip arthroplasty with use of the Metasul metal-on-metal articulation: Four to seven-year results. *J Bone Joint Surg Am* 2000;82:789-798.

48. Walker PS (ed): Friction and wear of artificial joints, in *Human Joints and Their Artificial Replacements*. Springfield, IL, Charles C Thomas, 1977, pp 368-442.

49. Boutin P, Christel P, Dorlot JM, et al: The use of dense alumina-alumina ceramic combination in total hip replacement. *J Biomed Mater Res* 1988;22:1203-1232.

50. Mittelmeier H, Heisel J: Sixteen-years' experience with ceramic hip prostheses. *Clin Orthop* 1992;282:64-72.

51. Nizard RS, Sedel L, Christel P, Meunier A, Soudry M, Witvoet J: Ten-year survivorship of cemented ceramic-ceramic total hip prosthesis. *Clin Orthop* 1992;282:53-63.

52. Clarke IC: Role of ceramic implants: Design and clinical success with total hip prosthetic ceramic-to-ceramic bearings. *Clin Orthop* 1992;282:19-30.

53. Clarke IC, Willmann G: Structural ceramics in orthopedics, in Cameron HU (ed): *Bone Implant Interface*. St. Louis, MO, Mosby Year Book, 1994, pp 203-252.

54. Garcia-Cimbrelo E, Martinez-Sayanes JM, Minuesa A, Munuera L: Mittelmeier ceramic-ceramic prosthesis after 10 years. *J Arthroplasty* 1996;11:773-781.

55. Meunier A, Nizard R, Bizot P, Sedel L: Clinical results of alumina-on-alumina couple in total hip replacement, in Jacobs JJ, Craig TL (eds): *Alternative Bearing Surfaces in Total Joint Replacement*. West Conshohocken, PA, ASTM, 1998, pp 213-234.

56. Mahoney OM, Dimon JH III: Unsatisfactory results with a ceramic total hip prosthesis. *J Bone Joint Surg Am* 1990;72:663-671.

57. Walter A: On the material and the tribology of alumina-alumina couplings for hip joint prostheses. *Clin Orthop* 1992;282:31-46.

58. Richter HG, Willmann G, Weick K: Improving the reliability of the ceramic-on-ceramic wear couple in THR, in Jacobs JJ, Craig TL (eds): *Alternative Bearing Surfaces in Total Joint Replacement*. West Conshohocken, PA, ASTM, 1998, pp 173-185.

59. Ueno M, Amino H, Okimatu H, Oonishi H: Wear, friction, and mechanical investigation and development of alumina-to-alumina combination total hip joint in Imura S, Wada M, Omori H (eds): *Joint Arthroplasty*. Tokyo, Japan, Springer, 1999, pp 119-131.

60. Willmann G: Ceramics for total hip replacement: What a surgeon should know. *Orthopedics* 1998;21:173-177.

61. Willmann G, Brodbeck A, Effenberger H, et al: Investigation of 87 retrieved ceramic femoral heads, in Puhl W (ed): *Bioceramics in Orthopaedics: New Applications*. Stuttgart, Germany, Ferdinand Enke Verlag, 1998, pp 13-18.

62. Taylor SK: In-vitro wear performance of a contemporary alumina:alumina bearing couple under

anatomically-relevant hip joint simulation, in Sedel S, Willmann G (eds): *Reliability and Long-term Results of Ceramics in Orthopaedics*. Stuttgart, Germany, Georg Thieme Verlag, 1999, pp 85-90.

63. Fisher J, Ingham E, Stone MH, et al: Wear and debris generation in artificial hip joints, in Sedel L, Willmann G (eds): *Reliability and Long-term Results of Ceramics in Orthopaedics*. Stuttgart, Germany, Georg Thieme Verlag, 1999, pp 78-81.

64. Oonishi H, Nishida M, Kawanabe K, et al: In-vitro wear of Al2O3/Al2O3 implant combination with over 10 million cycles duration. *Trans Orthop Res Soc* 1999;24:50.

65. Winter M, Griss P, Scheller G, Moser T: Ten- to 14-year results of a ceramic hip prosthesis. *Clin Orthop* 1992;282:73-80.

66. Nevelos JE, Fisher J, Ingham E, Doyle C, Nevelos AB: Examination of alumina ceramic components from Mittelmeier total hip arthroplasties. *Trans Orthop Res Soc* 1998;23:219.

67. Bergman NR, Young DA: The rationale, short-term outcome and early complications of a ceramic couple in total hip arthroplasty, in Sedel L, Willmann G (eds): *Reliability and Long-term Results of Ceramics in Orthopaedics*. Stuttgart, Germany, Georg Thieme Verlag, 1999, pp 52-56.

68. Yoon TR, Rowe SM, Jung ST, Seon KJ, Maloney WJ: Osteolysis in association with a total hip arthroplasty with ceramic bearing surfaces. *J Bone Joint Surg Am* 1998;80:1459-1468.

69. Boehler M, Knahr K, Plenk H Jr, Walter A, Salzer M, Schreiber V: Long-term results of uncemented alumina acetabular implants. *J Bone Joint Surg Br* 1994;76:53-59.

70. Fuchs GA: 2-4 year clinical results with a ceramic-on-ceramic articulation in a new modular THR-system, in Willmann G, Zweymuller K (eds): *Bioceramics in Hip Joint Replacement: Proceedings 5th International CeramTec Symposium*, Stuttgart. Germany, Georg Thieme, 2000, pp 39-46.

71. Allain J, Goutallier D, Voisin MC, Lemouel S: Failure of a stainless-steel femoral head of a revision total hip arthroplasty performed after a fracture of a ceramic femoral head: A case report. *J Bone Joint Surg Am* 1998;80:1355-1360.

72. Sedel L: Revision strategy for ceramic implant failures, in Sedel L, Willmann G (eds): *Reliability and Long-Term Results of Ceramics in Orthopaedics*. Stuttgart, Germany, Georg Thieme Verlag, 1999, pp 75-76.

73. Kempf I, Semlitsch M: Massive wear of a steel ball head by ceramic fragments in the polyethylene acetabular cup after revision of a total hip prosthesis with fractured ceramic ball. *Arch Orthop Trauma Surg* 1990;109:284-287.

74. Frohling M, Zichner L, Koch R: Revisionsstrategie bei der verwendung von keramikköpfen, in Sedel L, Willmann G (eds): *Reliability and Long-term Results of Ceramics in Orthopaedics*. Stuttgart, Germany, Georg Thieme Verlag, 1999, pp 72-74.

75. Fritsch EW, Gleitz M: Ceramic femoral head fractures in total hip arthroplasty. *Clin Orthop* 1996;328:129-136.

76. Piconi C, Labanti M, Magnani G, Caporale M, Maccauro G, Magliocchetti G: Analysis of a failed alumina THR ball head. *Biomaterials* 1999;20:1637-1646.

77. Christel P, Meunier A, Heller M, Torre JP, Peille CN: Mechanical properties and short-term in-vivo evaluation of yttrium-oxide-partially-stabilized zirconia. *J Biomed Mater Res* 1989;23:45-61.

78. Drouin JM, Cales B, Chevalier J, Fantozzi G: Fatigue behavior of zirconia hip joint heads: Experimental results and finite element analysis. *J Biomed Mater Res* 1997;34:149-155.

79. Cales B, Stefani Y: Yttria-stabilized zirconia for improved orthopaedic prostheses, in Wise DL, Trantolo DJ, Yaszemski MJ, Gresser JD, Schwartz ER (eds): *Encyclopedic Handbook of Biomaterials and Bioengineering Part B: Applications.* New York, NY, Marcel Dekker, 1995, pp 415-452.

80. Piconi C, Maccauro G: Zirconia as a ceramic biomaterial. *Biomaterials* 1999;20:1-25.

81. Birkby I, Harrison P, Stevens R: The effect of surface transformation on the wear behavior of zirconia TZP ceramics. *J European Ceramics Soc* 1989;5:37-45.

82. Piconi C, Burger W, Richter HG, et al: Y-TZP ceramics for artificial joint replacements. *Biomaterials* 1998;19:1489-1494.

83. Allain J, Le Mouel S, Goutallier D, Voison MC: Poor eight-year survival of cemented zirconia-polyethylene total hip replacements. *J Bone Joint Surg Br* 1999;81:835-842.

84. Cales B, Stefani Y, Lilley E: Long-term in vivo and in vitro aging of a zirconia ceramic used in orthopaedy. *J Biomed Mater Res* 1994;28:619-624.

85. Fruh HJ, Willmann G, Pfaff HG: Wear characteristics of ceramic-on-ceramic for hip endoprostheses. *Biomaterials* 1997;18:873-876.

86. Willmann G, Fruh HJ, Pfaff HG: Wear characteristics of sliding pairs of zirconia (Y-TZP) for hip endoprostheses. *Biomaterials* 1996;17:2157-2162.

87. Cales B, Chevalier J: Wear behavior of ceramic pairs compared on different testing configurations. in Jacobs JJ, Craig TL (eds): *Alternative Bearing Surfaces in Total Joint Replacement.* West Conshohocken, PA, ASTM, 1998, pp 186-196.

88. Affatato S, Testoni M, Cacciari GL, Toni A: Mixed-oxides prosthetic ceramic ball heads: Part 2. Effect of the ZrO2 fraction on the wear of ceramic on ceramic joints. *Biomaterials* 1999;20:1925-1929.

89. Affatato S, Testoni M, Cacciari GL, Toni A: Mixed oxides prosthetic ceramic ball heads: Part 1. Effect of the ZrO2 fraction on the wear of ceramic on polyethylene joints. *Biomaterials* 1999;20:971-975.

90. Kaddick C, Pfaff HG: Wear study in the alumina-zirconia system, in Sedel L, Willmann G (eds): *Reliability and Long-Term Results of Ceramics in Orthopaedics.* Stuttgart, Germany, Georg Thieme Verlag, 1999, pp 96-101.

91. McKellop H, Clarke I, Markolf K, Amstutz H: Friction and wear properties of polymer, metal, and ceramic prosthetic joint materials evaluated

92. Lancaster JG, Dowson D, Isaac GH, Fisher J: The wear of ultra-high molecular weight polyethylene sliding on metallic and ceramic counterfaces representative of current femoral surfaces in joint replacement. *Proc Inst Mech Eng [H]* 1997;211:17-24.

93. Bankston AB, Faris PM, Keating EM, Ritter MA: Polyethylene wear in total hip arthroplasty in patient-matched groups: A comparison of stainless steel, cobalt chrome, and titanium-bearing surfaces. *Arthroplasty* 1993;8:315-322.

94. Wroblewski BM: Wear of the high-density polyethylene socket in total hip arthroplasty and its role in endosteal cavitation. *Proc Inst Mech Eng [H]* 1997;211:109-118.

95. Furman BD, Lee CL, Block A, Lefebvre FK, Li S: A comparison of directly molded and machined retrieved acetabular cups of a single design. *Trans Orthop Res Soc* 1998;23:50.

96. Devane PA, Horne JG: Assessment of polyethylene wear in total hip replacement. *Clin Orthop* 1999;369:59-72.

97. McKellop HA, Sarmiento A, Schwinn CP, Ebramzadeh E: In vivo wear of titanium-alloy hip prostheses. *J Bone Joint Surg Am* 1990;72:512-517.

98. McKellop H, Rostlund T, Ebramzadeh E, Sarmiento A: Wear of titanium alloy in laboratory tests and in retrieved human joint replacements, in Brown SA, Lemons JE (eds): *Medical Applications of Titanium and Its Alloys: The Material and Biological Issues.* West Conshohocken, PA, ASTM, 1996, pp 266-293.

99. Agins HJ, Alcock NW, Bansal M, et al: Metallic wear in failed titanium-alloy total hip replacements: A histological and quantitative analysis. *J Bone Joint Surg Am* 1988;70:347-356.

100. Lombardi AV Jr, Mallory TH, Vaughn BK, Drouillard P: Aseptic loosening in total hip arthroplasty secondary to osteolysis induced by wear debris from titanium-alloy modular femoral heads. *J Bone Joint Surg Am* 1989;71:1337-1342.

101. McKellop HA, Rostlund TV: The wear behavior of ion-implanted Ti-6A1-4V against UHMW polyethylene. *J Biomed Mater Res* 1990;24:1413-1425.

102. Semlitsch M, Willert HG: Clinical wear behaviour of ultra-high molecular weight polyethylene cups paired with metal and ceramic ball heads in comparison to metal-on-metal pairings of hip joint replacements. *Proc Inst Mech Eng [H]* 1997;211:73-88.

103. Davidson JA, Poggie RA, Mishra AK: Abrasive wear of ceramic, metal, and UHMWPE bearing surfaces from third-body bone, PMMA bone cement, and titanium debris. *Biomed Mater Eng* 1994;4:213-229.

104. Mishra AK, Davidson JA, Poggie RA, Kovacs P, FitzGerald TJ: Mechanical and tribological properties and biocompatibility of diffusion hardened T-13Nb-13Zr: A new titanium alloy

for surgical implants, in Brown SA, Lemons JE (eds): *Medical Applications of Titanium and Its Alloys: The Material and Biological Issue.* West Conshohocken, PA, ASTM, 1996, pp 96-112.

105. Sauer WL, Anthony ME: Predicting the clinical wear performance of orthopaedic bearing surfaces, in Jacobs JJ, Craig TL (eds): *Alternative Bearing Surfaces in Total Joint Replacement.* West Conshohocken, PA, ASTM, 1998, pp 1-29.

106. Willmann G: New generation ceramics, in Willmann G, Zweymüller K (eds): *Bioceramics in Hip Joint Replacement: Proceedings of the 5th International CeramTec Symposium.* Stuttgart, Germany, Georg Thieme, 2000, pp 127-135.

107. Bragdon CR, O'Connor DO, Lowenstein JD, et al: Comparison of volumetric wear using 22mm, 26mm and 32mm femoral heads using a new hip simulator. *Trans Orthop Res Soc* 1998;23:53.

108. McKellop H, Lu B, Benya P:Friction, lubrication and wear of cobalt-chromium, alumina and zirconia hip prostheses compared on a joint simulator. *Trans Orthop Res Soc* 1992;17:402.

109. Li S, Burstein AH: Ultra-high molecular weight polyethylene: The material and its use in total joint implants. *J Bone Joint Surg Am* 1994;76:1080-1090.

110. Lewis G: Polyethylene wear in total hip and knee arthroplasties. *J Biomed Mater Res* 1997;38:55-75.

111. Kurtz SM, Muratoglu OK, Evans M, Edidin AA: Advances in the processing, sterilization, and cross-linking of ultra-high molecular weight polyethylene for total joint arthroplasty. *Biomaterials* 1999;20:1659-1688.

112. Fisher J, Reeves EA, Isaac GH, Saumm KA, Sanford WM: Comparison of the wear of aged and non-aged ultrahigh molecular weight polyethylene sterilized by gamma irradiation and by gas plasma, in *Fifth World Biomaterials Congress: Programme and Transactions.* Toronto, Canada, University of Toronto Press, 1996, p 971.

113. Goldman M, Pruitt L: Comparison of the effects of gamma radiation and low temperature hydrogen peroxide gas plasma sterilization on the molecular structure, fatigue resistance, and wear behavior of UHMWPE. *J Biomed Mater Res* 1998;40:378-384.

114. McNulty DE, Hastings RS, Swope SW, Huston DE:Sterilization methods and artificial aging of UHMWPE resins: The relation between resilience and oxidation. *Trans Orthop Res Soc* 1999;24:821.

115. Sutula LC, Collier JP, Saum KA, et al: Impact of gamma sterilization on clinical performance of polyethylene in the hip. *Clin Orthop* 1995;319:28-40.

116. Furman BD, Reish T, Li S: The effect of implantation on the oxidation of ultra high molecular weight polyethylene, in Merchant RE (ed): *Transactions: Twenty-Third Annual Meeting of the Society for Biomaterials.* Minneapolis, MN, Society for Biomaterials, 1997, p 427.

117. Pienkowski D, Patel A, Lee KY, et al: Solubility changes in shelf-aged ultra-high molecular weight polyethylene acetabular liners. *J Long Term Eff Med Implants* 1999;9:273-288.

118. Wang A, Essner A, Polineni VK, Stark C, Dumbleton JH: Lubrication and wear of ultra-high molecular weight polyethylene in total joint replacements. *Tribology* 1998;31:17-33.

119. McKellop H, Shen FW, Lu B, Campbell P, Salovey R: Development of an extremely wear-resistant ultra high molecular weight polyethylene for total hip replacements. *J Orthop Res* 1999;17:157-167.

120. Muratoglu OK, Bragdon CR, O'Connor DO, et al: Unified wear model for highly cross-linked ultra-high molecular weight polyethylenes (UHMWPE). *Biomaterials* 1999;20:1463-1470.

121. Gillis AM, Schmieg JJ, Bhattacharyya S, Li S:An independent evaluation of the mechanical, chemical and fracture properties of UHMWPE cross-linked by 34 different conditions, in LaBerge M, Agrawal C, Mauli CM (eds): *Transactions: Twenty-Fifth Annual Meeting of the Society for Biomaterials.* Minneapolis, MN, Society of Biomaterial, 1999, p 216.

122. Roe RJ, Grood ES, Shastri R, Gosselin CA, Noyes FR: Effect of radiation sterilization and aging on ultrahigh molecular weight polyethylene. *J Biomed Mater Res* 1981;15:209-230.

123. Eyerer P, Ke YC: Property changes of UHMW polyethylene hip cup endoprostheses during implantation. *J Biomed Mater Res* 1984;18:1137-1151.

124. Premnath V, Harris WH, Jasty M, Merrill EW: Gamma sterilization of UHMWPE articular implants: An analysis of the oxidation problem. Ultra high molecular weight poly ethylene. *Biomaterials* 1996;17:1741-1753.

125. Gillis AM, Furman BD, Li S: Influence of ultra high molecular weight polyethylene resin type and manufacturing method on real time oxidation. *Trans Orthop Res Soc* 1998;23:360.

126. Collier JP, Bargmann LS, Currier BH, Mayor MB, Currier JH, Bargmann BC: An analysis of Hylamer and polyethylene bearings from retrieved acetabular components. *Orthopedics* 1998;21:865-871.

127. Edidin A, Muth J, Spiegelberg S, Schaffner S: Sterilization of UHMWPE in nitrogen prevents oxidative degradation for more than ten years. *Trans Orthop Res Soc* 2000;25:1.

128. Greer KW, Schmidt MB, Hamilton JV: The hip simulator wear of gamma-vacuum, gamma-air, and ethylene oxide sterilized UHMWPE following a severe oxidative challenge. *Trans Orthop Res Soc* 1998;23:52.

129. Streicher RM: Influence of ionizing irradiation in air and nitrogen for sterilization of surgical grade polyethylene for implants. *Radiat Phys Chem* 1988;31:693-698.

130. Bapst JM, Valentine RH, Vasquez R: Wear simulation testing of direct compression molded UHMWPE irradiated in oxygenless packaging, in Merchant RE (ed): *Transactions: Twenty-Third Annual Meeting of the Society for Biomaterials.* Minneapolis, MN, Society for Biomaterials, 1997, p 72.

131. Sun DC, Wang A, Stark C, Dumbleton JH: The concept of stabilization in UHMWPE, in *Fifth World Biomaterials Congress: Programme and Transactions.* Toronto, Canada, University of Toronto Press, 1996, p 195.

132. McKellop H, Shen FW, Lu B, Campbell P, Salovey R: The effect of sterilization method and other modifications on the wear resistance of acetabular cups of ultra-high molecular weight polyethylene: A hip simulator study. *J Bone Joint Surg Am,* in press.

133. Currier BH, Currier JH, Collier JP, Mayor MB: Effect of fabrication method and resin type on performance of tibial bearings. *J Biomed Mater Res* 2000;53:143-51.

134. *"Arcom® Processed Polyethylene. A Technical Report."* Warsaw, IN, Biomet, 1996.

135. Walsh H, Gillis A, Furman B, Li S: Factors that determine the oxidation resistance of molded 1900: Is it the resin or the molding? *Trans Orthop Res Soc* 2000;25:543.

136. Grobbelaar CJ, du Plessis TA, Marais F: The radiation improvement of polyethylene prostheses: A preliminary study. *J Bone Joint Surg Br* 1978;60:370-374.

137. Grobbelaar CJ, Weber FA, Spirakis A, et al: Clinical experience with gamma irradiation-cross-linked polyethylene: A 14 to 20 year follow-up report. *SA Bone Joint & Joint Surg* 1999;9:140-147.

138. Oonishi H, Takayama Y, Tsuji E: Improvement of polyethylene by irradiation in artificial joints. *Radiat Phys Chem* 1992;39:495-504.

139. Oonishi H, Takayama Y, Tsuji E: The low wear of cross-linked polyethylene socket in total hip prostheses, in Wise DL, Trantolo DJ, Altobelli DE, Yaszemski MJ, Gresser JD, Schwartz ER (eds): *Encyclopedic Handbook of Biomaterials and Bioengineering: Part A. Materials.* New York, NY, Marcel Dekker, 1995, pp 1853-1868.

140. Oonishi H, Saito M, Kadoya Y: Wear of high-dose gamma irradiated polyethylene in total joint replacement: Long term radiological evaluation. *Trans Orthop Res Soc* 1998;23:97.

141. Wroblewski BM, Siney PD, Fleming PA: Low-friction arthroplasty of the hip using alumina ceramic and cross-linked polyethylene: A ten-year follow-up report. *J Bone Joint Surg Br* 1999;81:54-55.

142. McKellop H, Shen F-W, DiMaio W, Lancaster JG: Wear of gamma-cross-linked polyethylene acetabular cups against roughened femoral balls. *Clin Orthop* 1999;369:73-82.

143. DiMaio WG, Lilly WB, Moore WC, Saum KA: Low wear, low oxidation radiation cross-linked UHMWPE. *Trans Orthop Res Soc* 1998;23:363.

144. Hastings RS, Huston DE, Reber EW, DiMaio WG: Knee wear testing of a radiation cross-linked and remelted UHMWPE, in LaBerge M, Agrawal C, Mauli CM (eds): *Transactions: Twenty-Fifth Annual Meeting of the Society for Biomaterials.* Minneapolis, MN, Society for Biomaterials, 1999, p 328.

145. Bhateja SK, Duerst RW, Martens JA, Andrews EH: Radiation-induced enhancement of crystallinity in polymers. *J Macromol Sci-Revs Chem Phys* 1995;C35:581-659.

146. Essner A, Polineni VK, Wang A, Stark C, Dumbleton JH: Effect of femoral head surface roughness and cross-linking on the wear of UHMWPE acetabular cups, in Goodman SB (ed): *Transactions: Twenty-Fourth Annual Meeting of the Society for Biomaterials.* Minneapolis, MN, Society of Biomaterials, 1998, p 4.

147. Laurent MP, Yao JQ, Gilbertson LN, Swarts DF, Crowninshield RD: Wear of highly cross-linked UHMWPE acetabular liners under adverse conditions, in *Trans Sixth World Biomaterials Congress.* 2000, p 874.

148. Endo MM, Barbour PSM, Barton DC, et al: Comparative wear and debris generation of cross-linked and non-cross-linked ultrahigh molecular weight polyethylene under three different femoral counterface conditions, in *Trans Sixth World Biomaterials Congress.* 2000, p 836.

149. Greenwald AS, Ries MD, DuncanCP, Jacobs JJ, Stulberg BN: Abstract: New polys for old: Contribution or caveat? *67th Annual Meeting Proceedings.* Rosemont, IL, American Academy of Orthopaedic Surgeons, 2000, p 278.

150. Laurent MP, Yao JQ, Bhambri SK, et al: High cycle wear of highly cross-linked UHMWPE acetabular liners evaluated in a hip simulator. *Trans Orthop Res Soc* 2000;25:567.

151. Muratoglu OK, Bragdon CR, O'Connor DO, et al: The effect of temperature on radiation cross-linking of UHMWPE for use in total hip arthroplasty. *Trans Orthop Res Soc* 2000;25:547.

152. Muratoglu OK, Harris WH, Delaney J, et al: The development of an in vitro hip simulator model for fatigue failure: Application to conventional and highly cross-linked UHMWPE. *Trans Orthop Res Soc* 2000;25:548.

153. Manley MT, Capello WN, D'Antonio JA, Taylor SK, Wang A: Abstract: Reduction in wear in total hip replacement: Highly crosslinked polyethylene acetabular liners versus ceramic/ceramic bearings. *67th Annual Meeting Proceedings.* Rosemont, IL, American Academy of Orthopaedic Surgeons. 2000, p 275.

154. Muratoglu OK, Bragdon CR, O'Connor DO, et al: The comparison of the wear behavior of four different types of cross-linked acetabular components. *Trans Orthop Res Soc* 2000;25:566.

155. Streicher RM: Ionizing irradiation for sterilization and modification of high molecular weight polyethylenes. *Plastics and Rubber Processing and Applications* 1988;10:221-229.

156. Walsh HA, Furman BD, Naab S, Li S: Role of oxidation in the clinical fracture of acetabular cups. *Trans Orthop Res Soc* 1999;24:845.

157. McKellop HA: Wear assessment, in Callaghan JJ, Rosenberg AG, Rubash HE (eds): *The Adult Hip.* Philadelphia, PA, Lippincott-Raven, 1998, pp 231-246.

158. Xenos JS, Hopkinson WJ, Callaghan JJ, Heekin RD, Savory CG: Osteolysis around an uncemented cobalt chrome total hip arthroplasty. *Clin Orthop* 1995;317:29-36.

159. Devane PA, Bourne RB, Rorabeck CH, MacDonald S, Robinson EJ: Measurement of polyethylene wear in metal-backed acetabular cups II: Clinical application. *Clin Orthop* 1995;319:317-326.

160. Nashed RS, Becker DA, Gustilo RB: Are cementless acetabular components the cause of excess wear and osteolysis in total hip arthroplasty? *Clin Orthop* 1995;317:19-28.

161. Wan Z, Dorr LD: Natural history of femoral focal osteolysis with proximal ingrowth smooth stem implant. *J Arthroplasty* 1996;11:718-725.

Total Hip Arthroplasty in the Young Patient

Peter F. Sharkey, MD

Matthew S. Austin, MD

William Hozack, MD

Abstract

Total hip arthroplasty was originally indicated for older, sedentary patients because of concerns that catastrophic wear and failure would occur in younger and more active patients. With advances in implant design, tribology, and surgical technique, total hip arthroplasty has now become a viable option for younger patients seeking excellent pain relief and improvement in function. Long-term studies are needed to evaluate the outcome of hip arthroplasty in younger patients using the modern generation of implants and bearing surfaces.

Total hip arthroplasty was originally indicated for older, sedentary patients with intractable hip pain. Younger (age < 50 years), more active patients were offered arthrodesis as a treatment option because of the fear that implants in this patient population would experience catastrophic wear. Arthrodesis was successful in achieving pain relief; however, function was limited. In addition, progressive back and knee complications commonly occurred in patients who underwent the fusion procedure. The common diagnoses leading to end-stage arthritis in patients younger than 50 years include inflammatory arthritides, post-traumatic arthritis, septic arthritis, the sequelae of childhood diseases (Legg-Calvé-Perthes disease, slipped capital femoral epiphysis, and developmental hip dysplasia), and osteonecrosis.

Patients Younger Than 50 Years

The results of total hip arthroplasty in any age group must be carefully evaluated. Assumptions should not be made regarding outcomes of any procedure without evaluating the multiplicity of factors associated with a good or poor clinical outcome. The factors that are important to evaluate when considering the success of total hip arthroplasty include the length of follow-up, the definition of failure (revision, poor functional scores, and radiographic loosening), the method of obtaining fixation (cemented, cementless, or hybrid), the type of cup or stem, the underlying diagnosis, and the bearing surface used.

Cemented Total Hip Arthroplasty

Kerboull and associates[1] evaluated the results of 287 primary cemented total hip arthroplasties (average patient age, 40.1 years). At a mean follow-up of 14.5 years, the authors found a mean wear rate of 0.12 mm/yr; 25 hips (8.7%) required revision. Sixty-eight percent of the revisions were undertaken to treat aseptic loosening. The authors also evaluated a subset of patients at greater than 20-year follow-up. Using revision as an end point, these patients demonstrated a survival rate of 85.4%. Keener and associates[2] looked at the 25-year results of 42 patients. The overall survivorship was 69%. Aseptic loosening accounted for 79% of the 29 revisions. Loosening on the acetabular side was far more prevalent than loosening on the femoral side (18 of 23 patients).

Cementless Total Hip Arthroplasty

McAuley and associates[3] reviewed the long-term results of patients who were younger than 50 years at the time of the index procedure. The patient cohort consisted of 561 hips for which a press-fit acetabular component and an extensively porous-coated cobalt-chromium stem were used. The survivorship was 89% at 10-year and 60% at 15-year follow-up. An evaluation of a subset of patients who were younger than 40 years at the time of the initial implant showed that these patients trended toward slightly inferior outcomes, with 85% and 54% survival rates reported at 10- and 15-year follow-up, respectively. It is important to note that these rates were for revision carried out for any reason. A large number of revisions were done for polyethylene exchange; when these revisions are eliminated, the survivorship at 10- and 15-year follow-up improved to 95% and 83%, respectively. The mean polyethylene wear rate was 0.16 mm/yr. However, the wear rate in patients with revised hips was 0.29 mm/yr and 0.14 mm/yr in those with unrevised hips. This difference was statistically significant. Kim and associates[4] looked at the results of cementless total hip arthroplasty using a proximally coated femoral prosthesis. They followed 118 hips for a minimum of 8 years. The mean age of the patients was 46.8 years, and the most common diagnosis was osteonecrosis. In all patients, 22-mm heads with gamma-irradiated and ram-extruded polyethylene were used. Despite this poor combination, the wear rate was 0.12 mm/yr. Only one hip was revised to treat recurrent dislocation. No other revisions were reported. Capello and associates[5] reported a minimum 10-year follow-up of a proximally hydroxyapatite-coated femoral prosthesis. The rate of revision for aseptic loosening was 0.9%. All patients were younger than 50 years at the time of the primary procedure. Unfortunately, the stem was paired with a poor acetabular component that required a large number of acetabular

revisions. Crowther and Lachiewicz[6] studied 56 hips with a porous-coated acetabular component in patients younger than 50 years. They reported no revisions for aseptic loosening. Sporer and associates[7] reported no failures in 45 cementless cups in patients younger than 50 years; however, this component was paired with a poor cemented femoral component with a high failure rate. Cementless fixation is discussed in more detail in chapter 19.

Patients Younger Than 21 Years

Total hip replacement in patients younger than 21 years can be challenging because of poor bone quality secondary to systemic disease or medications. In addition, osseous deformities can complicate the insertion of the components. Furthermore, these patients tend to have had prior surgery on the hip that may have distorted the anatomy. Torchia and associates[8] reported 65 previous surgeries on 33 hips in a series of patients younger than 21 years. The diagnoses leading to hip replacement in patient population included juvenile rheumatoid arthritis, congenital hip dysplasia, slipped capital femoral epiphysis, trauma, tumor, spondyloepiphyseal dysplasia, sequelae of septic arthritis, Legg-Calvé-Perthes disease, osteonecrosis, ankylosing spondylitis, systemic lupus erythematosus, neurofibromatosis, and idiopathic protrusio acetabuli. The heterogenous etiology of hip disease makes interpreting the results of total hip arthroplasty in this population difficult. The authors used a variety of components, ranging from cemented Charnley prostheses to proximal femoral replacements. All components were inserted with cement. Forty-six percent of the total

hip arthroplasties in this group failed, 27% experienced failure by 10-year follow-up, and 45% experienced failure by 15-year follow-up. Seventy-six percent of failures occurred on the acetabular side. The patients with a higher probability of failure included those with a history of more than one previous procedure on the hip, unilateral surgery, posttraumatic osteoarthritis, absence of concomitant illnesses that limited use of the hip, moderate to high-demand manual labor, and weight more than 60 kg.

Bessette and associates[9] assessed a series of patients younger than 21 years at the time of initial total hip arthroplasty. A total of 15 hips were followed for an average of 13.6 years. Sixty-seven percent of the arthroplasties were functioning well at the conclusion of the study. All revisions were performed to treat aseptic loosening, with most of the revisions performed to treat loose acetabuli (four of five). The cup revisions were evenly divided between cemented and cementless components, and the single femoral revision was performed to treat aseptic loosening of a cemented femoral implant.

Juvenile Rheumatoid Arthritis and Osteonecrosis

Some studies have assessed a specific subset of young patients who have undergone hip replacement. Chmell and associates[10] reviewed 28 arthroplasties performed in patients with juvenile rheumatoid arthritis who were younger than 30 years. All components were inserted with cement. First-generation cementing technique was used in 47% of the procedures. Using revision as an end point, the 15-year survival rate (minimum 10-year follow-up) was 70% for the acetabular component and 85% for the femoral component.

Kim and associates[11] reviewed patients with osteonecrosis (average age, 47 years). All patients received a cementless acetabular component. The mean patient age at the time of arthroplasty was 47.3 years (age range, 26 to 58 years). Two thirds of the patients received a metaphyseal fitting cementless stem and one third received a cemented implant. No patients underwent revision to treat aseptic loosening of either the acetabular or femoral component.

Bearing Surface

Wear is a significant problem for young patients. The incidence of aseptic loosening is higher in this patient population presumably because of higher levels of activity. As a consequence, alternative bearing surfaces have been developed to decrease the amount of biologically active particle generation that can lead to osteolysis and aseptic loosening. These alternative surfaces include highly cross-linked polyethylene, metal-on-metal articulations, and ceramic-on-ceramic bearing surfaces (for additional information see chapter 18).

Highly Cross-Linked Polyethylene

Gamma radiation and electron beam radiation are used in conjunction with thermal treatment to induce cross-linking of polyethylene particles and reduce free radicals that oxidize and weaken the polyethylene. The highly cross-linked polyethylene is resistant to wear, particularly when the dose of radiation is increased from 0 to 5 Mrads.[12,13] However, too much radiation renders the material vulnerable to fatigue fracture.

Metal-on-Metal Articulations

Metal-on-metal articulations were first introduced with the McKee-

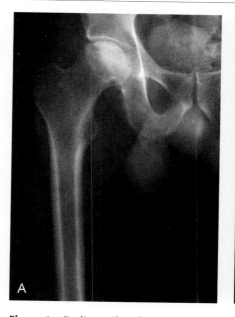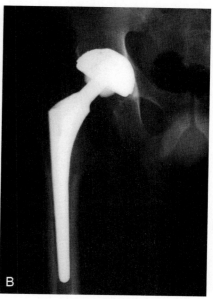

Figure 1 Radiographs of a 44-year-old man with stage IV osteonecrosis who underwent total hip arthroplasty using cementless components and ceramic-on-ceramic bearings. Preoperative radiograph **(A)** and postoperative radiograph **(B)** taken 64 months after surgery. Note that the inclination of the acetabular component is less than 45°.

Farrar hip replacement. The wear rate of these first-generation hips was extremely low, on the order of a few microns per year.[11] Unfortunately, the components were prone to seize and then consequently loosened. Currently, better manufacturing tolerances have taken advantage of the low wear rate of metal-on-metal articulations, while avoiding the problem of friction at the equator of the articulation. Metal-on-metal prostheses also offer the potential advantage of using large femoral heads to decrease dislocation rates without increasing wear. The main disadvantage of metal-on-metal articulations is the unknown consequences of metal debris generation. Serum, urine, and lymphatic accumulations of metal debris have been reported.[12,14-17]

Ceramic-on-Ceramic Bearings

Ceramic-on-ceramic bearings have been used since 1970.[12,18] Alumina-ceramic bearings have shown wear rates comparable to those of metal-on-metal articulations.[12] Ceramics are inert and do not cause concern for carcinogenesis as do metal bearings. The potential disadvantage of ceramic stems is associated with their brittle nature. Early studies showed failure rates as high as 13%.[12] However, stricter manufacturing tolerances have reduced the fracture rate to roughly 4 per 100,000 patients. Care must be taken when implanting these bearings to avoid chipping the liner. In addition, the acetabular shell must be inserted at less than 45° of abduction to better distribute the forces and to avoid striped wear.[12,19] (Figure 1). It is particularly important to note that substantial damage to the trunion may occur with use of a ceramic ball. The trunion should be carefully inspected at the time of revision, and consideration should be given to revising the entire stem if the Morse taper is significantly damaged. Hamadouche and associates[20] reported on a minimum 18.5-year follow-up of alumina-on-alumina total hip arthroplasty. One hundred eighteen consecutive total hip arthroplasties were performed with the use of a 32-mm head. A wear rate of 0.025 mm/yr was reported. No fractures of the alumina were noted. Osteolytic lesions were present in only 3 of 25 patients who required revision. Eighteen of the 25 revisions involved debonding of a cemented socket.

Summary
Total hip arthroplasty in young patients is a viable option for those with degenerative joint disease. The ultimate outcome of these patients is difficult to extrapolate from the available data. The diagnosis leading to total hip replacement is as varied as is the type of arthroplasty selected. Some young patients have undergone multiple previous procedures, some have deformities, some have been previously treated for sepsis, and some have idiopathic degenerative joint disease. Equally confounding is the fact that primary total hip arthroplasty in some series may involve a cementless tapered component, cemented components using first-generation or third-generation techniques, proximal femoral replacement for tumor, or custom prostheses to treat deformity. Similarly, the bearing surfaces may have been alumina-on-alumina, metal-on-metal, highly cross-linked polyethylene, nominally radiated polyethylene, or gamma-radiated polyethylene. Clearly, these different bearing surfaces cannot be judged on an equal playing field.

Thus, longer-term studies using accepted contemporary techniques are needed. Total hip arthroplasty is a viable option for young patients with disabling end-stage hip arthritis. Furthermore, long-term follow-up studies will be needed to assess the results of revision surgery in this population.

References

1. Kerboull L, Hamadouche M, Courpied JP, et al: Long-term results of Charnley-Kerboull hip arthroplasty in patients younger than 50 years. *Clin Orthop Relat Res* 2004;418:112-118.

2. Keener JD, Callaghan JJ, Goetz DD, et al: Twenty-five-year results after Charnley total hip arthroplasty in patients less than fifty years old: A concise follow-up of a previous report. *J Bone Joint Surg Am* 2003;85-A:1066-1072.

3. McAuley JP, Szuszczewicz ES, Young A, et al: Total hip arthroplasty in patients 50 years and younger. *Clin Orthop Relat Res* 2004;418:119-125.

4. Kim YH, Oh SH, Kim JS: Primary total hip arthroplasty with a second-generation cementless total hip prosthesis in patients younger than fifty years of age. *J Bone Joint Surg Am* 2003;85-A:109-114.

5. Capello WN, D'Antonio JA, Feinberg JR, et al: Ten-year results with hydroxyapatite-coated total hip femoral components in patients less than fifty years old: A concise follow-up of a previous report. *J Bone Joint Surg Am* 2003;85-A:885-889.

6. Crowther JD, Lachiewicz PF: Survival and polyethylene wear of porous-coated acetabular components in patients less than fifty years old: Results at nine to fourteen years. *J Bone Joint Surg Am* 2002;84-A:729-735.

7. Sporer SM, Callaghan JJ, Olejniczak JP, et al: Hybrid total hip arthroplasty in patients under the age of fifty: A five- to ten-year follow-up. *J Arthroplasty* 1998;13:485-491.

8. Torchia ME, Klassen RA, Bianco AJ: Total hip arthroplasty with cement in patients less than twenty years old: Long-term results. *J Bone Joint Surg Am* 1996;78:995-1003.

9. Bessette BJ, Fassier F, Tanzer M, Brooks CE: Total hip arthroplasty in patients younger than 21 years: A minimum 10-year follow-up. *Can J Surg* 2003;46:257-262.

10. Chmell MJ, Scott RD, Thomas WH: Total hip arthroplasty with cement for juvenile rheumatoid arthritis: Results at a minimum ten years in patients less than thirty years old. *J Bone Joint Surg Am* 1997;79:44-52.

11. Kim YH, Oh SH, Kim JS: Contemporary total hip arthroplasty with and without cement in patients with osteonecrosis of the femoral head. *J Bone Joint Surg Am* 2003;85-A:675-681.

12. Campbell P, Shen F-W, McKellop H: Biologic and tribiologic considerations of alternative bearing surfaces. *Clin Orthop Relat Res* 2004;418:98-111.

13. McKellop HA: Bearing surfaces in THRs: State of the art and future developments. *Instr Course Lect* 2001;50:165-179.

14. Jacobs JJ, Skipor AK, Doorn PF, et al: Cobalt and chromium concentrations in patients with metal on metal total hip replacements. *Clin Orthop Relat Res* 1996;329(suppl):S256-S263.

15. MacDonald SJ, McCalden RW, Chess DG, et al: Metal-on-metal versus polyethylene in hip arthroplasty: A randomized clinical trial. *Clin Orthop Relat Res* 2003;406:282-296.

16. Schaffer AW, Pilger A, Engelhart C, et al: Increased blood cobalt and chromium after total hip replacement. *J Toxicol Clin Toxicol* 1999;37:839-844.

17. Sunderman FW Jr, Hopfer SM, Switt T, et al: Cobalt, chromium and nickel concentrations in body fluids of patients with porous-coated knee or hip prostheses. *J Orthop Res* 1989;7:307-315.

18. Sedel L: Evolution of alumina-on-alumina implants: A review. *Clin Orthop Relat Res* 2000;379:48-54.

19. Garino JP: Modern ceramic-on-ceramic total hip systems in the United States: Early results. *Clin Orthop Relat Res* 2000;379:41-47.

20. Hamadouche M, Boutin P, Daussange J, et al: Alumina-on-alumina total hip arthroplasty: A minimum 18.5-year follow-up study. *J Bone Joint Surg Am* 2002;84-A:69-77.

Bearing Surface Options for Total Hip Replacement in Young Patients

Christian Heisel, MD
Mauricio Silva, MD
Thomas P. Schmalzried, MD

Abstract

Encouraging results and new implant developments have allowed total hip replacement to be performed in increasingly younger and more active patients. In young patients, however, outcomes are not comparable to those seen in older patients. The inflammatory reaction to polyethylene wear particles is one of the main causes of aseptic loosening and subsequent revision surgery and can limit the longevity of an arthroplasty in young and active patients.

The wear resistance of polyethylene has been improved by cross-linking; however, greater degrees of cross-linking are associated with progressive decreases in other material properties, which theoretically increase the risk of component failure from very high or localized stresses. Ceramic femoral heads have been associated with lower in vivo polyethylene wear rates, which have been variable and up to 50% lower than with metallic heads. Metal-on-metal bearings have been reintroduced with improved materials, design, and manufacturing, although theoretical concerns remain regarding long-term exposure to metal particles and ions. Improved ceramic-on-ceramic bearings also are available and have the lowest wear rates. They offer a very small risk of in vivo fracture; however, they are the most expensive bearing option and wear rate is more sensitive to implant position. Long-term clinical studies are needed to show a reduction in revision surgery associated with the use of this current generation of bearings. The use of any of these bearings has specific benefits and risks that should be considered on a patient-by-patient basis.

Total hip arthroplasty is one of the most successful and cost-effective surgical interventions in medicine[1] and is the most effective treatment of osteoarthritis of the hip joint. Long-term studies of selected patient cohorts[2-4] and the Scandinavian hip registries[5,6] have demonstrated high survivorship rates after more than 20 years. On the basis of this success, total hip replacement is being performed on increasingly younger and more active patients. However, there are at least two problems that a young or active patient faces with regard to the prosthetic joint. First, the use of the implant is more intense in proportion to the patient's physical activities.[7] Second, the patient's life expectancy is longer and the potential total number of loading cycles is increased proportionally.

Patient-related factors contribute to implant wear regardless of the type of bearing.[8] Higher patient activity levels result in higher wear rates.[8] Follow-up studies of young patients have demonstrated a relationship between the amount of wear and the age of the patient,[9,10] the revision rate,[11] osteolysis,[9,12,13] and aseptic loosening.[12] The overall rate of survival of total hip arthroplasty implants in young patients is reduced compared with that in average patient groups.[3] The survival rate of artificial joints in patients younger than 50 years of age is approximately 80% after 10 years or more, regardless of the fixation technique and bearing combination.[11,12,14-18] To our knowledge, only one recent study, by Kim and associates,[10] demonstrated a survival rate of 99% after 10 years in patients younger than 50 years of age.

In chronological order, the cate-

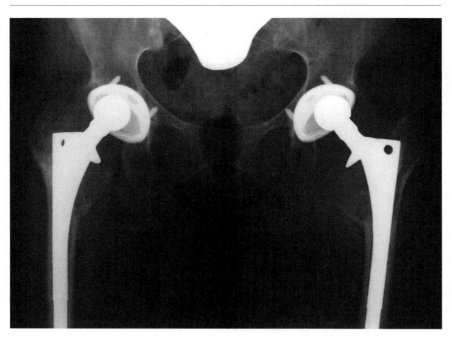

Figure 1 Radiograph made 8 years after total hip replacement in a 50-year-old woman. A high degree of polyethylene wear and associated osteolysis is seen.

gorical factors limiting the function and longevity of a total hip prosthesis are the surgical technique, fixation of the implant to the bone, osteolysis (often associated with wear of the bearing), fatigue failure of the implants, and long-term skeletal remodeling. No implant system can overcome inadequate surgical technique. A sound biomechanical construct is the foundation of a well-functioning prosthesis. The next challenge is to obtain and maintain satisfactory fixation. As physical activity increases, the stresses on the fixation interfaces and the implants also increase. The durability of implant fixation in young patients has been improved by cementless fixation.[19] Osteolysis associated with polyethylene wear has become the limiting factor[20,21] (Figure 1). Except in cases where the bearing actually wears through, wear is clinically important only if it induces progressive osteolysis. Hips are generally not revised as a result of wear; they are revised because of osteolysis associated with wear (and the generation of wear particles).

Polyethylene, ceramic, and metal wear particles incite an inflammatory response that can result in periprosthetic bone resorption (osteolysis).[22-26] Bearing wear, osteolysis, and aseptic loosening can limit the durability of a prosthetic hip joint, irrespective of the combination of materials used,[27,28] given that the biomechanical reconstruction and fixation are satisfactory.

New bearings for total hip arthroplasty have been introduced with the aim of reducing the number of biologically active wear particles. There are two approaches: one is to improve the wear resistance of polyethylene through cross-linking,[29] and the other is to avoid polyethylene and use alternative bearings. The latter approach has fueled the development and reintroduction of new ceramic-on-ceramic and metal-on-metal bearings. The goal of all bearing combinations is to reduce wear to less than a clinically relevant level, that is, a level that does not induce osteolysis or another outcome that necessitates revision surgery. Although the use of surrogate variables such as wear rates to predict the outcome of a total joint arthroplasty may be helpful as a prognostic tool, this should be done with caution.

Tribology: Wear and Lubrication

Tribology is defined as the science of surfaces interacting under an applied load and in relative motion (as in bearings or gears). It includes the study of friction, lubrication, and wear. Wear is the removal of material, with the generation of wear particles that results from relative motion between two apposed surfaces under load. The primary wear mechanisms are adhesion, abrasion, and fatigue. Adhesion involves bonding of the surfaces when they are pressed together under load. Sufficient relative motion results in material being pulled away from one or more surfaces, usually from the weaker material. Abrasion is a mechanical process in which asperities on the harder surface cut and plow through the softer surface, resulting in removal of material. When local stresses exceed the fatigue strength of a material, that material fails after a certain number of loading cycles, with release of material from the surface.[28]

The conditions under which the prosthesis was functioning when the wear occurred have been termed the wear modes.[30] Mode 1 wear results from the motion of two primary bearing surfaces against each other, as intended. Mode 2 refers to the condition of a primary bearing surface moving against a secondary surface that was not intended to come into contact with the first. Usually, this mode of wear occurs after excessive wear in mode 1. An example would be when a femoral component penetrates through a modular polyethylene liner and articulates with the metal backing. Mode 3 refers to the condition of the primary surfaces moving against each other, but with third-body particles interposed. In mode 3, the contaminant particles directly abrade one or both of the primary bearing surfaces. This is known as three-body abrasion or three-body wear. The primary bearing surfaces may be transiently or permanently roughened by this interaction, leading to a higher mode 1 wear rate. Mode 4 wear refers to two secondary (nonprimary) surfaces rubbing together. Examples of mode 4 wear include wear due to relative motion of the outer surface of a modular polyethylene component against the metal support, so-called backside wear, fretting between a metallic substrate and a fixation screw, or fretting and corrosion of modular taper connections and extra-articular sources. Particles produced by mode 4 wear can migrate to the primary bearing surfaces, inducing three-body wear (mode 3).[30]

Lubrication has a major influence on the amount of abrasive and, especially, adhesive wear. The tribologic performance of a joint depends on the fluid film covering its surfaces.[31] A high ratio of fluid-film thickness to surface roughness (λ ratio) is desirable to reduce friction and wear. A λ ratio equal to or less than unity describes boundary lubrication. With an increasing λ ratio, friction is reduced and the bearing reaches a state of mixed lubrication. A value of more than 3 represents fluid-film lubrication.[32,33] Fluid-film lubrication completely separates the surfaces of a bearing. This occurs when the lubricating film is thicker than the height of the asperities on the bearing surfaces. In this situation the load is carried by the fluid, and wear of the bearing is minimal. Mixed film lubrication separates the surfaces only partially and is represented by a λ ratio of more than 1 and less than 3. For a given load and sliding velocity, fluid-film thickness is dependent on the properties of the fluid, the bearing materials, the macrogeometry of the bearing (which is a function of diameter and radial clearance), and the surface microtopography (surface finish).[34]

Cross-Linked Polyethylene Acetabular Bearings

Ultra-high molecular weight polyethylene has been the preferred acetabular bearing material for more than 30 years. The aggregate clinical experience indicates a low probability of gross material failure of this application and, despite evidence of systemic distribution, there are no clinically apparent systemic consequences. The fundamental limitation is wear resistance.

Ethylene is a gaseous hydrocarbon composed of two carbon atoms and four hydrogen atoms: C_2H_4. Polyethylene is a long-chain polymer of ethylene molecules in which all of the carbon atoms are linked, each of them holding its two hydrogen atoms.[35] The mechanical properties of ultra-high molecular weight polyethylene are strongly related to its chemical structure, molecular weight, crystalline organization, and thermal history.[36]

The microstructure of ultra-high molecular weight polyethylene is a two-phase viscoplastic solid consisting of crystalline domains embedded within an amorphous matrix.[36,37] Connecting the crystalline domains are bridging tie molecules that provide improved stress transfer and physical strength.[37] Ultra-high molecular weight polyethylene is defined as polyethylene with an average molecular weight of greater than 3 million g/mol.[36] The ultra-high molecular weight polyethylene currently used in orthopaedic applications[36,38] has a molecular weight of 3 to 6 million g/mol, a melting point of 125°C to 145°C, and a density of 0.930 to 0.945 g/cm^3. Ticona (Summit, NJ) and Basell Polyolefins (Wilmington, DE) supply ultra-high molecular weight polyethylene resins to orthopaedic manufacturers. Calcium stearate is an additive in the manufacturing process of many polyethylene resins; it acts as a corrosion inhibitor,[36,39] whitening agent,[38] and lubricant to facilitate the extrusion process.[36,39,40] In general, both Ticona and Basell resin powders consist of numerous fused, spheroidal ultra-high molecular weight polyethylene particles, but a fine network of submicrometer-sized fibrils that interconnect the microscopic spheroids characterizes Ticona resins. Ticona resins have a mean particle size of approximately 140 μm, whereas Basell resins have a mean particle size of approximately 300 μm.[36]

Cross-linking has been used to improve the wear resistance of polyethylene and can be accomplished with use of peroxide chemistry, variable-dose ionizing radiation, or electron beam irradiation.[41] Cross-linking occurs when free radicals, located on the amorphous regions of polyethylene molecules, react to form a covalent bond between adjacent polyethylene molecules. It is believed that cross-linking of the polyethylene molecules resists intermolecular mobility, making the polyethylene more resistant to deformation and wear in the plane perpendicular to the primary molecular axis. This has been demonstrated to

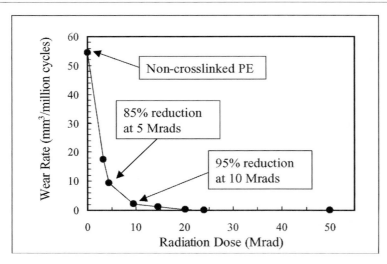

Figure 2 Wear rate of polyethylene (PE) acetabular components in a hip simulator as a function of radiation dose.[29] 1 Mrad = 10,000 Gy. (Reproduced with permission from McKellop H, Shen FW, Campbell P, Salovey R: Development of an extremely wear resistant ultra high molecular weight polyethylene for total hip replacements. *J Orthop Res*1999;17;157-167.)

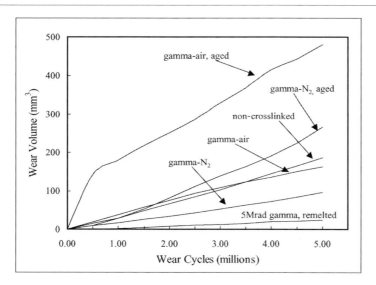

Figure 3 Wear of polyethylene acetabular components in a hip simulator as a function of manufacturing and sterilization method. Wear rate increases with higher levels of oxidation.[46] Gamma = gamma irradiation, and 1 Mrad = 10,000 Gy. (Reproduced with permission from McKellop H, Shen F W, Lu B, Campbell P, Salovey R: Effect of sterilization method and other modifications on the wear resistance of acetabular clips mode of ultra-high molecular weight polyethylene. *J Bone Joint Surg Am* 2000;82: 1708-1725.)

dramatically reduce wear from crossing-path motion, as occurs in acetabular components.[42,43] Cross-linking has a detrimental effect on yield strength, ultimate tensile strength, and elongation to break.[29] The decrease in these properties is proportional to the degree of cross-linking. This fact has generated debates on the optimal degree of cross-linking. Hip simulator studies have indicated that cross-linking can reduce the type of wear that occurs in acetabular components by more than 95%[29,44,45] (Figure 2).

Clinical and laboratory research has revealed that sterilization methods can dramatically affect the in vivo performance of a polyethylene component[46] (Figure 3). Polyethylene components can be sterilized with gamma irradiation, gas plasma, or ethylene oxide. Gamma irradiation in an air environment was the industry standard since the early 1970s; the doses range between 2.5 and 4 Mrad (1 Mrad = 10^6 radiation absorbed dose = 10^4 Gy) and are most commonly between 3.0 and 3.5 Mrad (30,000 to 35,000 Gy). Gamma radiation breaks covalent bonds, including those in the polyethylene molecules. This produces unpaired electrons from the broken covalent bonds, called free radicals. These highly reactive moieties can combine with oxygen (if present) during the irradiation process, during shelf storage, and in vivo.

Oxidation of the polyethylene molecule is a chemical reaction that results in chain scission (fragmentation and shortening of the large polymer chains) and introduction of oxygen into the polymer.[38] The net result lowers the molecular weight of the polymer; reduces its yield strength, ultimate tensile strength, elongation to break (makes it more brittle), and toughness; and increases its density (lowers its volume).[47-50]

In general, oxidation and cross-linking are competing reactions. As cross-linking increases, oxidation decreases and vice versa.[51,52] In components subjected to gamma irradiation in air, the relative amount of oxidation and cross-linking varies with the depth from the surface of the component.[52] This results in a corresponding variation in the wear resistance of the material as a function of the depth from the surface.[51] Once implanted, the component is exposed to dissolved oxygen in body fluids. Free radicals in the polyethylene will react with the available oxygen over time. Relatively little is known about the rate of oxidation of polyethylene in vivo. It appears that it is lower than that in vitro, but there is debate about how much lower, and it is likely that several factors affect the rate of oxidation.

Methods have been developed to produce components with increased wear resistance due to cross-linking that do not oxidize on the shelf or in the body. Free radicals created in polyethylene by ionizing radiation can be driven to a cross-linking reaction by heating the polymer to above the melting temperature (125°C to 135°C).[29] Components made from such remelted material have no residual free radicals; thus, there is no potential for oxidation when the component is subsequently sterilized by ethylene oxide or gas plasma. Remelting does, however, induce changes in the crystalline structure of the material that are associated with a decrease in some material properties. This fact has resulted in controversy regarding the relative detriment of remelting compared with that of retention of some residual free radicals.

The manufacturing processes of the currently available products—Marathon (DePuy, Warsaw, IN), Longevity (Zimmer, Warsaw, IN), Durasul (Centerpulse Orthopaedics, Austin, TX), Crossfire (Stryker Howmedica Osteonics, Allendale, NJ), and XLPE (Smith and Nephew Orthopaedics, Memphis, TN)—differ with regard to the dose and type of irradiation (gamma or electron beam), thermal stabilization (remelting or annealing), machining, and fi-

nal sterilization.[53] For this reason, each material should be considered separately, and the specific wear characteristics of each should be established through clinical studies.

A revision for any reason is the primary definition of failure of a total hip arthroplasty. Unfortunately, often a long follow-up period is required to demonstrate statistical and practical differences among implant systems. Shorter-term in vivo wear studies may help to predict long-term outcomes. Increased volumetric wear has been associated with component loosening and osteolysis.[54-58] The association between volumetric wear and periprosthetic bone resorption appears to be related to the number and size of polyethylene wear particles that are generated and are released into the effective joint space.[59] On this basis, a lower wear rate may not necessarily be clinically preferred if a higher number of biologically active wear particles are generated.

Penetration of the femoral head into the acetabular polyethylene is due to a combination of creep and wear. Because of creep, short-term linear penetration rates tend to be higher than those seen over the longer term. Because creep decreases exponentially with time, it is generally accepted that most of the linear penetration that occurs after the first 1 or 2 years is caused by wear.[60,61]

Data from clinical trials with small patient groups have shown a reduction in wear rate associated with cross-linking.[60,62-64] Martell and associates[65] evaluated 74 patients at a minimum of 2 years postoperatively. Thirty-five patients had a polyethylene acetabular liner that had been gamma irradiated in air (the historical standard), and 39 had a liner that had been cross-linked with 3 Mrad (30,000 Gy) of gamma radiation in

nitrogen and then heat annealed. Radiographs were analyzed with a computer-assisted, two-dimensional digital edge detection technique.[66] The hips treated with the historical standard had a mean volumetric wear rate of 94 ± 78 mm^3/yr compared with a mean of 54 ± 70 mm^3/yr in the hips with the cross-linked polyethylene ($P < 0.05$). The degree of clinical wear reduction associated with the intentionally cross-linked material was very similar to the degree of wear reduction seen in a hip-wear simulator study comparing these same acetabular components.[65] In another clinical study, Martell and Incavo[67] compared 24 liners made of highly cross-linked polyethylene (Crossfire; gamma irradiation to 7.5 Mrad [75,000 Gy], heat-annealed at 120°C, and sterilized with 2.5 to 3.5 Mrad [25,000 to 35,000 Gy] of gamma radiation while packaged in nitrogen) with 25 standard polyethylene liners that had been sterilized in the same manner. After 2 years of follow-up, the cross-linked polyethylene showed a significant (53%) reduction in linear wear (0.094 compared with 0.202 mm/yr; $P = 0.008$).

Digas and associates[68] initiated a prospective study comparing a cemented, highly cross-linked polyethylene acetabular component (Durasul; electron beam radiation to 9.5 Mrad [95,000 Gy] at 125°C, remelted at 150°C for 2 hours, and sterilized with ethylene oxide) with a cemented polyethylene component that had been sterilized with gamma irradiation in nitrogen. The in vivo wear in 33 patients followed for a minimum of 2 years was measured with radiostereometric analysis. In the 15 patients with the cross-linked polyethylene there was less three-dimensional femoral head penetration (0.18 compared with 0.20 mm/yr) but the difference was not significant. The fact that there was not more of a difference in the linear penetration in this short-term study is not surprising given that the creep rates of the two polymers are about the same.[68] Another conclusion that could be reached on the basis of those data are that the clinical performance of moderately cross-linked polyethylene with little oxidation (the "standard" polyethylene) is quite good.

In another study, (TP Schmalzried, MD, C Heisel, MD, Cambridge, MA, unpublished data, 2002) 24 hips received a modular polyethylene liner sterilized with gamma radiation in air (Enduron, DePuy, Warsaw, IN) in combination with a cementless acetabular component, and 30 hips received the same acetabular component with a cross-linked polyethylene liner (Marathon; gamma irradiation to 5 Mrad [50,000 Gy], remelted at 155°C for 24 hours, machined from the center of a ram-extruded bar, and sterilized with gas plasma). The patients treated with the cross-linked polyethylene were younger and more active than the patients treated with the conventional polyethylene (mean ages, 59 and 74 years, $P < 0.0001$). After a minimum of 2 years of follow-up, the conventional polyethylene liners had a mean volumetric wear rate of 88 ± 79 mm^3/yr, with 104 mm^3/yr in the men and 74 mm^3/yr in the women. The cross-linked liners had a mean volumetric wear rate of 21 ± 23 mm^3/yr, with 28 mm^3/yr in the men and 15 mm^3/yr in the women. The difference between the conventional and cross-linked liners was significant ($P = 0.0001$). Some of the reduction in linear penetration observed in this study may have been due to a reduction in conformational change (backside bedding-in) between the modular acetabular liner and the metal shell. Adjusted for the measured activity, the volumetric wear rate per million cycles was 48 mm^3 for the conventional polyethylene liners and 10 mm^3 for the cross-linked polyethylene liners ($P = 0.0004$). Hip simulator studies with those materials have shown wear rates of 36.8 mm^3 and 5 mm^3, respectively, per million cycles.[43,46] The reductions of wear of cross-linked polyethylene per million cycles in vivo (79%) and in vitro (86%) were similar. The increased wear resistance of cross-linked polyethylene is fueling an increase in the use of larger-diameter heads. This trend is driving debates on the minimum thickness needed for cross-linked polyethylene components and the degree of increase in volumetric wear with larger-diameter heads.

Polyethylene Wear Particles

The number, shape, and size of polyethylene wear particles are multifactorial: they are a function of the modes and mechanisms of wear that produce them, the stresses on the bearing surface, the motions, and the polyethylene molecular orientation. Most of the polyethylene wear particles produced in a prosthetic joint are micrometers to submicrometers in size and are produced in mode 1, in very large quantities, by well-functioning joints.[30] The predominant wear mechanisms appear to involve microadhesion and microabrasion with the generation of many polyethylene particles of less than 1 μm in length. The resultant wear damage is predominantly burnishing and scratching.[30]

Techniques have been developed to isolate and analyze wear particles generated in vivo by retrieving them from periprosthetic tissues.[30,59,69-73] The concentration of debris particles from prosthetic joints is directly related to the duration of implantation[74] and can extend into the billions per gram of tissue.[70-72,75] So far, these data are available only for conventional polyethylene because of the limited number of retrieved samples of cross-linked polyethylene.[27,76,77]

Substantial differences between the wear particles from cross-linked and non–cross-linked polyethylenes have been found in vitro (Figure 4). Cross-linked polyethylene releases a relatively high number of submicrometer and nanometer-sized polyethylene particles and relatively fewer particles that are several micrometers in dimension.[78-81] These submicrometer particles induce a greater inflammatory response in vitro than do larger particles.[79-82] Additionally, the cellular response is dependent on the shape of the particles: elongated particles generate a more severe inflammatory reaction than do globular particles.[83]

Illgen and associates[80] tried to correlate volumetric wear with biologic activity in vitro. They compared the wear of a cross-linked polyethylene (Longevity; electron beam irradiation to 9 Mrad [90,000 Gy] and gas plasma sterilization) with that of a conventional polyethylene (gamma irradiation in nitrogen), as measured in a hip simulator, and then tested the biologic activity of the isolated particles in cell cultures. They found a reduced relative biologic activity of the cross-linked polyethylene particles. Because the number, size, and shape of the particles released by the cross-linked polyethylene liners depend on the material used,[82] the mode of cross-linking,[78] and patient-related wear factors, only clinical studies of each specific cross-linked polyethylene can answer the question of whether cross-linked polyethylene offers a favorable benefit-to-risk ratio.

Although the short-term clinical data on cross-linked polyethylene are encouraging, it will be possible to draw stronger conclusions after minimum 5-year clinical data have been compiled and retrieval data have become available. The central issue is not linear penetration or wear rate, but the development of osteolysis, loosening, or the need for revision surgery for any reason related to the bearing.

Ceramic Femoral Heads

Another approach to reducing polyethylene wear is to improve the wear characteristics of the femoral head. In a hip simulator study, McKellop and associates[43] demonstrated that decreased surface roughness reduces polyethylene wear. As an alternative to metallic (cobalt-chromium) heads, ceramic heads are manufactured in many variations and sizes. The ceramic materials are much harder and can be polished to a lower surface roughness (made smoother) than metal heads. Alumina (Al_2O_3) or zirconia (ZrO_2) heads have both a high hardness and a high strength, which make them more difficult to scratch, and this can reduce abrasive wear.[31,84,85] Another important issue is the better wettability of the material. Ceramics are more hydrophilic and have improved lubrication and lower friction. Hip simulator and clinical studies have indicated that the wear of a ceramic-on-polyethylene bearing is at least equivalent to[61,86-88] or less than[60,89-91] that of a metal-on-polyethylene bearing. Wear reduction of up to 50% has been reported.[31,84,89-91]

Ceramics are brittle materials, creating the possibility of a fracture of a ceramic head. A review of more than 500,000 current-generation alumina femoral heads indicated a fracture rate of 0.004% (4:100,000).[92]

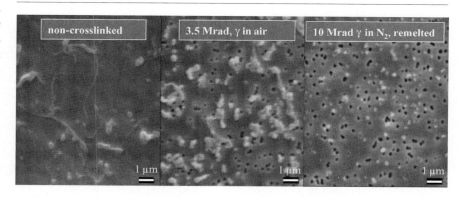

Figure 4 Shape and size of polyethylene particles isolated from hip-simulator studies. Non-cross-linked polyethylene produces a large amount of particles that are elongated fibrils. A substantial reduction in particle size is seen between the non-cross-linked polyethylene (left) and the partially cross-linked polyethylene (3.5 Mrad [35,000 Gy]) (center). Partially cross-linked polyethylene produces mostly round particles of submicrometer size and fibrils of up to a few micrometers in size. Highly cross-linked polyethylene (10 Mrad [100,000 Gy]) (right) shows predominantly round particles in the submicrometer size range (×10,000).

Even if the number of unreported cases is assumed to be three times higher,[92] the fracture rate of ceramic heads is still much lower than that of femoral stems, which is approximately 0.27% (270:100,000).[93] Following a specific change in their manufacturing process in 1998, zirconia heads (Prozyr) from one manufacturer (Saint-Gobain Céramiques Avancées Desmarquest, Vincennes CEDEX, France, www.prozyr.com) had an increased rate of fracture. It is important to recognize that the risk of fracture of alumina and zirconia heads from other manufacturers was not affected by this change.

Zirconia has a higher hardness and burst strength than alumina, but it is not thermostable. It can undergo phase transformation, probably as a result of its reduced heat conductivity.[53,94] A practical effect of this material property is that zirconia femoral heads should not be sterilized in an autoclave. Usually yttrium oxide (Y_2O_3) is added to improve the material properties of zirconia. A new approach is the use of so-called zirconia-toughened aluminas.[95,96]

Mixing of the two materials achieves a composite with the high strength of zirconia and the thermal stability of alumina. Additional studies must be performed to evaluate the possible benefits of these composites.

Metal-on-Metal Bearings

Early loosening of prostheses with a metal-on-metal bearing was initially assumed to be due to the bearing but has now been recognized as being due to suboptimal implant design, inconsistent manufacturing, and surgical technique.[53,97-100] A review of the 15- to 20-year results showed that the survivorship of metal-on-metal hip prostheses is comparable with that of Charnley and other metal-on-polyethylene prostheses.[101] The failures were not due to the wear properties of the bearing.[97,98,102-108] Retrieval studies have indicated that the metal-on-metal McKee-Farrar prostheses produced substantially less wear than did the conventional metal-on-polyethylene bearings.[32,53,109] Hip simulator studies of metal-on-metal bearings have shown a substantial (up to 200-fold)

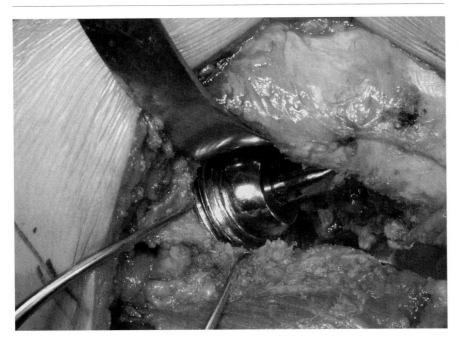

Figure 5 A modern metal-on-metal modular articulation. Modularity increases reconstructive options but can also be a source of metal particles and ions. The larger-diameter articulation (36 mm in this example) reduces wear and increases the range of motion.

reduction in volumetric wear rates compared with those of conventional polyethylene articulations.[110-117] Consequently, there is renewed interest in metal-on-metal bearings for total hip arthroplasty, and there has been a revival of research on and development of metal-on-metal bearings, initially in Europe[118-120] and later in the United States.[121,122]

In 1988, Müller and Weber reintroduced the metal-on-metal bearing, and the development of this cobalt-chromium alloy bearing was sold under the brand name Metasul (Centerpulse Orthopaedics). With more than a decade of experience with second-generation metal-on-metal bearings, more than 160,000 Metasul bearings have been implanted, and this bearing technology has also been extended to large-diameter surface-replacement components.[99,123]

The interplay of materials, macro-geometry (diameter and radial clearance), microgeometry (surface topography), and lubrication influences the wear of metal-on-metal bearings to a far greater degree than it influences the wear of metal-on-polyethylene bearings.[124] Mixed film lubrication appears to be the surgical mechanism in most metal-on-metal hip joints. Fluid-film lubrication is encouraged by making the femoral head as large as practically possible (doing so increases the sliding velocity and pulls more fluid into the articulation), the clearance as small as practically possible, and the surface as smooth as practically possible. With metal-on-metal bearings, in contrast to polyethylene bearings, a larger-diameter bearing actually produces lower wear rates than does a smaller-diameter bearing with similar manufacturing parameters.[33,125]

The clinical outcomes associated with contemporary total hip systems with metal-on-metal bearings have generally been good.[119-121] We are not aware of any reports of revisions for a problem directly attributable to the metal-on-metal articulation, we know of no evidence of runaway wear, and few metal particles have been seen in histologic sections.[119,120,123] There have, however, been revisions as a result of infection, heterotopic ossification, instability, impingement, and aseptic loosening. Impingement wear can be a source of metallosis, especially if a titanium-alloy neck impinges on a cobalt-chromium acetabular articulation.[126] Larger-diameter bearings have a greater arc of motion, which decreases the risk of impingement (Figure 5).

Sieber and associates[127] reported on 118 Metasul components (65 heads and 53 cups) retrieved because of dislocation (24%), loosening of the stem (17%), loosening of the cup (28%), or other reasons such as heterotopic ossification or infection (31%). None was revised because of osteolysis. The mean time to revision was 22 months (range, 2 to 98 months). An update on this experience included 297 retrieved heads or cups (U Wyss, C Rieker, Cambridge, MA, unpublished data, 2002). The time between implantation and revision in this group ranged from 1 to 117 months, and the distribution of indications for the revisions was similar (dislocation in 21%, loosening of any component in 39%, and other reasons in 40%). The mean annual linear wear rates in the two studies were found to decrease with the time from the insertion of the implant: they were 25 and 35 μm in the running-in period (conditioning phase), decreasing to a steady state of about 5 μm after the third year in both studies. The volumetric wear rate after the running-in period was estimated to be 0.3 mm³/yr, leading to the conclusion that these metal-on-metal bearings have a volumetric wear rate more than 100 times lower than that of conventional polyethylene bearings.

Osteolysis has been rare in clinical reports on hips with second-generation metal-on-metal bearings followed for 2.2 to 5 years.[119-121,123] Beaulé and associates,[128] however, reported a case of progressive diaphyseal osteolysis occurring within 2 years postoperatively in a patient with a well-fixed cementless total hip prosthesis with a Metasul bearing. Histologic analysis showed minimal wear of the bearing surface and only a small number of inflammatory cells in the tissues. Because there was no evidence of a foreign body reaction, it was hypothesized that the osteolysis was secondary to transmission of joint fluid pressure rather than induced by particles.[129]

In the initial US experience, 74 Metasul bearings, in Weber cemented cups, were implanted with a variety of femoral components. After follow-up periods of up to 4 years (average, 2.2 years), the clinical results were good to excellent and no hip prosthesis had loosened. Twenty-seven of the patients had a metal-on-polyethylene bearing prosthesis of similar design in the contralateral hip, and none of those patients could detect a difference between the two hips.[121] Complete clinical and radiographic data on 56 patients (56 hips), followed for 4 to 6.8 years (average, 5.2 years), have also been reported.[131] Good to excellent clinical results were found in 99%. One patient required acetabular revision because of loosening secondary to suboptimal cementing technique. There were no loose or revised femoral components or radiographically apparent osteolysis.[130]

Metal Wear Particles and Ion Release

Wear particles from metal-on-metal bearings measure nanometers in the linear dimension and are substantially smaller than polyethylene wear particles.[25,131] The size of metal particles, as demonstrated by scanning electron microscopy studies, ranges from 0.1 to 5 μm. Scanning electron microscopy studies suggested that large metallic particles observed with light microscopy were agglomerates of smaller particles.[131,132]

Little is known about the rates of metallic particle production in vivo, lymphatic transport of metallic particles from the joint, or systemic dissemination.[133,134] On the basis of information on volumetric wear rates and average particle size, it has been estimated that 6.7×10^{12} to 2.5×10^{14} metal particles are produced per year, which is 13 to 500 times the number of polyethylene particles produced per year by a typical metal-on-polyethylene joint.[131] The aggregate surface area of these metal wear particles is substantial and may have both local and systemic effects. Surface area has been identified as a variable affecting the macrophage response to particles.[135] However, the local tissue reaction around a metal-on-metal prosthesis, indicated by the number of histiocytes, is about one grade lower than that around a metal-on-polyethylene prosthesis.[131,133] Several hypotheses have been proposed to explain this discrepancy.[131] Because metal particles are considerably smaller than polyethylene particles, histiocytes can store a larger number of metal particles; therefore, the total number of histiocytes required to store the metal particles is lower. Very small particles may enter macrophages by pinocytosis instead of phagocytosis, which may alter the cellular response

to the particles. There may be a difference between metal wear particles and polyethylene wear particles with regard to the relative proportion that are retained locally as opposed to distributed systemically. Dissolution of metal particles results in elevation of the cobalt and chromium ion concentrations in erythrocytes, serum, and urine.[136]

It is important to recognize that there may be several sources of metal particle and ion generation in modern total hip replacements. Studies have shown systemic dissemination of soluble and particulate corrosion products from modular junctions, resulting in the presence of metallic particles in the lymph nodes, liver, and spleen.[137-141] In patients without a metallic implant, the levels of serum and urine cobalt and chromium are undetectable or nearly undetectable,[138] whereas the levels of metal ions in erythrocytes, serum, and urine are elevated in patients with a metal-on-metal bearing. It appears that the ion levels are higher in the short term and decrease over time. This finding is consistent with a conditioning phase or running-in period of the bearing.[142] Because wear of a metal-on-metal bearing cannot generally be measured on a radiograph, erythrocyte, serum, and urine metal-ion concentrations may be useful indicators of patient activity and the tribologic performance of these bearings. Unfortunately, the toxicologic importance of these elevations in trace metal levels has not been established yet.

Delayed-type hypersensitivity, an immune response resulting from exposure to metal ions such as nickel, chromium, and cobalt, may develop in a small number of susceptible patients. Recently, some authors (AP Davies, HG Willert, PA Campbell, PC Case, New Orleans, LA, unpub-

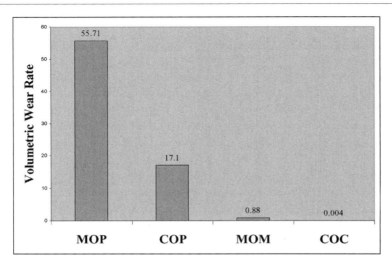

Figure 6 Wear rates (in cubic millimeters per year) of different bearing combinations tested in a hip simulator.[115] MOP = metal-on-polyethylene, COP = ceramic-on-polyethylene, MOM = metal-on-metal, and COC = ceramic-on-ceramic. (Reproduced with permission from Greenwald A S, Garino J P: Alternative bearing surfaces: The odd, the bad, and the ugly. *J Bone Joint Surg Am* 2001;83:68-72.)

lished data, 2003) have described specific histologic changes in the tissues around revised metal-on-metal prostheses.[143-145] They found lymphocytic infiltrations in the subsurface layer of the lining tissues, which were either diffuse or aggregated around small postcapillary vessels. The tissues from patients with a metal-on-metal implant also showed ulcerations of the pseudosynovial surface compared with those from patients with a metal-on-polyethylene implant. Interestingly, all of these changes were less obvious in tissues retrieved from patients with a McKee-Farrar or loose cemented curved cobalt-chromium stem than they were in tissues retrieved from patients with a modern metal-on-metal bearing.[144] There seems to be no correlation between the amount of metal debris and the occurrence or extent of the immunologic reaction (AP Davies, HG Willert, PA Campbell, PC Case, New Orleans, LA, unpublished data, 2003). These immunologic reactions are termed "aseptic lymphocytic vasculitis-associated lesions." The clinical relevance of these findings is not yet clear because only a small number of patients with a metal-on-metal bearing have had to have a revision so far and only a fraction of the revised cases have shown these histologic changes.

Clinically, delayed-type hypersensitivity may present as unexplained pain associated with aseptic effusions and interfacial loosening. It is unclear whether delayed-type hypersensitivity contributes to aseptic loosening or whether implant loosening contributes to delayed-type hypersensitivity.[134,143,146-152] In vitro studies have also demonstrated that polyethylene particles cause a greater inflammatory response in general but cobalt-chromium particles have higher toxicity.[134,153-155]

There remains a theoretical increase in the risk of cancer with metal-on-metal bearings.[141,156-163] The aggregate clinical data have not indicated such an increase in risk, but the most patients in the reports presenting those data were followed for less than 10 years. The latency period of known carcinogens, such as tobacco, asbestos, and ionizing radiation, is several decades. Longer follow-up of large groups of patients is needed to better assess the risk of cancer with any implant system.[164] Because the goal of more wear-resistant bearings is to reduce the need for a revision, theoretical risks should be weighed against the known risks of revision total hip replacement. In the Medicare population, the 90-day mortality rate following revision total hip arthroplasty was reported to be 2.6%, which is substantially higher than that following primary total hip arthroplasty and is directly related to the revision procedure.[165]

Ceramic-on-Ceramic Bearings

Ceramic-on-ceramic bearings have demonstrated the lowest in vivo wear rates to date of any bearing combination[112,166] (Figure 6). The same principles of friction and lubrication reported for metal-on-metal bearings apply to ceramic-on-ceramic bearings. However, ceramics have two important properties that make them an outstanding material with regard to friction and wear. First, ceramics are hydrophilic, permitting a better wettability of the surface. This ensures that the synovial fluid film is uniformly distributed over the entire bearing surface area. Second, ceramics have a greater hardness than metal and can be polished to a much lower surface roughness. Although the better wettability results in a fluid film that is slightly thinner than that found with metal-on-metal bearings, it is compensated for by the reduced size of the asperities on the surface. Overall, this results in a favorable higher λ ratio and in a reduced coefficient of friction. This bearing combination is the most likely to achieve true fluid-film lubrication.[33] However, because of the hardness of ceramics, the wear characteristics are sensitive to design, manufacturing, and implantation variables. Rapid wear has also been observed, generally associated with suboptimal positioning of the implants.[167,168]

Ceramic-on-ceramic bearings currently in clinical use are made of alumina. Developments in the production process (sintering) have improved the quality of the material.[169] Modern alumina ceramics have a low porosity, low grain size, high density, and high purity. Thus, hardness, fracture toughness, and burst strength are increased.[169-171] There have been in vitro tests using zirconia and alumina-zirconia composites to improve wear characteristics,[95,96] but these mixed oxides must be studied further before clinical trials can be conducted.

The US experience with ceramic-on-ceramic bearings was initially limited to the Autophor/Xenophor prostheses, which were conceived and introduced in Europe by Mittelmeier.[172,173] The clinical results with the Autophor prosthesis were generally less satisfactory than those with established metal-on-polyethylene designs, and ceramic-on-ceramic implants were never widely used in the United States.[174] Previous studies (mostly from Europe) showed prosthetic survival rates of 75% to 84% after 10 years[168,175,176] and 68% after 20 years.[18] For patients 50 years of age and younger, the prosthetic survival rates were 84% after 10 years, 80% after 15 years,[176] and 61% after 20 years.[18]

Similar to the situation with metal-on-metal bearings, the per-ception of which was based on the clinical performance of the McKee-Farrar prosthesis,[97] the perception of the performance of ceramic-on-ceramic bearings has been complicated by the fact that the Autophor stem and socket had features that are now recognized as suboptimal.[167] Follow-up studies showed very low in vivo wear rates,[18,177,178] but failures occurred as a result of inferior implant design and fixation technique.[171,179] The current generation of ceramic-on-ceramic bearings is frequently being used in implant systems that have demonstrated long-term successful fixation and excellent clinical results with a metal-on-polyethylene bearing.

Two prospective, randomized multicenter trials are being performed in the United States, with more than 300 patients enrolled in each study. Garino[180] reported the experience with the Transcend system (Wright Medical Technology, Arlington, TN). A modular cementless acetabular component with either a cemented or a cementless stem was implanted in 333 hips. After a follow-up of 18 to 36 months (mean, 22 months), 98.8% of the implants were still in situ. In the second trial, the ABC System (Stryker Howmedica Osteonics) was implanted in 349 hips.[181,182] D'Antonio and Capello[181] evaluated the most recent results of the six participating surgeons with the highest number of enrolled patients. This subgroup consisted of 207 patients with 222 hips followed for a mean of 48 months. Five hips had been revised, and 97.7% of the implants were in place. An additional, nonrandomized arm of this multicenter study (J D'Antonio, W Capello, M Manley, B Bierbaum, Rochester, MN, unpublished data, 2002) consisted of 209 patients treated with the Trident system (Stryker Howmedica Osteonics). One hundred seventy-five of these patients had been followed for a minimum of 2 years, and the revision rate in that group was 1.7% (three revisions).

One potential complication with these implants that a surgeon should recognize is chipping of the liner during insertion. This happened in three cases (1%)[180] treated with the Transcend system and in nine (2.6%) treated with the ABC system (J D'Antonio, W Capello, M Manley, B Bierbaum, Rochester, MN, unpublished data, 2002). The Trident bearing has a metal-backed ceramic insert with an elevated titanium liner rim, and no intraoperative chipping of that liner was reported.[181]

Including the original study groups and additional implantations, at the time of this writing, 1,361 ceramic inserts have been implanted in these studies and there have been no failures due to the bearing.[180,181] No fractures of the implanted liners or ceramic heads have been reported. The incidence of fractures of current-generation ceramic heads[93] is 4 in 100,000. It is too early to make a comparable statement about the acetabular inserts as more data on a higher number of implants are needed. Results from the multicenter studies are encouraging, with no liner fractures reported to date.

Ceramic Wear Particles

Ceramic materials may have better biocompatibility than metal alloys,[183] but the relative size, shape, number, reactivity, and distribution (local compared with systemic) of the respective wear particles have not been fully determined. Hatton and associates[184] reported a bimodal size range of particles isolated from tissue around failed ceramic-on-ceramic total hip replacements. They found a

Table 1
Alternate Bearing Combinations for Total Hip Arthroplasty

Bearing Material	Benefits	Risks
Cross-linked polyethylene	High wear resistance, no toxicity, relatively low cost, multiple liner options (elevated rim, etc)	Reduction in other material properties (gross material failure), increased bioactivity of wear particles
Metal-on-metal	Very high wear resistance, favors larger diameters (reduces wear), long in vivo experience	Increased ion levels, delayed-type hypersensitivity, carcinogenesis
Ceramic-on-ceramic	Highest wear resistance, no toxicity, long in vivo experience	Position sensitivity, liner chipping, fracture risk

large amount of small particles between 5 and 90 nm (mean, 24 nm) but also larger particles between 0.05 and 3.2 μm. Ceramic debris may not be bioinert as initially assumed because osteolysis has been described in some patients with a ceramic-on-ceramic bearing.[26,185] Recently, some studies have demonstrated inflammatory and cytotoxic reactions on the cellular level, but the relationship to material, size, and particle number remains uncertain.[184,186-188] It seems that there is less inflammatory reaction than that found with metal-on-metal or metal-on-polyethylene bearings in well-functioning prostheses.[189] Ion toxicity is not an issue with ceramics because of their high corrosion resistance.[189]

Summary

Cross-linked polyethylene, metal-on-metal, and ceramic-on-ceramic bearings have all demonstrated lower in vivo wear rates than conventional metal-on-polyethylene couples. The degree of wear reduction is promising, but it may not directly translate into greater longevity of a total hip replacement in all patients. Continued close follow-up is needed to demonstrate a favorable benefit-to-risk ratio based on a reduction in the number of revision operations (Table 1). The use of any of these bearings has specific benefits and risks that should be considered on a patient-by-patient basis.

References

1. Garellick G, Malchau H, Herberts P, Hansson E, Axelsson H, Hansson T: Life expectancy and cost utility after total hip replacement. *Clin Orthop* 1998;346:141-151.

2. Charnley J: The long-term results of low-friction arthroplasty of the hip performed as a primary intervention. *J Bone Joint Surg Br* 1972;54:61-76.

3. Older J: Charnley low-friction arthroplasty: A worldwide retrospective review at 15 to 20 years. *J Arthroplasty* 2002;17:675-680.

4. Wroblewski BM: 15-21-year results of the Charnley low-friction arthroplasty. *Clin Orthop* 1986;211:30-35.

5. Havelin LI, Engesaeter LB, Espehaug B, Furnes O, Lie SA, Vollset SE: The Norwegian Arthroplasty Register: 11 years and 73,000 arthroplasties. *Acta Orthop Scand* 2000;71:337-353.

6. Malchau H, Soderman P, Herberts P: Abstract: Swedish hip registry. Results with 20-year follow up with validation clinically and radiographically. *67th Annual Meeting Proceedings*. Rosemont, IL, American Academy of Orthopaedic Surgeons, 2000, p 276.

7. Silva M, Shepherd EF, Jackson WO, Dorey FJ, Schmalzried TP: Average patient walking activity approaches 2 million cycles per year: Pedometers under-record walking activity. *J Arthroplasty* 2002;17:693-697.

8. Schmalzried TP, Shepherd EF, Dorey FJ, et al: Wear is a function of use, not time. *Clin Orthop* 2000;381:36-46.

9. Berger RA, Jacobs JJ, Quigley LR, Rosenberg AG, Galante JO: Primary cementless acetabular reconstruction in patients younger than 50 years old: 7- to 11-year results. *Clin Orthop* 1997; 344:216-226.

10. Kim YH, Oh SH, Kim JS: Primary total hip arthroplasty with a second-generation cementless total hip prosthesis in patients younger than fifty years of age. *J Bone Joint Surg Am* 2003;85:109-114.

11. Devitt A, O'Sullivan T, Quinlan W: 16- to 25-year follow-up study of cemented arthroplasty of the hip in patients aged 50 years or younger. *J Arthroplasty* 1997;12:479-489.

12. Callaghan JJ, Forest EE, Olejniczak JP, Goetz DD, Johnston RC: Charnley total hip arthroplasty in patients less than fifty years old: A twenty to twenty-five-year follow-up note. *J Bone Joint Surg Am* 1998;80:704-714.

13. Dumbleton JH, Manley MT, Edidin AA: A literature review of the association between wear rate and osteolysis in total hip arthroplasty. *J Arthroplasty* 2002;17: 649-661.

14. Dorr LD, Kane TJ III, Conaty JP: Long-term results of cemented total hip arthroplasty in patients 45 years old or younger: A 16-year follow-up study. *J Arthroplasty* 1994;9:453-456.

15. Sullivan PM, MacKenzie JR, Callaghan JJ, Johnston RC: Total hip arthroplasty with cement in patients who are less than fifty years old: A sixteen to twenty-two-year follow-up study. *J Bone Joint Surg Am* 1994;76:863-869.

16. Collis DK: Long-term (twelve to eighteen-year) follow-up of cemented total hip replacements in patients who were less than fifty years old: A follow-up note. *J Bone Joint Surg Am* 1991; 73:593-597.

17. Duffy GP, Berry DJ, Rowland C, Cabanela ME: Primary uncemented total hip arthroplasty in patients < 40 years old: 10- to 14-year results using first-generation proximally porous-coated implants. *J Arthroplasty* 2001;16:140-144.

18. Hamadouche M, Boutin P, Daussange J, Bolander ME, Sedel L: Alumina-on-alumina total hip arthroplasty: A minimum 18.5-year follow-up study. *J Bone Joint Surg Am* 2002;84:69-77.

19. Engh CA, Hopper RH Jr: Porous-coated total hip arthroplasty in the young. *Orthopedics* 1998;21:953-956.

20. Engh CA Jr, Claus AM, Hopper RH Jr, Engh CA: Long-term results using the

anatomic medullary locking hip prosthesis. *Clin Orthop* 2001;393:137-146.

21. Hartley WT, McAuley JP, Culpepper WJ, Engh CA Jr, Engh CA Sr: Osteonecrosis of the femoral head treated with cementless total hip arthroplasty. *J Bone Joint Surg Am* 2000;82:1408-1413.

22. Bauer TW: Particles and periimplant bone resorption. *Clin Orthop* 2002;405:138-143.

23. Bohler M, Kanz F, Schwarz B, et al: Adverse tissue reactions to wear particles from Co-alloy articulations, increased by alumina-blasting particle contamination from cementless Ti-based total hip implants: A report of seven revisions with early failure. *J Bone Joint Surg Br* 2002;84:128-136.

24. Harris WH: The problem is osteolysis. *Clin Orthop* 1995;311:46-53.

25. Doorn PF, Campbell PA, Amstutz HC: Metal versus polyethylene wear particles in total hip replacements: A review. *Clin Orthop* 1996;329(suppl):S206-S216.

26. Yoon TR, Rowe SM, Jung ST, Seon KJ, Maloney WJ: Osteolysis in association with a total hip arthroplasty with ceramic bearing surfaces. *J Bone Joint Surg Am* 1998;80:1459-1468.

27. Schmalzried TP, Jasty M, Rosenberg A, Harris WH: Polyethylene wear debris and tissue reactions in knee as compared to hip replacement prostheses. *J Appl Biomater* 1994;5:185-190.

28. Schmalzried TP, Callaghan JJ: Wear in total hip and knee replacements. *J Bone Joint Surg Am* 1999;81:115-136.

29. McKellop H, Shen FW, Lu B, Campbell P, Salovey R: Development of an extremely wear resistant ultra high molecular weight polyethylene for total hip replacements. *J Orthop Res* 1999;17:157-167.

30. McKellop HA, Campbell P, Park SH, et al: The origin of submicron polyethylene wear debris in total hip arthroplasty. *Clin Orthop* 1995;311:3-20.

31. Dowson D: A comparative study of the performance of metallic and ceramic femoral head components in total replacement hip joints. *Wear* 1995;190:171-183.

32. Medley JB, Bobyn JD, Krygier JJ, Chan FW, Tanzer M, Roter GE: Elastohydrodynamic lubrication and wear of metal-on-metal hip implants, in Rieker C, Oberholzer S, Wyss U (eds): *World Tribology Forum in Arthroplasty*. Bern, Switzerland, Hans Huber, 2001, pp 125-136.

33. Dowson D: New joints for the Millennium: Wear control in total replacement hip joints. *Proc Inst Mech Eng [H]* 2001;215:335-358.

34. Schey JA: Systems view of optimizing metal on metal bearings. *Clin Orthop* 1996;329(suppl):S115-S127.

35. *Plastics and Polyolefins: Petrothene polyolefins. A Processing Guide.* New York, NY, National Distillers and Chemical Corporation, 1965, pp 6-12.

36. Kurtz SM, Muratoglu OK, Evans M, Edidin AA: Advances in the processing, sterilization, and crosslinking of ultra-high molecular weight polyethylene for total joint arthroplasty. *Biomaterials* 1999;20:1659-1688.

37. Ayers DC: Polyethylene wear and osteolysis following total knee replacement. *Instr Course Lect* 1997;46:205-213.

38. Li S, Burstein AH: Ultra-high molecular weight polyethylene: The material and its use in total joint implants. *J Bone Joint Surg Am* 1994;76:1080-1090.

39. Willie BM, Gingell DT, Bloebaum RD, Hofmann AA: Possible explanation for the white band artifact seen in clinically retrieved polyethylene tibial components. *J Biomed Mater Res* 2000;52:558-566.

40. Tanner MG, Whiteside LA, White SE: Effect of polyethylene quality on wear in total knee arthroplasty. *Clin Orthop* 1995;317:83-88.

41. Silva M, Schmalzried TP: Polyethylene in total knee arthroplasty, in Callaghan JJ, Rosenberg AG, Rubash HE, Simonian PT, Wickiewicz TL (eds): *The Adult Knee.* Philadelphia, PA, Lippincott Williams and Wilkins, 2003, pp 279-288.

42. Baker DA, Hastings RS, Pruitt L: Study of fatigue resistance of chemical and radiation cross-linked medical grade ultrahigh molecular weight polyethylene. *J Biomed Mater Res* 1999;46:573-581.

43. McKellop H, Shen FW, DiMaio W, Lancaster JG: Wear of gamma-cross-linked polyethylene acetabular cups against roughened femoral balls. *Clin Orthop* 1999;369:73-82.

44. Wang A, Essner A, Polineni V, Sun D, Stark C, Dumbleton J: Wear mechanisms and wear testing of ultra-high molecular weight polyethylene in total joint replacements, in *Polyethylene Wear in Orthopaedic Implants Workshop.* Minneapolis, MN, Society for Biomaterials, 1997, pp 4-18.

45. Jasty M, Bragdon C, O'Connor DO, Muratoglu O, Permnath V, Merrill E: Marker improvement in the wear resistance of a new form of UHMWPE in a physiologic hip simulator. *Trans Soc Biomater* 1997;20:157.

46. McKellop H, Shen FW, Lu B, Campbell P, Salovey R: Effect of sterilization method and other modifications on the wear resistance of acetabular cups made of ultra-high molecular weight polyethylene: A hip-simulator study. *J Bone Joint Surg Am* 2000;82:1708-1725.

47. McKellop HA, Shen FW, Campbell P, Ota T: Effect of molecular weight, calcium stearate, and sterilization methods on the wear of ultra high molecular weight polyethylene acetabular cups in a hip joint simulator. *J Orthop Res* 1999;17:329-339.

48. Rose RM, Crugnola A, Ries M, Cimino WR, Paul I, Radin EL: On the origins of high in vivo wear rates in polyethylene components of total joint prostheses. *Clin Orthop* 1979;145:277-286.

49. Sutula LC, Collier JP, Saum KA, et al: Impact of gamma sterilization on clinical performance of polyethylene in the hip. *Clin Orthop* 1995;319:28-40.

50. Collier JP, Sperling DK, Currier JH, Sutula LC, Saum KA, Mayor MB: Impact of gamma sterilization on clinical performance of polyethylene in the knee. *J Arthroplasty* 1996;11:377-389.

51. McKellop H, Shen F, Yu Y, Lu B, Salovey R, Campbell P: Effect of sterilization method and other modifications on the wear resistance of UHMWPE acetabular cups, in *Polyethylene Wear in Orthopaedic Implants Workshop.* Minneapolis, MN, Society for Biomaterials, 1997, pp 20-31.

52. Shen FW, McKellop HA: Interaction of oxidation and crosslinking in gamma-irradiated ultrahigh molecular-weight polyethylene. *J Biomed Mater Res* 2002;61:430-439.

53. McKellop HA: Bearing surfaces in total hip replacements: State of the art and future developments. *Instr Course Lect* 2001;50:165-179.

54. Morrey BF, Ilstrup D: Size of the femoral head and acetabular revision in total hip-replacement arthroplasty. *J Bone Joint Surg Am* 1989;71:50-55.

55. Schmalzried TP, Kwong LM, Jasty M, et al: The mechanism of loosening of cemented acetabular components in total hip arthroplasty: Analysis of specimens retrieved at autopsy. *Clin Orthop* 1992;274:60-78.

56. Cates HE, Faris PM, Keating EM, Ritter MA: Polyethylene wear in cemented metal-backed acetabular cups. *J Bone Joint Surg Br* 1993;75:249-253.

57. Schmalzried TP, Guttmann D, Grecula M, Amstutz HC: The relationship between the design, position, and articular wear of acetabular components inserted without cement and the development of pelvic osteolysis. *J Bone Joint Surg Am* 1994;76:677-688.

58. Nashed RS, Becker DA, Gustilo RB: Are cementless acetabular components the cause of excess wear and osteolysis in total hip arthroplasty? *Clin Orthop* 1995;317:19-28.

59. Schmalzried TP, Jasty M, Harris WH: Periprosthetic bone loss in total hip arthroplasty: Polyethylene wear debris and the concept of the effective joint space. *J Bone Joint Surg Am* 1992;74:849-863.

60. Wroblewski BM, Siney PD, Dowson D, Collins SN: Prospective clinical and joint simulator studies of a new total hip arthroplasty using alumina ceramic heads and cross-linked polyethylene cups. *J Bone Joint Surg Br* 1996;78:280-285.

61. Devane PA, Horne JG: Assessment of polyethylene wear in total hip replacement. *Clin Orthop* 1999;369:59-72.

62. Grobbelaar CJ, Weber FA, Spirakis A, Du Plessis TA, Cappaert G, Cakic JN: Clinical experience with gamma irradiation-crosslinked polyethylene: A 14 to 20 year follow-up report. *J Bone Joint Surg* 1999;9(suppl):140-147.

63. Oonishi H, Kadoya Y, Masuda S: Gammairradiated cross-linked polyethylene in total hip replacements: Analysis of retrieved sockets after long-term implantation. *J Biomed Mater Res* 2001;58:167-171.

64. Sakoda H, Voice AM, McEwen HM, et al: A comparison of the wear and physical properties of silane cross-linked polyethylene and ultra-high molecular weight polyethylene. *J Arthroplasty* 2001;16:1018-1023.

65. Martell J, Edidin A, Dumbleton J: Preclinical evaluation followed by randomized clinical study of a crosslinked polyethylene for total hip arthroplasty at two year follow-up. *Trans Orthop Res Soc* 2001;26:163.

66. Martell JM, Berdia S: Determination of polyethylene wear in total hip replacements with use of digital radiographs. *J Bone Joint Surg Am* 1997;79:1635-1641.

67. Martell JM, Incavo SJ: Clinical performance of a highly crosslinked polyethylene at two years in total hip arthroplasty: A randomized prospective trial. *Trans Orthop Res Soc* 2003;28:1431.

68. Digas G, Karrholm J, Malchau H, et al: RSA evaluation of wear of conventional versus highly cross-linked polyethylene acetabular components in vivo. *Trans Orthop Res Soc* 2003;28:1430.

69. Campbell P, Ma S, Yeom B, McKellop H, Schmalzried TP, Amstutz HC: Isolation of predominantly submicron-sized UHMWPE wear particles from periprosthetic tissues. *J Biomed Mater Res* 1995;29:127-131.

70. Hirakawa K, Bauer TW, Stulberg BN, Wilde AH: Comparison and quantitation of wear debris of failed total hip and total knee arthroplasty. *J Biomed Mater Res* 1996;31:257-263.

71. Maloney WJ, Smith RL, Schmalzried TP, Chiba J, Huene D, Rubash H: Isolation and characterization of wear particles generated in patients who have had failure of a hip arthroplasty without cement. *J Bone Joint Surg Am* 1995;77:1301-1310.

72. Margevicius KJ, Bauer TW, McMahon JT, Brown SA, Merritt K: Isolation and characterization of debris in membranes around total joint prostheses. *J Bone Joint Surg Am* 1994;76:1664-1675.

73. Shanbhag AS, Jacobs JJ, Glant TT, Gilbert JL, Black J, Galante JO: Composition and morphology of wear debris in failed uncemented total hip replacement. *J Bone Joint Surg Br* 1994;76:60-67.

74. Hirakawa K, Bauer TW, Stulberg BN, Wilde AH, Borden LS: Characterization of debris adjacent to failed knee implants of 3 different designs. *Clin Orthop* 1996;331:151-158.

75. Tipper JL, Ingham E, Hailey JL, et al: Quantitative comparison of polyethylene wear debris, wear rate and head damage in retrieved hip prostheses. *Trans Orthop Res Soc* 1997;22:355.

76. Schmalzried TP, Campbell P: Isolation and characterization of debris in membranes around total joint prostheses. *J Bone Joint Surg Am* 1995;77:1625-1626.

77. Schmalzried TP, Campbell P, Schmitt AK, Brown IC, Amstutz HC: Shapes and dimensional characteristics of polyethylene wear particles generated in vivo by total knee replacements compared to total hip replacements. *J Biomed Mater Res* 1997;38:203-210.

78. Ries MD, Scott ML, Jani S: Relationship between gravimetric wear and particle generation in hip simulators: Conventional compared with cross-linked polyethylene. *J Bone Joint Surg Am* 2001;83(suppl 2):116-122.

79. Endo M, Tipper JL, Barton DC, Stone MH, Ingham E, Fisher J: Comparison of wear, wear debris and biological activity of moderately crosslinked and non-crosslinked polyethylenes in hip prostheses. *Proc Inst Mech Eng [H]* 2002;216:111-122.

80. Illgen RL, Laurent MP, Watanuki M, et al: Highly crosslinked vs. conventional polyethylene particles: An in vitro comparison of biologic activities. *Trans Orthop Res Soc* 2003;28:1438.

81. Ingram JH, Fisher J, Stone M, Ingham E: Effect of crosslinking on biological activity of UHMWPE wear debris. *Trans Orthop Res Soc* 2003;28:1439.

82. Ingram J, Matthews JB, Tipper J, Stone M, Fisher J, Ingham E: Comparison of the biological activity of grade GUR 1120 and GUR 415HP UHMWPE wear debris. *Biomed Mater Eng* 2002;12:177-188.

83. Yang SY, Ren W, Park Y, et al: Diverse cellular and apoptotic responses to variant shapes of UHMWPE particles in a murine model of inflammation. *Biomaterials* 2002;23:3535-3543.

84. Skinner HB: Ceramic bearing surfaces. *Clin Orthop* 1999;369:83-91.

85. Cuckler JM, Bearcroft J, Asgian CM: Femoral head technologies to reduce polyethylene wear in total hip arthroplasty. *Clin Orthop* 1995;317:57-63.

86. Kim YH, Kim JS, Cho SH: A comparison of polyethylene wear in hips with cobalt-chrome or zirconia heads: A prospective, randomised study. *J Bone Joint Surg Br* 2001;83:742-750.

87. Sychterz CJ, Engh CA Jr, Young AM, Hopper RH Jr, Engh CA: Comparison of in vivo wear between polyethylene liners articulating with ceramic and cobalt-chrome femoral heads. *J Bone Joint Surg Br* 2000;82:948-951.

88. Bigsby RJ, Hardaker CS, Fisher J: Wear of ultrahigh molecular weight polyethylene acetabular cups in a physiological hip joint simulator in the anatomical position using bovine serum as a lubricant. *Proc Inst Mech Eng [H]* 1997;211:265-269.

89. Oonishi H, Wakitani S, Murata N, et al: Clinical experience with ceramics in total

hip replacement. *Clin Orthop* 2000; 379:77-84.

90. Clarke IC, Gustafson A: Clinical and hip simulator comparisons of ceramic-on-polyethylene and metal-on-polyethylene wear. *Clin Orthop* 2000;379:34-40.

91. Zichner LP, Willert HG: Comparison of alumina-polyethylene and metal-polyethylene in clinical trials. *Clin Orthop* 1992;282:86-94.

92. Willmann G: Ceramic femoral head retrieval data. *Clin Orthop* 2000;379:22-28.

93. Heck DA, Partridge CM, Reuben JD, Lanzer WL, Lewis CG, Keating EM: Prosthetic component failures in hip arthroplasty surgery. *J Arthroplasty* 1995;10:575-580.

94. Lu Z, McKellop H: Frictional heating of bearing materials tested in a hip joint wear simulator. *Proc Inst Mech Eng [H]* 1997;211:101-108.

95. Affatato S, Goldoni M, Testoni M, Toni A: Mixed oxides prosthetic ceramic ball heads: Part 3. Effect of the ZrO2 fraction on the wear of ceramic on ceramic hip joint prostheses: A long-term in vitro wear study. *Biomaterials* 2001;22:717-723.

96. Affatato S, Testoni M, Cacciari GL, Toni A: Mixed-oxides prosthetic ceramic ball heads: Part 2. Effect of the ZrO2 fraction on the wear of ceramic on ceramic joints. *Biomaterials* 1999;20:1925-1929.

97. Schmalzried TP, Peters PC, Maurer BT, Bragdon CR, Harris WH: Long-duration metal-on-metal total hip arthroplasties with low wear of the articulating surfaces. *J Arthroplasty* 1996;11:322-331.

98. Schmalzried TP, Szuszczewicz ES, Akizuki KH, Petersen TD, Amstutz HC: Factors correlating with long term survival of McKee-Farrar total hip prostheses. *Clin Orthop* 1996; 329(suppl):S48-S59.

99. Amstutz HC, Grigoris P: Metal on metal bearings in hip arthroplasty. *Clin Orthop* 1996;329(suppl):S11-S34.

100. Amstutz HC: History of metal-on-metal articulations including surface arthroplasty of the hip, in Rieker C, Oberholzer S, Wyss U (eds): *World Tribology Forum in Arthroplasty*. Bern, Switzerland, Hans Huber, 2001, pp 113-123.

101. Jacobsson SA, Djerf K, Wahlstrom O: Twenty-year results of McKee-Farrar versus Charnley prosthesis. *Clin Orthop* 1996;329(suppl):S60-S68.

102. Zahiri CA, Schmalzried TP, Ebramzadeh E, et al: Lessons learned from loosening of the McKee-Farrar metal-on-metal total hip replacement. *J Arthroplasty* 1999;14:326-332.

103. August AC, Aldam CH, Pynsent PB: The McKee-Farrar hip arthroplasty: A long-term study. *J Bone Joint Surg Br* 1986;68:520-527.

104. Visuri T: Long-term results and survivorship of the McKee-Farrar total hip prosthesis. *Arch Orthop Trauma Surg* 1987;106:368-374.

105. Ahnfelt L, Herberts P, Malchau H, Andersson GB: Prognosis of total hip replacement: A Swedish multicenter study of 4,664 revisions. *Acta Orthop Scand Suppl* 1990;238:1-26.

106. Jacobsson SA, Djerf K, Wahlstrom O: A comparative study between McKee-Farrar and Charnley arthroplasty with long-term follow-up periods. *J Arthroplasty* 1990;5:9-14.

107. Higuchi F, Inoue A, Semlitsch M: Metal-on-metal CoCrMo McKee-Farrar total hip arthroplasty: Characteristics from a long-term follow-up study. *Arch Orthop Trauma Surg* 1997;116:121-124.

108. Brown SR, Davies WA, DeHeer DH, Swanson AB: Long-term survival of McKee-Farrar total hip prostheses. *Clin Orthop* 2002;402:157-163.

109. Schmidt M, Weber H, Schon R: Cobalt chromium molybdenum metal combination for modular hip prostheses. *Clin Orthop* 1996;329(suppl):S35-S47.

110. McKellop H, Park SH, Chiesa R, et al: In vivo wear of three types of metal on metal hip prostheses during two decades of use. *Clin Orthop* 1996; 329(suppl):S128-S140.

111. Anissian HL, Stark A, Gustafson A, Good V, Clarke IC: Metal-on-metal bearing in hip prosthesis generates 100-fold less wear debris than metal-on-polyethylene. *Acta Orthop Scand* 1999;70:578-582.

112. Clarke IC, Good V, Williams P, et al: Ultra-low wear rates for rigid-on-rigid bearings in total hip replacements. *Proc Inst Mech Eng [H]* 2000;214:331-347.

113. Brill W: Comparison of different bearing surfaces in new and retrieved total hip prostheses, in Rieker C, Oberholzer S, Wyss U (eds): *World Tribology Forum in Arthroplasty*. Bern, Switzerland, Hans Huber, 2001, pp 105-109.

114. Firkins PJ, Tipper JL, Ingham E, Stone MH, Farrar R, Fisher J: A novel low wearing differential hardness, ceramic-on-metal hip joint prosthesis. *J Biomech* 2001;34:1291-1298.

115. Greenwald AS, Garino JP: Alternative bearing surfaces: The good, the bad, and the ugly. *J Bone Joint Surg Am* 2001;83(suppl 2):68-72.

116. Rieker C, Shen M, Kottig P: In-vivo tribological performance of 177 metal-on-metal hip articulations, in Rieker C, Oberholzer S, Wyss U (eds): *World Tribology Forum in Arthroplasty*. Bern, Switzerland, Hans Huber, 2001, pp 137-142.

117. Scholes SC, Green SM, Unsworth A: The wear of metal-on-metal total hip prostheses measured in a hip simulator. *Proc Inst Mech Eng [H]* 2001;215:523-530.

118. Müller ME: The benefits of metal-on-metal total hip replacements. *Clin Orthop* 1995;311:54-59.

119. Weber BG: Experience with the Metasul total hip bearing system. *Clin Orthop* 1996;329(suppl):S69-S77.

120. Wagner M, Wagner H: Medium-term results of a modern metal-on-metal system in total hip replacement. *Clin Orthop* 2000;379:123-133.

121. Hilton KR, Dorr LD, Wan Z, McPherson EJ: Contemporary total hip replacement with metal on metal articulation. *Clin Orthop* 1996;329(suppl):S99-S105.

122. Schmalzried TP, Fowble VA, Ure KJ, Amstutz HC: Metal on metal surface replacement of the hip: Technique, fixation, and early results. *Clin Orthop* 1996;329(suppl):S106-S114.

123. Wagner M, Wagner H: Preliminary results of uncemented metal on metal stemmed and resurfacing hip replacement arthroplasty. *Clin Orthop* 1996;329(suppl):S78-S88.

124. Silva M, Schmalzried TP: Alternate bearing materials: Metal-on-metal, in Shanbhag A, Rubash HE, Jacobs JJ (eds): *Joint Replacements and Bone Resorption: Pathology, Biomaterials and Clinical Practice*. New York, NY, Marcel Dekker, 2003, in press.

125. Smith SL, Dowson D, Goldsmith AA: The effect of diametral clearances, motion and loading cycles upon lubrication of metal-on-metal hip replacements. *Proc Inst Mech Eng [C]* 2001;215:1-5.

126. Iida H, Kaneda E, Takada H, Uchida K, Kawanabe K, Nakamura T: Metallosis due to impingement between the socket and the femoral neck in a metal-on-metal bearing total hip prosthesis: A case report. *J Bone Joint Surg Am* 1999;81:400-403.

127. Sieber HP, Rieker CB, Kottig P: Analysis of 118 second-generation metal-on-metal retrieved hip implants. *J Bone Joint Surg Br* 1999;81:46-50.

128. Beaulé PE, Campbell P, Mirra J, Hooper JC, Schmalzried TP: Osteolysis in a cementless, second generation metal-on-metal hip replacement. *Clin Orthop* 2001;386:159-165.

129. Schmalzried TP, Akizuki KH, Fedenko AN, Mirra J: The role of access of joint fluid to bone in periarticular osteolysis: A report of four cases. *J Bone Joint Surg Am* 1997;79:447-452.

130. Dorr LD, Wan Z, Longjohn DB, Dubois B, Murken R: Total hip arthroplasty with use of the Metasul metal-on-metal articulation: Four to seven-year results. *J Bone Joint Surg Am* 2000;82:789-798.

131. Doorn PF, Campbell PA, Worrall J, Benya PD, McKellop HA, Amstutz HC: Metal wear particle characterization from metal on metal total hip replacements: Transmission electron microscopy study of periprosthetic tissues and isolated particles. *J Biomed Mater Res* 1998;42:103-111.

132. Hanlon J, Ozuna R, Shortkroff S, Sledge CB, Thornhill TS, Spector M: Analysis of metallic wear debris retrieved at revision arthroplasty, in *Implant Retrieval Symposium of The Society for Biomaterials*. St. Charles, IL, Society for Biomaterials, 1992.

133. Doorn PF, Mirra JM, Campbell PA, Amstutz HC: Tissue reaction to metal on metal total hip prostheses. *Clin Orthop* 1996;329(suppl):S187-S205.

134. Merritt K, Brown SA: Distribution of cobalt chromium wear and corrosion products and biologic reactions. *Clin Orthop* 1996;329(suppl):S233-S243.

135. Shanbhag AS, Jacobs JJ, Black J, Galante JO, Glant TT: Macrophage particle interactions: Effect of size, composition and surface area. *J Biomed Mater Res* 1994;28:81-90.

136. MacDonald SJ, McCalden RW, Chess DG, et al: Metal-on-metal versus polyethylene in hip arthroplasty: A randomized clinical trial. *Clin Orthop* 2003;406:282-296.

137. Archibeck MJ, Jacobs JJ, Black J: Alternate bearing surfaces in total joint arthroplasty: Biologic considerations. *Clin Orthop* 2000;379:12-21.

138. Jacobs JJ, Urban RM, Gilbert JL, et al: Local and distant products from modularity. *Clin Orthop* 1995;319:94-105.

139. Shea KG, Lundeen GA, Bloebaum RD, Bachus KN, Zou L: Lymphoreticular dissemination of metal particles after primary joint replacements. *Clin Orthop* 1997;338:219-226.

140. Urban RM, Jacobs JJ, Tomlinson MJ, Black J, Turner TM, Galante JO: Particles of metal alloys and their corrosion products in the liver, spleen and para-aortic lymph nodes of patients with total hip replacement prostheses. *Trans Orthop Res Soc* 1995;20:241.

141. Urban RM, Jacobs JJ, Tomlinson MJ, Gavrilovic J, Black J, Peoc'h M: Dissemination of wear particles to the liver, spleen, and abdominal lymph nodes of patients with hip or knee replacement. *J Bone Joint Surg Am* 2000;82:457-476.

142. Firkins PJ, Tipper JL, Saadatzadeh MR, et al: Quantitative analysis of wear and wear debris from metal-on-metal hip prostheses tested in a physiological hip joint simulator. *Biomed Mater Eng* 2001;11:143-157.

143. Willert HG, Buchhorn GH, Fayyazi A, Lohmann CH: Histopathological changes in tissues surrounding metal/metal joints: Signs of delayed type hypersensitivity (DTH)?, in Rieker C, Oberholzer S, Wyss U (eds): *World Tribology Forum in Arthroplasty*. Bern, Switzerland, Hans Huber, 2001, pp 147-166.

144. Willert H-G, Buchhorn GH, Fayyazi A, Lohmann CN: Histopathological changes around metal/metal joints indicate delayed type hypersensitivity: Primary results of 14 cases. *Osteologie* 2000;9:2-16.

145. Al-Saffar N: Early clinical failure of total joint replacement in association with follicular proliferation of B-lymphocytes: A report of two cases. *J Bone Joint Surg Am* 2002;84:2270-2273.

146. Amstutz HC, Campbell P, McKellop H, et al: Metal on metal total hip replacement workshop consensus document. *Clin Orthop* 1996;329(suppl):S297-S303.

147. Hallab N, Merritt K, Jacobs JJ: Metal sensitivity in patients with orthopaedic implants. *J Bone Joint Surg Am* 2001;83:428-436.

148. Dowd JE, Cha CW, Trakru S, Kim SY, Yang IH, Rubash HE: Failure of total hip arthroplasty with a precoated prosthesis: 4- to 11-year results. *Clin Orthop* 1998;355:123-136.

149. Bentley G, Duthie RB: A comparative review of the McKee-Farrar and Charnley total hip prostheses. *Clin Orthop* 1973;95:127-142.

150. Elves MW, Wilson JN, Scales JT, Kemp HB: Incidence of metal sensitivity in patients with total joint replacements. *Br Med J* 1975;4:376-378.

151. Yang J, Merritt K: Detection of antibodies against corrosion products in patients after Co-Cr total joint replacements. *J Biomed Mater Res* 1994;28:1249-1258.

152. Jazrawi LM, Kummer FJ, Di Cesare PE: Hard bearing surfaces in total hip arthroplasty. *Am J Orthop* 1998;27:283-292.

153. Howie DW, Rogers SD, McGee MA, Haynes DR: Biologic effects of cobalt chrome in cell and animal models. *Clin Orthop* 1996;329(suppl):S217-S232.

154. Brown SA, Farnsworth LJ, Merritt K, Crowe TD: In vitro and in vivo metal ion release. *J Biomed Mater Res* 1988;22:321-338.

155. Merritt K, Crowe TD, Brown SA: Elimination of nickel, cobalt, and chromium following repeated injections of high dose metal salts. *J Biomed Mater Res* 1989;23:845-862.

156. Clark CR: A potential concern in total joint arthroplasty: Systemic dissemination of wear debris. *J Bone Joint Surg Am* 2000;82:455-456.

157. Dobbs HS, Minski MJ: Metal ion release after total hip replacement. *Biomaterials* 1980;1:193-198.

158. Case CP, Langkamer VG, James C, et al: Widespread dissemination of metal debris from implants. *J Bone Joint Surg Br* 1994;76:701-712.

159. Lidor C, McDonald JW, Roggli VL, Vail TP: Wear particles in bilateral internal iliac lymph nodes after loosening of a painless unilateral cemented total hip arthroplasty. *J Urol* 1996;156:1775-1776.

160. Jacobs JJ, Hallab NJ, Urban R, Skipor A: Systemic implications of total joint replacement, in Rieker C, Oberholzer S, Wyss U (eds): *World Tribology Forum in Arthroplasty*. Bern, Switzerland, Hans Huber, 2001, pp 77-82.

161. Visuri T, Koskenvuo M: Cancer risk after Mckee-Farrar total hip replacement. *Orthopedics* 1991; 14:137-142.

162. Visuri T, Pukkala E: Does metal-on-metal total hip prosthesis have influence on cancer?, in Rieker C, Oberholzer S, Wyss U (eds): *World Tribology Forum in Arthroplasty*. Bern, Switzerland, Hans Huber, 2001, pp 181-187.

163. Visuri T, Pukkala E, Paavolainen P, Pulkkinen P, Riska EB: Cancer risk after metal on metal and polyethylene on metal total hip arthroplasty. *Clin Orthop* 1996;329(suppl):S280-S289.

164. Tharani R, Dorey FJ, Schmalzried TP: The risk of cancer following total hip or knee arthroplasty. *J Bone Joint Surg Am* 2001;83:774-780.

165. Mahomed NN, Barrett JA, Katz JN, et al: Rates and outcomes of primary and revision total hip replacement in the United States medicare population. *J Bone Joint Surg Am* 2003;85:27-32.

166. Boutin P, Christel P, Dorlot JM, et al: The use of dense alumina-alumina ceramic combination in total hip replacement. *J Biomed Mater Res* 1988;22:1203-1232.

167. Clarke IC: Role of ceramic implants: Design and clinical success with total hip prosthetic ceramic-to-ceramic bearings. *Clin Orthop* 1992;282:19-30.

168. Winter M, Griss P, Scheller G, Moser T: Ten- to 14-year results of a ceramic hip prosthesis. *Clin Orthop* 1992;282:73-80.

169. Bierbaum BE, Nairus J, Kuesis D, Morrison JC, Ward D: Ceramic-on-ceramic bearings in total hip arthroplasty. *Clin Orthop* 2002;405:158-163.

170. Bizot P, Nizard R, Lerouge S, Prudhommeaux F, Sedel L: Ceramic/ceramic total hip arthroplasty. *J Orthop Sci* 2000;5:622-627.

171. Sedel L: Evolution of alumina-on-alumina implants: A review. *Clin Orthop* 2000;379:48-54.

172. Mittlemeier H: Abstract: Eight years of clinical experience with self-locking ceramic hip prosthesis, "Autophor." *J Bone Joint Surg Br* 1984;66:300.

173. Mittelmeier H, Heisel J: Sixteen-years' experience with ceramic hip prostheses. *Clin Orthop* 1992;282:64-72.

174. Mahoney OM, Dimon JH III: Unsatisfactory results with a ceramic total hip prosthesis. *J Bone Joint Surg Am* 1990;72:663-671.

175. Nizard RS, Sedel L, Christel P, Meunier A, Soudry M, Witvoet J: Ten-year survivorship of cemented ceramic-ceramic total hip prosthesis. *Clin Orthop* 1992;282:53-63.

176. Bizot P, Banallec L, Sedel L, Nizard R: Alumina-on-alumina total hip prostheses in patients 40 years of age or younger. *Clin Orthop* 2000;379:68-76.

177. Jazrawi LM, Bogner E, Della Valle CJ, et al: Wear rates of ceramic-on-ceramic bearing surfaces in total hip implants: A 12-year follow-up study. *J Arthroplasty* 1999;14:781-787.

178. Prudhommeaux F, Hamadouche M, Nevelos J, Doyle C, Meunier A, Sedel L: Wear of alumina-on-alumina total hip arthroplasties at a mean 11-year follow-up. *Clin Orthop* 2000;379:113-122.

179. Boehler M, Plenk H Jr, Salzer M: Alumina ceramic bearings for hip endoprostheses: The Austrian experiences. *Clin Orthop* 2000;379:85-93.

180. Garino JP: Modern ceramic-on-ceramic total hip systems in the United States: Early results. *Clin Orthop* 2000;379:41-47.

181. D'Antonio J, Capello W: Alumina ceramic bearings for total hip arthroplasty. *Semin Arthroplasty*, in press.

182. D'Antonio J, Capello W, Manley M, Bierbaum B: New experience with alumina-on-alumina ceramic bearings for total hip arthroplasty. *J Arthroplasty* 2002;17:390-397.

183. Christel PS: Biocompatibility of surgical-grade dense polycrystalline alumina. *Clin Orthop* 1992;282:10-18.

184. Hatton A, Nevelos JE, Nevelos AA, Banks RE, Fisher J, Ingham E: Alumina-alumina artificial hip joints: Part I. A histological analysis and characterisation of wear debris by laser capture microdissection of tissues retrieved at revision. *Biomaterials* 2002;23:3429-3440.

185. Wirganowicz PZ, Thomas BJ: Massive osteolysis after ceramic on ceramic total hip arthroplasty: A case report. *Clin Orthop* 1997;338:100-104.

186. Hatton A, Nevelos JE, Matthews JB, Fisher J, Ingham E: Effects of clinically relevant alumina ceramic wear particles on TNF-alpha production by human peripheral blood mononuclear phagocytes. *Biomaterials* 2003;24:1193-1204.

187. Lohmann CH, Dean DD, Koster G, et al: Ceramic and PMMA particles differentially affect osteoblast phenotype. *Biomaterials* 2002; 23:1855-1863.

188. Germain MA, Hatton A, Williams S, et al: Comparison of the cytotoxicity of clinically relevant cobalt-chromium and alumina ceramic wear particles in vitro. *Biomaterials* 2003;24:469-479.

189. Bos I, Willmann G: Morphologic characteristics of periprosthetic tissues from hip prostheses with ceramic-ceramic couples: A comparative histologic investigation of 18 revision and 30 autopsy cases. *Acta Orthop Scand* 2001;72:335-342.

Soft-Tissue Balancing of the Hip: The Role of Femoral Offset Restoration

Mark N. Charles, MD
Robert B. Bourne, MD
J. Roderick Davey, MD
A. Seth Greenwald, D. Phil. (Oxon)
Bernard F. Morrey, MD
Cecil H. Rorabeck, MD

Abstract

Inadequate soft-tissue balancing is a major yet often underemphasized cause of failure for primary and revision total hip arthroplasty. Accordingly, contemporary cemented and cementless hip prostheses have been designed with consideration of this issue, and this has substantially increased the long-term survival of total hip replacements. Therefore, it is important for orthopaedic surgeons to be familiar with the rationale, biomechanical principles, and clinical implications associated with soft-tissue balancing of the hip as well as strategies to avoid inadequate soft-tissue balancing and systematic techniques to restore adequate soft-tissue tensioning during total hip arthroplasty.

Sir John Charnley was one of the first orthopaedic surgeons to address the issue of soft-tissue tensioning in total hip arthroplasty. However, it has only been over the past 10 to 15 years that the orthopaedic community has had an increasing awareness of and interest in this concept.[1-4] Charnley described the importance of restoring femoral offset by one of several methods: medializing the acetabular component, avoiding excessive anteversion of the femoral component, completing the femoral neck osteotomy at an appropriate level, maintaining a 135° neck-shaft angle, and when indicated, advancing the greater trochanter.[5] The goal of Charnley's philosophy was to increase the abductor moment arm and hence restore more normal biomechanics to the affected hip joint.

Although the concept is well understood, the precise definition of femoral offset has varied. The simplest and most frequently used measurement of femoral offset is the perpendicular distance between the center of the femoral head and a line drawn down the center of the femoral shaft (Figure 1). However, for the purpose of understanding the force alterations that occur with alteration of offset, the perpendicular distance from the line of action of the abductor muscles to the center of the femoral head is the most effective variable for the numerical calculation. The variable that is most frequently altered to effect a change in this dimension and the strongest determinant of offset is the neck-shaft angle. Traditionally, total hip implants have had a relatively high neck-shaft angle, averaging 135°, despite earlier studies[6] demonstrating the mean angle of the normal hip to be closer to 125°.

There is a large body of evidence supporting the concept that femoral offset should be restored.[5,7-9] In particular, the relationship between underrestoration of femoral offset and compromised abductor function has been well established. For example, clinical studies have demonstrated an increase in the prevalence of limp, fatigue, and dependence on walking aids when offset was not fully restored.[10-12] Furthermore, the inability to restore femoral offset adequately has been correlated with increased resultant forces across the hip joint and their associated deleterious effects on wear rates. For example, Sakalkale and associates[13] compared polyethylene wear between sides in 17 patients with bilateral replacement in whom the two components were

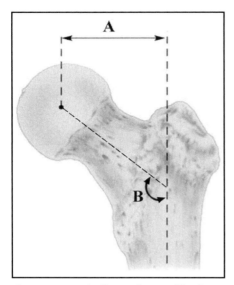

Figure 1 Femoral offset is illustrated by the perpendicular distance A from the center of the femoral head to the long axis of the femur. The neck-shaft angle is represented by angle B, which subtends the long axis of the femoral neck and the long axis of the femoral shaft.

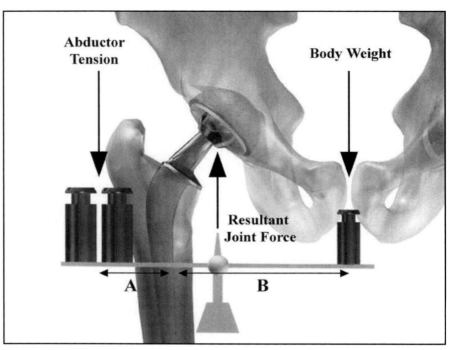

Figure 2 Illustration of the hip joint as it acts as a fulcrum balancing the force of body weight with the force generated by the hip abductors.

similar except for the offset: one hip in each patient had been replaced with a femoral prosthesis with a standard offset and the other had been replaced with a high-offset implant. At more than 5 years postoperatively, the linear wear rate averaged 0.21 mm/yr for the standard offset components and 0.01 mm/yr for the high-offset components.

Dennis and associates[14] used fluoroscopy to study in vivo the role of relevant soft-tissue structures in stabilizing the femoral head within the acetabulum. They examined 10 normal hips (five with an unconstrained total hip replacement and five with a constrained total hip replacement) while patients actively abducted the hip. Measurement of the images demonstrated no separation between the femoral head and acetabulum in the normal hips or in those with a constrained total hip replacement. However, all five patients with an unconstrained prosthesis had separation of the femoral head from the acetabulum,

which averaged 3.3 mm. The authors concluded that the soft-tissue envelope that surrounds the hip exerts a resistive force that prevents the femoral head from subluxating within the acetabulum. Therefore, preservation of these structures is important when total hip replacement is performed.[9]

Biomechanical Principles

The hip joint functions effectively as a fulcrum, resulting in a state of equilibrium between body weight and the opposing hip abductors.[5,15,16] The outcome of this interplay of opposing forces is the ability to maintain a level pelvis throughout the gait cycle.

The length of the lever arm that acts between the femoral head and the insertion of the hip abductors (A in Figure 2) is markedly smaller than that between the femoral head and body weight (B in Figure 2). Therefore, the abductors must generate a force that is larger than body weight to compensate for their mechani-

cal disadvantage. Gait analyses and free body diagrams have shown this discordant biomechanical relationship to translate into significantly higher ($P < 0.05$) joint-reaction forces in total hip replacements without restoration of femoral offset.[17] Conversely, an increase in femoral offset increases the lever arm of the abductor muscles, thereby reducing the abductor muscle force required for normal gait. This in turn minimizes the resultant reactive force across the hip joint and hence results in lower rates of polyethylene wear. Furthermore, the lateralized position of the femoral shaft relative to the hip center tends to decrease the prevalence of femoropelvic impingement while concomitantly improving soft-tissue tensioning (Figure 3).

In view of these facts, an understanding of the forces that act across the hip joint provides the surgeon with the capacity to address the factors that may contribute to inadequate soft-tissue tensioning during total hip replacement.

Femoral Offset

The shape and geometry of the proximal part of the femur have been studied by several investigators.[6,18] In a study of 50 consecutive patients scheduled for total hip arthroplasty, Davey[19] obtained standard radiographs of the hip, applied templates, and measured femoral offset after adjustment for magnification. The average offset was 43.9 mm, but the range was 27 to 57 mm. These results are consistent with others reported in the literature.[4,6,16,20]

Several factors determine the amount of offset of the femur. Large femora tend to have more offset than smaller ones. Noble and associates[6] found the average neck-shaft angle to be 124.7°, with a range of 105.7° to 154.5°. They concluded that hips with a varus neck-shaft angle tend to have greater femoral offset and hips with a valgus neck-shaft angle tend to have less femoral offset.

Offset of a femoral component, as with offset of the native femur, can be measured from the center of rotation of the femoral head to the long axis of the stem. Femoral component offset depends on both the length of the femoral neck and the neck-shaft angle of the prosthesis.

Reduced offset in a reconstructed hip may result from use of a femoral component with less offset than was present in the native hip of the patient, from a valgus position of the femoral stem relative to the femoral shaft, or from use of a short-necked modular head. Such a decrease in femoral offset medializes the locus of the abductor muscle insertion, decreases the abductor moment arm, and therefore increases both the resultant force across the hip joint and the energy required for normal gait.

Theoretic Considerations

The effect of femoral offset has been discussed at both the theoretic and clinical levels. Despite this, there is a paucity of clinical studies in which the theoretic information has been applied in a manner

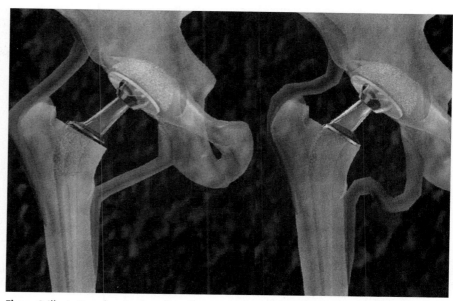

Figure 3 Illustration showing how lateralization of the femoral shaft restores offset, reduces femoropelvic impingement, and increases abductor tension.

that provides insight or offers a basis for decision making regarding surgical technique and implant design.[7] As noted previously, offset may be defined in several ways, but increasing any of the parameters mentioned above has two benefits: (1) contractile efficiency is enhanced by an increase in the resting length of the muscle, and (2) the mechanical advantage of the muscle is improved by an increase in the lever arm of muscle action.

Clinical Implications

Three aspects of the function of a joint arthroplasty are at least theoretically influenced by femoral offset. These aspects are strength, motion, and stability.

The increase in the moment created by lengthening of the functional lever arm (Figure 4) increases strength and therefore lessens the joint reactive forces. This in turn decreases rates of wear and aseptic loosening, as reported by Sakalkale and associates.[13] The increased abductor strength also decreases the prevalence of a Trendelenburg gait and enhances stability at the hip joint. The latter concept is supported by the obser-

vation of a sixfold increase in implant dislocation in association with trochanteric nonunion.[21] Finally, it has been theorized that the displacement of the femur with reference to the socket and pelvis that occurs with increased femoral offset increases motion. This lessens the likelihood of impingement and thus provides a second explanation and basis for enhanced stability.[6]

Davey and associates[22] investigated the effect of increased femoral offset on the distribution of strain in the bone and cement mantle while determining the abductor and resultant forces in a cemented total hip model. Cadaveric femora were harvested and were tested in a materials testing machine (MTS Systems, Minneapolis, MN) in a position simulating single limb stance. Static vertical loads of 600 N were applied to the femora. Abductor and resultant forces along with strain in the cement mantle and in the proximal part of the femur were recorded as offset was increased from 33 to 53 mm. When the femoral offset was increased by 10 mm, the abduction force decreased by approxi-

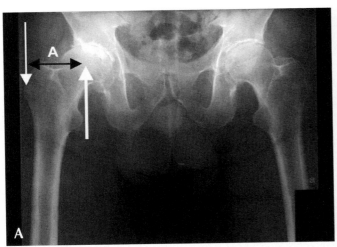
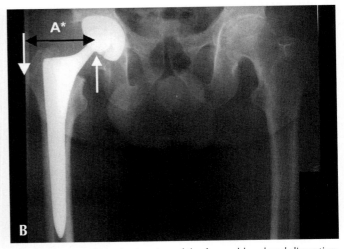

Figure 4 A, Radiograph showing severe osteoarthritis of the right hip associated with superolateral migration of the femoral head and disruption of the Shenton line (A) in a 67-year-old male patient. **B,** Radiograph of the same patient after total hip arthroplasty shows a high-offset femoral component and that the joint center has been displaced medially coincident with an increase in the abductor lever arm (A*) and a corresponding reduction in the joint reactive force.

mately 10% and this was associated with a 10% decrease in force transmission at the acetabulum. These results concur with Charnley's biomechanical calculations regarding offset.[5]

Implications With Regard to Implant Design

Manufacturers have considered the implication of precisely restoring femoral offset when designing femoral implants. An anatomic study of the proximal part of the femur indicated that if a prosthetic implant system has a single neck-shaft angle, up to 67% of patients will not have accurate restoration of the biomechanical center of the hip or femoral offset.[23] Furthermore, it was noted that eight different neck-shaft angles would have to be available to restore the anatomy accurately in only 50% of patients. The inference of this finding is that a greater variety of implant sizes might be necessary to restore proper hip balance. Noble and associates[6] called attention to the need for a greater selection of femoral shaft sizes and diameters to accommodate and restore the neck-shaft angle in a manner that approximates normal.

All of these factors influence the production and use of total hip components with regard to implant design, shape, and size variation. Clinicians should consider these variables when making decisions about implant selection and surgical technique.

Effects on the Prosthesis

The strength of the prosthesis is determined by several factors, including type of metal alloy, geometry, presence of porous coating, size, and modularity. The orthopaedic industry must test using American Society for Testing and Materials standards (ASTM, West Conshohocken, PA) and ISO standards (International Organization for Standardization, Geneva, Switzerland) to ensure that components can withstand the potential increase in forces as offset is increased. Increasing offset increases the bending moment of the implant. One factor limiting the potential to manufacture more anatomic components is the increased prevalence of fractures of prostheses with lower neck-shaft angles. This is a consequence of the higher offset, which in turn increases the bending

moment of the implant. Furthermore, the use of weaker metal alloys in first-generation implants compounded this unfavorable biomechanical relationship.[4,6,18]

To examine this issue further, Davey and associates[24] and O'Connor and associates[25] measured strain at the base of the neck of titanium prostheses with increasing offset in a cementless total hip implant model. The strain increased in a linear fashion with increases in offset. However, even at the maximum offset tested (58 mm), the stress in the titanium stem was only 27% of the fatigue stress.

The increased bending moment may also contribute to increased micromotion, which could affect bone ingrowth and the longevity of fixation of both cemented and cementless hip replacements. The effect of offset on micromotion of both cemented and cementless femoral components has been investigated in cadaveric femora.[24,25] An MTS extensometer (MTS Systems) was used to measure movement between the prosthesis and the bone in five cadaveric femora with a cementless replacement and five with a cemented implant. A static vertical load of 600 N was applied to the femora, and both axial and transverse movement of the prosthesis was recorded. Testing was performed in a position simulating single-limb stance and repeated in a position simulating stair climbing.

Micromotion in the transverse plane increased from an average of 38.3 μm with an offset of 28 mm to an average of 75.0 μm with an offset of 53 mm in the cementless model, and it increased from an average of 15.0 μm with an offset of 28 mm to an average of 23.5 μm with an offset of 53 mm in the cemented model. The increase in transverse micromotion in the stair climbing position was somewhat concerning, especially with the cementless prostheses. This increased micromotion could possibly decrease or prevent bone ingrowth, leading to early failure of the implant. However, the effect of increased offset on bone growth into a femoral component cannot be assessed in a cadaver model. The influence of the transverse motion must be studied in an in vivo model subjecting components to rotational forces and allowing osseous ingrowth.[24] Accordingly, a canine cementless total hip replacement model, with biomechanical, radiographic, and histomorphometric analyses, was used to assess the effect of increased femoral offset in vivo.[26] Right-sided cementless total hip arthroplasties were performed on 12 skeletally mature dogs randomized into two groups: those treated with a normal (17-mm) offset femoral component and those treated with an increased (22-mm) offset component. The animals were killed at 14 weeks after implantation. Proximal femoral bone strains under an axial load of 120 N were recorded, decalcified sections of the proximal part of the femora were examined, and fine-detail microradiographs were made. Increasing femoral component offset reduced the hip abductor force and hip reaction force but did not significantly affect bone strains. Radiographs showed no changes in the specimens with an increased-offset implant compared with those with a regular-offset component. Bone ingrowth also was not adversely affected by an increase in femoral offset. These biomechanical studies support the use of an increased-offset femoral component with cementless fixation.

How to Increase Femoral Offset
There are five ways to increase femoral offset. The first four are based on altering the geometry of the femoral component or the proximal femoral anatomy. They are: increasing the length of the femoral neck, decreasing the neck-shaft angle, medializing the femoral neck while concomitantly increasing femoral neck length, and trochanteric advancement. The fifth method involves alteration of the geometry of the acetabular liner. It is clear, from a clinical perspective, that the surgeon should be able to recognize the implications of the different techniques for varying offset.

Femoral Component
Increasing Neck Length
Increasing the length of the femoral neck or head increases the resting length of the hip abductors and, depending on the angle of the femoral neck, increases their contractile efficiency while concomitantly lengthening the abductor lever arm. Unfortunately, an increase in the neck length also increases the limb length, resulting in a limb-length discrepancy. This is an undesirable clinical outcome in most patients (Figure 5).

Decreasing Neck-Shaft Angle
Decreasing the neck-shaft angle reduces the height of the femoral head, and thus the limb length, while increasing offset. This construct directly increases the magnitude of the abductor lever arm. It also has the positive effect of increasing abductor tension, making the muscles more efficient. However, this change in implant dimension has the negative effect of increasing the rotational torque

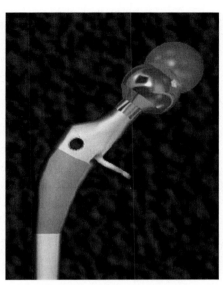

Figure 5 Illustration showing that increasing the length of the femoral neck or head increases the resting length of the hip abductors, and thereby increases their contractile efficiency while concomitantly lengthening the abductor lever arm.

imparted to the implant from out-of-plane forces. The greater varus neck-shaft angle results in an increased torsional (or out-of-plane) force that tends to rotate the femoral component, especially with activities involving load transmission during hip flexion and extension such as stair climbing. The impact of this change is calculated with the equation: $I = mr^2$, where I reflects the magnitude of the out-of-plane rotation; r is the radius, or distance, of the offset; and m is the mass or applied force. It should be noted that the offset dimension is squared, thus increasing axial torque at a rate that is greater than the rate at which abduction strength is enhanced (Figure 6).

Medializing the Femoral Neck While Concomitantly Lengthening the Femoral Neck (Dual or High-Offset Femoral Components)
Dual or high-offset femoral components either vary the neck-shaft angle of the implant or medialize the neck to vary offset. This geometry maintains the neck-

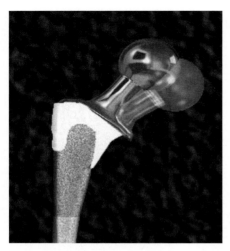

Figure 6 Illustration showing that decreasing the neck-shaft angle reduces the height of the femoral head and thus the limb length while increasing offset. This construct directly increases the magnitude of the abductor lever arm. It also has the positive effect of increasing abductor tension, making the muscles more efficient.

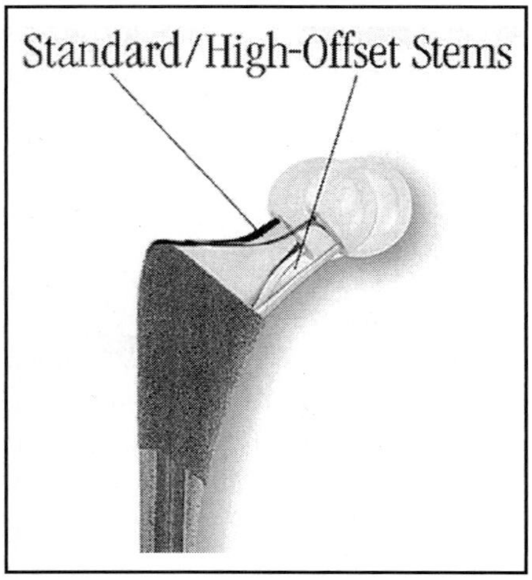

Standard/High-Offset Stems

Figure 7 Illustration comparing standard and high-offset stems. Dual or high-offset femoral components either vary the neck-shaft angle of the implant or medialize the neck to vary offset. This geometry maintains the neck-shaft angle relationship while concomitantly restoring offset.

shaft angle relationship while concomitantly restoring offset. A major advantage of this technique is that it can be used to enhance abductor tensioning without substantially affecting limb length (Figure 7). Therefore, medialization and concomitant lengthening of the femoral neck represents the basis for the dual or high-offset femoral design.

Trochanteric Osteotomy
In this instance, offset is defined as the distance from the center of the head to the attachment of the abductor muscles or as the perpendicular distance from the center of the head to the line of action of the abductor muscles. Because this definition differs from the usual definition of femoral offset, it may better be termed abductor offset. Trochanteric osteotomy provides a biomechanical advantage by laterally and distally advancing the point of insertion of the abductors. It has a positive effect in that it increases the strength of the abductors and hence decreases the likelihood of a Trendelenburg gait. The

increased mechanical advantage decreases the resultant moment arm and thus decreases the compressive force across the joint. This lessens the likelihood of wear and loosening. However, the procedure does not improve motion or lessen the likelihood of impingement.

Acetabular Component
Modular offset (lateralized) liners have been shown to increase offset while preserving limb length. The offset may be altered by modifying the relationship of the articulation at the socket so that the center of rotation at the hip is translated both laterally and inferiorly.[2] A laterally displaced socket increases the abductor tension, which is a desirable outcome. However, it also increases the body weight lever arm (Figure 2), which is considered an adverse outcome. The impact of the latter increase is greater because body weight acts at a perpendicular distance to the increments of lateral displacement. On the other hand, improvement of the moment arm depends

on the angle of the line of displacement. In other words, the adverse effect is a 1:1 ratio, whereas the beneficial effect is less than a 1:1 ratio and is proportional to the line of pull of the abductors. Accordingly, lateralized liners are typically used when the surgeon has tried a high-offset femoral component but additional offset is needed to restore the abductor tension and thereby enhance hip stability (Figure 8).

Method of Restoration of Femoral Offset
Templating is typically performed on radiographs of the contralateral, normal hip because one of the primary goals of surgery is to restore normal biomechanical properties to the affected joint. In particular, when a patient has unilateral disease, the normal joint can be used to measure the optimal amount of femoral offset that should be reproduced. Three radiographs—an AP view of the pelvis, an AP view centered at the hip, and a lateral view of the hip joint—are essential for accurate templating. Furthermore, if there is any evidence of deformity, previous fracture, or previous surgical interventions, a 3-ft (0.9-m) standing radiograph from the hip to the ankle joint may be helpful for surgical planning. When a patient has had a previous fracture-dislocation of the acetabulum, Judet radiographs and/or CT images should be made to assess the location and degree of bone loss.[3]

Templating permits the surgeon to quantify several important parameters, including the patient's bone stock, component sizes, anticipated depth of seating of the femoral component within the canal, potential limb-length discrepancy, optimal level of proximal femoral resection, and anticipated position of the acetabular component. Together these variables will determine the new center of rotation of the joint. The basic principle of templating is to reproduce the normal anatomic center of rotation and restore femoral offset while maintaining equal limb lengths.

Limb Length

Although there are several methods for measuring limb length radiographically, two techniques are used more commonly than others. The first method consists of drawing a horizontal line through two points located at the inferior aspect of the ischial tuberosities. Alternatively, a horizontal line can be drawn between the inferior aspects of the acetabular teardrops, which may be more reliable points of reference than the ischia. The teardrop is a more discrete anatomic structure, and therefore its vertical position is not affected as much by rotation of the pelvis.[27] A vertical line is then extended perpendicularly from the horizontal reference to the estimated center of each femoral head. The difference in length between the two vertical lines (A–B) represents an estimate of the limb-length discrepancy (Figure 9). Alternatively, two lines can be drawn through the center of the lesser trochanter of each femur and parallel to the ischial line. The net difference in height between the lesser trochanter and ischium or femoral head and ischium is then measured. Finally, all measurements should be reduced by a factor of approximately 20% to account for the enlargement of the osseous anatomy on the radiographs.[28] Therefore, in this example, increasing the neck length in the affected right hip by the distance A–B and then multiplying this value by 0.80 (to account for the 20% magnification) should equalize the limb lengths for determinations of limb lengths; radiographic measurements should be adjusted on the basis of the findings of the relevant clinical examination. For example, a unilateral adduction contracture will result in a perceived increase in limb length on the affected side, whereas a fixed flexion contracture tends to result in an overestimation of any shortening that may be present. Furthermore, PA

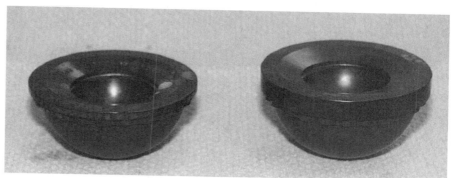

Figure 8 Photograph comparing standard (left) and offset (lateralized) (right) modular liners. It has been shown that a modular offset (lateralized) liner increases offset while preserving limb length. The offset may be altered by modifying the relationship of the articulation at the socket such that the center of rotation at the hip is translated both laterally and inferiorly.[2] A laterally displaced socket increases the abductor tension.

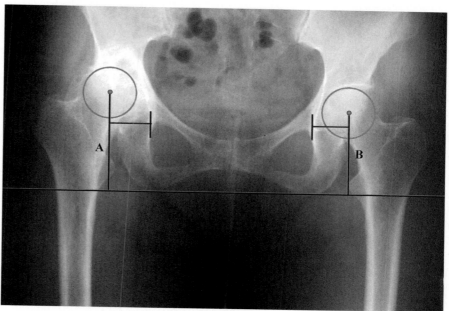

Figure 9 Radiographic assessment of limb-length discrepancy. A horizontal line is drawn through two points located at the most inferior aspect of the ischial tuberosities. A vertical line is then extended perpendicularly from the horizontal reference to the estimated center of each femoral head. The difference in length between the two vertical lines (A–B) represents the estimated limb-length discrepancy.

positioning of the osseous landmarks can be used for templating and determinations of limb lengths. Accordingly, one of the most important questions that the clinician should ask the patient is what is his or her perceived limb-length discrepancy (if any).[3]

Acetabular Component

Templating typically is begun on the acetabular side of the joint, with the more normal hip used as a reference. The orientation of the acetabular shell is typically 45° relative to the horizontal plane (on the AP radiograph) and in approximately

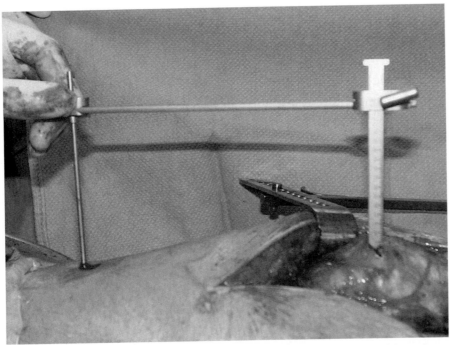

Figure 10 Photograph of a jig, which measures femoral offset and limb length and depends on a fixed reference point. The proximal reference consists of a Steinmann pin placed into the tubercle of the iliac crest through a percutaneous stab wound. A second point is then marked on the lateral aspect of the greater trochanter. With the hip in full extension, limb length and femoral offset can then be precisely measured and adjusted.

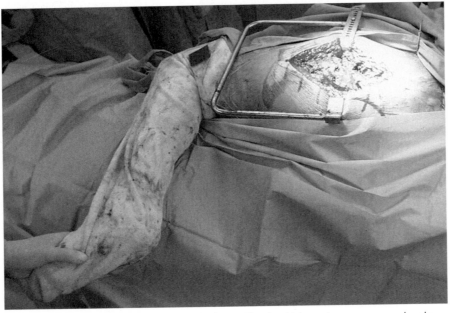

Figure 11 Photograph illustrating the dropkick test. The dropkick test is a maneuver whereby the hip is held in extension while the knee is concomitantly flexed to 90°. If the extremity has been overlengthened, the extensor mechanism becomes excessively taut and may manifest as a tendency for the knee to passively swing into extension when the leg is released.

20° of anteversion (on the lateral radiograph). The apex of the acetabular component should be positioned just lateral to the teardrop.

An appropriately sized acetabular component should be covered at its superolateral margin by host bone with avoidance of excessive overhang or underhang. Finally, if the acetabular component is to be fixed with cement, a minimum of 2 mm should be allowed between the acetabular template and the host bone for an adequate cement mantle. The template that satisfies all of these criteria is then selected, positioned, and marked at its center, which will represent the new center of rotation for the joint.

Femoral Component

After the center of rotation of the acetabular component has been established, the femoral template is superimposed on the radiograph. An AP radiograph with the femur internally rotated approximately 20° (so that the true neck-shaft angle is in the same plane as the radiograph) provides the surgeon with the most representative view of the proximal femoral anatomy. The optimal component size is then established from the radiograph by matching the geometry of the implant to that of the host bone. The various implant designs will influence the type and size of the components that are selected. For example, for cemented femoral prostheses, a minimum of 2 to 3 mm of cement mantle is required to provide adequate fixation, whereas for proximally coated implants, metaphyseal fit and fill are of greatest importance. Moreover, the manufacturers of extensively porous-coated prostheses advocate a minimum of 4 to 5 cm of cortical interdigitation ("scratch fit") to obtain adequate torsional stability and minimize subsidence.

Once the appropriate type and size of the femoral component have been determined, the template should be positioned so that it is parallel to the anatomic axis of the proximal part of the femur, with particular care taken to avoid varus or valgus malalignment. If no limb-length discrepancy is present, the surgeon should align the center of the appropriate femoral head template with the anticipated center of rotation previously marked on the radiograph. However, if the affected hip is short, then the head center should be positioned above the anticipated center of rotation by a distance that is equal to the measured limb-length discrepancy (A-B).

Finally, the neck length is marked and measured relative to its distance above the lesser trochanter. The optimal neck length can then be determined intraoperatively by testing various head lengths. If the center of the trial femoral head is positioned medial to the planned center of rotation, femoral offset will necessarily be increased and the joint reactive forces acting at the hip will be correspondingly reduced. Conversely, if the femoral head center lies lateral to the center of rotation, offset will be reduced, resulting in lower abductor strength and increased joint reaction force. Clearly, this latter scenario should be avoided whenever possible.[3,29]

Intraoperative Measurements
Limb Length and Femoral Offset

To equalize limb lengths and restore offset, the surgeon should first measure the limb length and femoral offset on the affected side before dislocation and again with the trial implants in place. A jig that measures both of these parameters depends on a fixed reference point. The proximal reference consists of a Steinmann pin placed into the tubercle of the iliac crest through a percutaneous stab wound. A second point is then marked on the lateral aspect of the greater trochanter. With the hip in full extension, limb length and offset can then be precisely measured (Figure 10) and may be adjusted as required.[8]

As discussed previously, there are four ways to effectively restore femoral

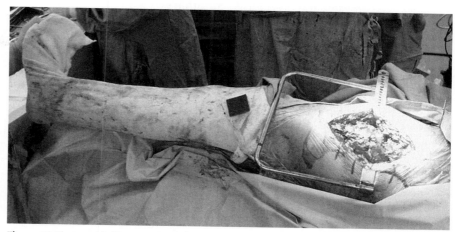

Figure 12 Photograph illustrating stability testing in full extension with concomitant maximal external rotation of the hip.

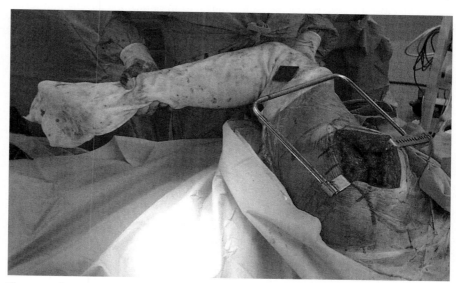

Figure 13 Photograph illustrating stability testing in 90° of flexion of both the hip and knee with concomitant maximal internal rotation of the hip.

offset intraoperatively. Of these methods, only the medialized high-offset femoral component design was found to not appreciably alter limb length. Accordingly, in the absence of a limb-length discrepancy, these two techniques are the authors' preferred system for restoring femoral offset.

Special Tests

In addition to modifying the geometry of the femoral or acetabular component,

preoperative templating, and intraoperative measurement of offset and limb length, there are several intraoperative maneuvers that can be used to assess both soft-tissue tensioning and limb lengths. Typically, all of these techniques are performed with the trial components. This affords the surgeon the flexibility to adjust length or offset by using various combinations of sizes and offset designs to obtain an optimal clinical result. Specifically, these maneuvers consist of the shuck test, dropkick test, leg-to-leg comparison, and additional stability tests.

Shuck Test. The shuck test facilitates an assessment of stability by distracting the hip joint through the application of in-line traction in a distal direction. This maneuver allows a subjective determination of the overall soft-tissue tension around the hip joint. By testing various combinations of neck offsets (high or standard), neck lengths, and possibly liners (standard or lateralized), the surgeon can assess which trial components provide optimal tensioning of the soft-tissue structures.[7]

Dropkick Test. The dropkick test is a maneuver whereby the hip is held in extension while the knee is concomitantly flexed to 90°. If the extremity has been overlengthened, the extensor mechanism becomes excessively taut and this may manifest itself as a tendency for the knee to passively swing into extension when the leg is released (Figure 11).

Leg-to-Leg Comparison. During patient positioning, it is essential that the patient's contralateral heel and knee are palpable through the drapes so that a side-to-side comparison of the treated and untreated limbs can be performed both prior and subsequent to insertion of the trial components. This technique serves as yet another means of assessing and comparing limb lengths in the operating room.

Additional Tests. Additional tests include an assessment of stability both in extension with concomitant maximal external rotation (Figure 12) and in 90° of flexion of the hip and knee with concomitant maximal internal rotation[7] (Figure 13). It is important to note that, under all circumstances, the establishment of hip stability must take precedence over equalization of limb lengths and restoration of femoral offset. Accordingly, as a component of obtaining informed consent, it is imperative that the surgeon discuss the potential of limb-length discrepancy with the patient.

Summary

Several clinical advantages are associated with the reproduction of normal femoral offset during total hip arthroplasty. These include improved abductor strength,[30] enhanced stability,[31] greater range of motion,[30] and reduced rates of aseptic loosening[20] and polyethylene wear.[13] Normal femoral offset is often attained with the use of a high-offset femoral component. However, as the neck-shaft angle decreases and offset increases, the design must incorporate a shape that resists axial torque because axial torque adversely increases exponentially with a decreasing neck-shaft angle. The optimal amount of alteration of the neck-shaft angle to minimize the adverse impact of out-of-plane force has not been documented. Simply increasing neck length has the adverse effect of also increasing limb length, which is not an acceptable compromise under most circumstances. With regard to the techniques for restoring femoral offset, several basic steps must be considered. These include preoperative templating, intraoperative determinations of limb length and femoral offset, and a thorough understanding of the various intraoperative options and special tests that can be used to achieve appropriate soft-tissue balancing during total hip arthroplasty.

References

1. Alberton GM, High WA, Morrey BF: Dislocation after revision total hip arthroplasty: An analysis of risk factors and treatment options. *J Bone Joint Surg Am* 2002;84:1788-1792.
2. Berry DJ: Unstable total hip arthroplasty: Detailed overview. *Instr Course Lect* 2001;50:265-274.
3. Blackley HR, Howell GE, Rorabeck CH: Planning and management of the difficult primary hip replacement: Preoperative planning and technical considerations. *Instr Course Lect* 2000;49:3-11.
4. Blaimont P, Delronge G, Smeyers B, Halleux P, Lasudry N, Sintzoff S: Anatomical and extensometric study concerning the collar support and the prosthetic sleeve: Basis of the conception of an anatomic prosthesis. *Acta Orthop Belg* 1993;59(suppl 1):170-181.
5. Charnley J: *Low Friction Arthroplasty of the Hip: Theory and Practice.* New York, NY, Springer, 1979, pp 336-344.
6. Noble PC, Alexander JW, Lindahl LJ, Yew DT, Granberry WM, Tullos HS: The anatomic basis of femoral component design. *Clin Orthop* 1988;235:148-165.
7. Bourne RB, Rorabeck CH: Soft tissue balancing: The hip. *J Arthroplasty* 2002;17(suppl 1):17-22.
8. Dolhain P, Tsigaras H, Bourne RB, Rorabeck CH, MacDonald S, McCalden R: The effectiveness of dual offset stems in restoring offset during total hip replacement. *Acta Orthop Belg* 2002;68:490-499.
9. Mahoney CR, Pellicci PM: Complications in primary total hip arthroplasty: Avoidance and management of dislocations. *Instr Course Lect* 2003;52:247-255.
10. Rothman RH: The effect of varying femoral offset on component fixation in cemented total hip arthroplasty. *63rd Annual Meeting Proceedings.* Rosemont, IL, American Academy of Orthopaedic Surgeons, 1993.
11. Devane PA, Horne JG: Assessment of polyethylene wear in total hip replacement. *Clin Orthop* 1999;369:59-72.
12. Devane PA, Robinson EJ, Bourne RB, Rorabeck CH, Nayak NN, Horne JG: Measurement of polyethylene wear in acetabular components inserted with and without cement: A randomized trial. *J Bone Joint Surg Am* 1997;79:682-689.
13. Sakalkale DP, Sharkey PF, Eng K, Hozack WJ, Rothman RH: Effect of femoral component offset on polyethylene wear in total hip arthroplasty. *Clin Orthop* 2001;388:125-134.
14. Dennis DA, Komistek RD, Northcut EJ, Ochoa JA, Ritchie A: "In vivo" determination of hip joint separation and the forces generated due to impact loading conditions. *J Biomech* 2001;34:623-629.
15. Radin EL: Biomechanics of the human hip. *Clin Orthop* 1980;152:28-34.
16. Johnston RC, Brand RA, Crowninshield RD: Reconstruction of the hip: A mathematical approach to determine optimum geometric relationships. *J Bone Joint Surg Am* 1979;61:639-652.
17. Greenwald AS: Biomechanical factors in THR offset restoration. *70th Annual Meeting Proceedings.* Rosemont, IL, American Academy of Orthopaedic Surgeons, 2003.
18. Rubin PJ, Leyvraz PF, Aubaniac JM, Argenson JN, Esteve P, de Roguin B: The morphology of the proximal femur: A three-dimensional radiographic analysis. *J Bone Joint Surg Br* 1992;74:28-32.
19. Davey JR: Implant issues in using high offset femoral stems. *70th Annual Meeting Proceedings.* Rosemont, IL, American Academy of Orthopaedic Surgeons, 2003.
20. Hodge WA, Andriacchi TP, Galante JO: A relationship between stem orientation and function following total hip arthroplasty. *J Arthroplasty* 1991;6:229-235.

21. Woo RY, Morrey BF: Dislocations after total hip arthroplasty. *J Bone Joint Surg Am* 1982;64:1295-1306.

22. Davey JR, O'Connor DO, Burke DW, Harris WH: Femoral component offset: Its effect on strain in bone-cement. *J Arthroplasty* 1993;8: 23-26.

23. Massin P, Geais L, Astoin E, Simondi M, Lavaste F: The anatomic basis for the concept of lateralized femoral stems: A frontal plane radiographic study of the proximal femur. *J Arthroplasty* 2000;15:93-101.

24. Davey J, O'Connor D, Burke DW: Femoral component offset: Its effect on micromotion strain in the cement, bone, and prosthesis. *Orthop Trans* 1989;13:566.

25. O'Connor DO, Davey JR, Zalenski E, Burke DW, Harris WH: Femoral component offset: Its effect on micromotion in stance and stair-climbing loading. *Orthop Trans* 1989;13: 394-395.

26. Wong P, Otsuka N, Davey JR, Fornasier VL, Binnington AG: The effect of femoral component offset in uncemented total hip arthroplasty. *Annual Meeting Proceedings of the Canadian Orthopaedic Association.* Montreal, Quebec, Canadian Orthopaedic Association, 1993.

27. Goodman SB, Adler SJ, Fyhrie DP, Schurman DJ: The acetabular teardrop and its relevance to acetabular migration. *Clin Orthop* 1988;236:199-204.

28. Woolson ST, Hartford JM, Sawyer A: Results of a method of leg-length equalization for patients undergoing primary total hip replacement. *J Arthroplasty* 1999;14:159-164.

29. D'Antonio JA: Preoperative templating and choosing the implant for primary THA in the young patient. *Instr Course Lect* 1994;43: 339-346.

30. McGrory BJ, Morrey BF, Cahalan TD, An KN, Cabanela ME: Effect of femoral offset on range of motion and abductor muscle strength after total hip arthroplasty. *J Bone Joint Surg Br* 1995;77:865-869.

31. Fackler CD, Poss R: Dislocation in total hip arthroplasties. *Clin Orthop* 1980;151:169-178.

Developments in Spinal and Epidural Anesthesia and Nerve Blocks for Total Joint Arthroplasty: What Is New and Exciting in Pain Management

Eugene R. Viscusi, MD
Javad Parvizi, MD
T. David Tarity, BS

Abstract

The decision to use regional or general anesthesia for patients undergoing total joint arthroplasty continues to be controversial. Recent reviews of the literature support the growing trend for the use of regional anesthesia with a multifaceted approach, spanning nuances in block placement as well as pharmacologic agents and delivery systems. Innovative developments offer appealing options and encouraging results for the management of pain after major orthopaedic procedures. The ultimate decision, although varied, requires careful preoperative planning and protocols to ensure adequate pain control and patient satisfaction.

Since the dawn of modern anesthesia techniques, there has been controversy regarding the benefits and shortcomings of regional versus general anesthesia. During the past decade, extensive literature confirming the benefits of regional anesthesia, particularly for patients undergoing total joint arthroplasty, have shifted the preferred modality toward regional anesthesia.[1] Regional anesthesia produces nearly ideal surgical conditions, including profound muscle relaxation, controlled reduction of blood pressure, and better control of postoperative pain.[2] Neuraxial techniques have also been shown to offer protection against deep venous thrombosis[3-5] and less consumption of opioids during the perioperative and postoperative rehabilitation periods.[6-8] The advent of vigorous anticoagulation protocols aimed at reducing the risk of thromboembolic events has placed some constraints on the use of regional anesthesia. The most feared complication resulting from the coadministration of anticoagulants and spinal or epidural anesthesia/analgesia is the development of a spinal hematoma that may lead to irreversible spinal cord ischemia and neurologic damage.[9]

Perioperative and postoperative pain, if mismanaged, may contribute to the surgical stress response leading to hypercoagulability, pulmonary or urinary problems, hyperdynamic circulation, increased oxygen consumption, and less than sufficient rehabilitation that contributes to poor outcomes.[10,11] This chapter highlights the current trends and emerging technologies in the field of regional anesthesia for pain management after total joint arthroplasty.

Spinal (Intrathecal) Analgesia

Spinal anesthesia, with the addition of spinal morphine, is a relatively simple anesthetic technique that provides excellent surgical conditions and extended postoperative analgesia.[12] Intrathecal morphine (typical dose, 0.2 to 0.5 mg) is combined with local anesthetic at the time of spinal injection. At the authors' institution, intrathecal morphine 0.2 mg is most commonly combined with isobaric bupivacaine 7.5 to 15 mg. Intrathecal morphine is reported to provide between 12 and 20 hours of pain relief. Most anesthesiologists believe smaller doses of morphine provide the best ratio of analgesia to adverse effects, although at least one recent study found that 0.5 mg of morphine produced better analgesia than 0.2 mg, with a similar profile of adverse effects.[13] Spinal anesthesia/analgesia is most commonly delivered through the placement of a small-bore 24- to 27-gauge spinal needle. The use of pencil-point needles, such as the Sprotte Pencil Point Spinal Needle (Pajunk GmbH, Geisingen, Germany), significantly reduces the incidence of postdural puncture headache (spinal headache). The coagulation profile of the patient must be normal before spinal injection to reduce the risk of epidural hematoma. Hematoma may result from traumatic needle/catheter placement, sustained anticoagulation with an indwelling epidural catheter, and with epidural catheter removal.[9] Dose intervals and coagulation monitoring must be coordinated with the anesthesiology/acute pain team to optimize safety. The American Society of Regional Anesthesia has published guidelines for neuraxial anesthesia and anticoagulation therapy.[14]

Typical opioid adverse effects such as nausea, vomiting, pruritus, respiratory depression, and hypotension have been reported with this combination.[10] All patients receiving opioids require monitoring for respiratory depression. Standard monitoring of patients who have received spinal or epidural opioids at the authors' institution includes hourly assessment of respiratory rate and sedation for 24

hours. Standing orders and protocols facilitate the management of these conditions. Strategies to reduce "breakthrough" pain typically use a multimodal approach, including both opioid and nonopioid analgesics (acetaminophen, cyclo-oxygenase-2 selective inhibitors, and nonselective anti-inflammatory drugs). Supplemental opioids such as intravenous patient-controlled analgesia can be safely coadministered with intrathecal morphine with proper patient surveillance. Appropriate monitoring and treatment of adverse effects allows this technique to be a useful tool for pain control, particularly for patients undergoing total hip arthroplasty.

Epidural Anesthesia and Analgesia

For patients undergoing total joint arthroplasty, some practitioners prefer epidural anesthesia. Similar to spinal anesthesia, epidural anesthesia offers reasonable muscle relaxation and controlled reduction in blood pressure, but it also provides extended duration of anesthesia delivered by means of an indwelling epidural catheter. Postoperatively, the catheter may be used for continuous analgesia. A recent meta-analysis concluded that continuous epidural analgesia provided better postoperative analgesia when compared with parenteral opioids regardless of agent, location of catheter placement, and type and time of pain assessment.[15] Typical infusions consist of local anesthetic (bupivacaine or ropivacaine) and/or opioid (morphine, fentanyl, or hydromorphone). Reports in the literature suggest significantly improved pain control with a mixture of local anesthetics and opioids after major orthopaedic surgery.[16-18] Epidural local anesthetic can contribute to postoperative hypotension and motor impairment. Hypotension is exacerbated by hypo-

volemia. Motor weakness is usually easily managed with adjustment of the rate of epidural infusion. Hypotension results from sympathetic chain blockade, which accompanies sensory and motor blockade.[18] Hypotension usually responds to appropriate fluid management. Epidural opioids may cause the typical opioid-related adverse effects. Standing orders for treatment of nausea, vomiting, and pruritus are generally effective. Epidural opioids, such as intrathecal morphine, can cause respiratory depression and hence require similar respiratory monitoring. Epidural catheters are not recommended for use with the most aggressive anticoagulation regimens because of the potential for epidural hematoma formation.

Continuous epidural analgesia via a catheter is a relatively burdensome technique, with a reported failure rate of approximately 30%.[19,20] Catheter, tubing, and epidural pumps often impede patient activity and may be cumbersome, especially during physical therapy. Catheter systems also require a considerable amount of maintenance by a knowledgeable and dedicated nursing staff. Furthermore, the possibility for programming and medication errors with epidural and intravenous patient-controlled analgesia pumps should not be discounted. The adequacy of analgesia and signs of epidural hematoma should be monitored at regular intervals. Although highly effective, epidural analgesia is labor intensive and generally requires an acute pain management team.

Combined Spinal-Epidural Anesthesia

Combined spinal-epidural anesthesia, most commonly administered via a needle through a needle approach, was first described in 1982[21] and has continued to gain popularity for use in patients undergoing orthopaedic surgery. After an epidural needle is introduced into the epidural space, a spinal needle is advanced though the epidural needle, and a standard spinal anesthetic is performed. The spinal needle is then removed, and an epidural catheter is advanced into the epidural space.

Other techniques of delivering combined spinal-epidural anesthesia include a two-needlestick approach in which an epidural catheter placement at L1-L2 is followed by placement of a subarachnoid needle at L3-L4[22] and the combined needle approach, which consists of joining a spinal needle along the length of an epidural needle with particular attention to ensure dural puncture separate from epidural catheter placement.[23,24]

A review of the various combined spinal-epidural anesthesia techniques by Cook[24] provides technical details as well as the causes of failure and failure rates associated with each method. Recent reports suggest a failure rate of the spinal component of the needle-through-needle approach to administering combined spinal-epidural anesthesia to be approximately 5%.[25,26] There has also been a reported failure rate of epidural analgesia for postoperative analgesia after combined spinal-epidural anesthesia ranging between 18% to 22% compared with a failure rate of 6% to 8% for epidurals alone.[24] The advantages of the combined spinal-epidural anesthesia technique include spinal anesthesia for surgery with the potential to use the epidural catheter if the surgery outlasts the spinal anesthetic. Moreover, the epidural catheter is available for postoperative analgesia. Despite the advantages of this technique, the

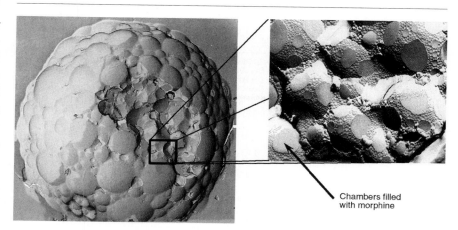

Figure 1   DepoDur scanning electron micrograph. Inset (*arrow*) shows chambers filled with morphine. (Courtesy of SkyePharma, London, England.)

epidural catheter cannot be tested at the time of placement, leading to a potentially nonfunctioning catheter and consequently a dissatisfied patient. All cautions related to epidural and spinal catheters apply to the combined spinal-epidural anesthesia technique; hence, this type of anesthesia should be administered by experienced clinicians.

Extended Release Epidural Morphine

The US Food and Drug Administration has recently approved a novel formulation of extended-release epidural morphine (EREM) known as DepoDur (SkyePharma, London, England) (Figure 1). This formulation consists of a lyposomal carrier (DepoFoam, SkyePharma) with preservative-free morphine. EREM is injected via a standard lumbar epidural injection for postoperative analgesia; however, an indwelling epidural catheter is not used with this preparation. EREM has been studied in patients undergoing hip and knee arthroplasty and demonstrated a 48-hour period of analgesia.[27] In a hip arthroplasty study, patients who received EREM showed a significant reduction in the need for supplemen-

tal analgesia (Figure 2). In the same study, patients who received EREM had significantly better pain intensity scores compared with intravenous patient-controlled analgesia alone. This technique offers the advantage of catheter-free and pump-free pain relief and is particularly appealing for patients receiving anticoagulation therapy.[28] The absence of an epidural catheter reduces the risk of epidural hematoma formation with anticoagulation. Adverse effects are similar to those of standard opioid therapy; careful monitoring by a knowledgeable staff is mandated. The absence of external paraphernalia should facilitate patient mobility and reduce the burden of care related to catheter maintenance. Furthermore, additional considerations of the decreased burden of use for the patient, nursing staff, and pain management team add to the appeal of this novel analgesic.

Single-Injection Peripheral Nerve Blocks and Continuous Peripheral Nerve Blocks

Peripheral neural blockade can be used as a sole anesthetic technique for patients undergoing total joint arthroplasty. In a comparison with intravenous patient-controlled anal-

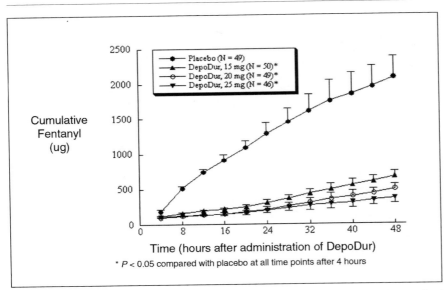

Figure 2   Graph showing cumulative fentanyl usage over 48 hours (mean, standard error) during hip arthroplasty. (Courtesy of SkyePharma.)

gesia using morphine after undergoing total knee arthroplasty, continuous lumbar plexus anesthesia (3-in-1 block) provided better pain relief and faster knee rehabilitation with fewer adverse events.[29] A prospective study by Singelyn and Gouverneur comparing a 3-in-1 block and patient-controlled analgesia with morphine after total hip arthroplasty found comparable pain relief with fewer technical problems and adverse effects with 3-in-1 block administration.[30] This approach completely eliminates central neuraxial manipulation and any potential for related problems such as epidural hematoma formation. Peripheral blocks are used more often as effective adjunctive analgesic techniques, particularly after total knee arthroplasty.[31] A recent study concluded that combining femoral nerve block with epidural analgesia after total knee arthroplasty significantly improved pain control compared with epidural anesthesia alone.[32] Furthermore, in a recent meta-analysis, Richman and associates[33] concluded that continuous peripheral nerve block analgesia significantly reduced opioid consumption and opioid-related adverse effects compared with opioid analgesia.

The blocks of interest for total joint arthroplasty involve the major plexi of the lower extremity: the lumbar plexus (L2, L3, and L4) and the lumbosacral plexus (L5, S1, S2, and S3). Blocks of the lumbar plexus will provide analgesia to the hip and anteromedial aspect of the knee. The lumbosacral plexus provides analgesia to the posterolateral aspect of the knee and the remainder of the leg below the knee. L2, L3, and L4 can be blocked posteriorly through the posterior lumbar plexus block or anteriorly by a femoral block. L5, S1, S2, and S3 can be blocked at the sciatic nerve posteriorly or in the popliteal fossa. The latter block is particularly useful for foot and ankle surgery and less commonly used for adult reconstruction.

Single-injection perineural local anesthetic blocks have the potential to provide extended analgesia after surgery. Depending on the specific local anesthetic used, analgesia may last 12 to 24 hours. In many circumstances, however, this duration of action fails to provide adequate analgesia as a sole strategy. Similar to epidural analgesia, single-injection blocks and continuous catheter blocks may provide less than complete analgesia, although continuous catheter systems have been demonstrated to markedly prolong the duration of pain relief compared with single-injection peripheral blocks.[6,34] Moreover, femoral nerve blocks have been found to provide incomplete anesthesia to the obturator nerve.[35] The short duration of single-injection perineural local anesthetic blocks can be overcome by catheter insertion and continuous infusion of perineural local anesthetic as well as parenteral opioids and nonopioid analgesics. Hence, additional analgesics should be available and ordered as part of a multimodal analgesia plan.

Standard inpatient infusion pumps may be used. Additionally, a variety of disposable electronic and mechanical pumps are available if the practitioner wishes to send the patient home with a continuous infusion of local anesthetic. These techniques provide localized analgesia, without the potential adverse effect of hypotension that may accompany epidural analgesia. Furthermore, an attractive quality of this approach is a localized motor block limited to one extremity.

The addition of a perineural catheter delivery system introduces some problems, although fewer problems occur than with an epidural catheter. With anticoagulation, perineural catheters may present some risk for bleeding and potential hematoma formation. Although not

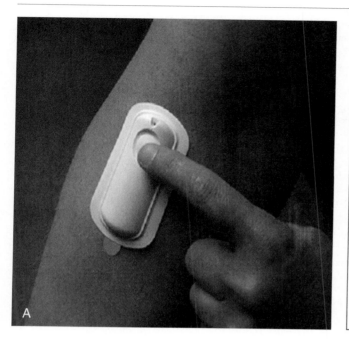
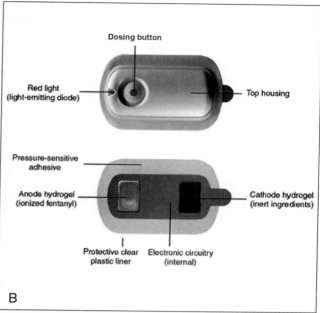

Figure 3 **A,** Photograph showing use of the patient-activated fentanyl iontophoretic transdermal system (Fentanyl Iontophoretic Transdermal System [IONSYS™], ALZA Corporation, Mountain View, CA). **B,** Illustration showing the components of the Fentanyl Iontophoretic Transdermal System (IONSYS™). (Courtesy of ALZA Corporation.)

as catastrophic as an epidural hematoma, several case reports have documented injury from psoas compartment hematomas.[36-38] As with any catheter delivery system, there is a slight chance of infection and other catheter-related problems. These problems include potential bleeding, increased systemic absorption of local anesthetic, and increased burden of care. Local anesthetic toxicity is rare, but potentially a risk. If patients are to be sent home with a catheter and infusion device, surveillance and follow-up is mandatory. In addition, patients should be instructed to avoid potential injury of the insensate limb. As with neuraxial techniques, there is a rare incidence of nerve injury associated with peripheral nerve blocks. Peripheral nerve blocks and particularly continuous blocks with indwelling catheters require particular skills from the anesthesia and acute pain team.

Intra-articular and Incisional Local Anesthetic Infusions

Wound infiltration of local anesthetic can provide short-term cutaneous analgesia. A catheter can be placed in the incision to provide an extended infusion of local anesthetic; however, catheter precautions apply with this technique. Intra-articular local anesthetic, with or without a catheter, has been reported to have mixed results after total joint replacement because of the complexity and severity of pain associated with these procedures.[39] After total knee arthroplasty, some studies advocate local anesthetic infusion with anesthetics, epinephrine, and morphine, which has been shown to result in increased flexion and reduced hospital stays.[40,41] These techniques are best reserved for procedures with less resulting pain or as a multimodal approach for pain management because the duration of this type of analgesia is short-lived.

Patient-Activated Transdermal Analgesia

Intravenous patient-controlled analgesia is used routinely as an adjunct to many of the techniques described. Although it is an effective method of delivering pain relief, problems frequently occur such as intravenous tube infiltration, pump malfunction, kinking of intravenous tubing, and interference with patient activity. Intravenous patient-controlled analgesia also has been implicated in medication errors that may lead to patient harm.[42] As a result, a novel iontophoretic patient-activated device has been developed to address some of these issues[43] (Figure 3). The device is the size of a credit card, uses no needle, and is patient activated. This device can be applied to the upper arm or the chest and is designed to manage moderate to severe pain requiring opioid analgesia. The system delivers a preprogrammed amount of fentanyl hydrochloride over 10 minutes for a total of 80 doses or for 24 hours.[44] In a double-blind, placebo-controlled trial, the iontophoretic fentanyl hydrochloride patient-administered transdermal analgesic system demonstrated superiority over placebo for acute postoperative pain management.[45] A recent study comparing this iontophoretic transdermal system (IONSYS, ALZA Corporation, Mountain View, CA) with standard morphine intravenous patient-controlled analgesia demonstrated therapeutic equivalence.[46] When approved, this system may be a useful adjuvant for total joint arthroplasty analgesia.

Summary

Regional anesthesia is an important part of the current approach to providing analgesia to patients who have undergone total joint arthroplasty. Multimodal analgesic regimens incorporate various agents and techniques, whose aim is to thwart pain at multiple sites of action. When considering the analgesic options, it is important to consider the implications of anticoagulation, ease of use, and burden of care. Less invasive delivery systems that provide continuous analgesia and are compatible with aggressive anticoagulation regimens may facilitate rehabilitation and ultimately improve patient outcomes. Moreover, emerging technologies may soon address currently unmet needs.

References

1. Borghi B, Laici C, Iuorio S, et al: Epidural vs general anaesthesia. [In Italian.] *Minerva Anestesiol* 2002;68:171-177.

2. Liu SS, Strodtbeck WM, Richman JM, Wu CL: A comparison of regional versus general anesthesia for ambulatory anesthesia: A meta-analysis of randomized controlled trials. *Anesth Analg* 2005;101:1634-1642.

3. Modig J: The role of lumbar epidural anaesthesia as antithrombotic prophylaxis in total hip replacement. *Acta Chir Scand* 1985;151:589-594.

4. Davis FM, Laurenson VG, Gillespie WJ, Wells JE, Foate J, Newman E: Deep vein thrombosis after total hip replacement: A comparison between spinal and general anaesthesia. *J Bone Joint Surg Br* 1989;71:181-185.

5. Sharrock NE, Cazan MG, Hargett MJ, Williams-Russo P, Wilson PD Jr: Changes in mortality after total hip and knee arthroplasty over a ten-year period. *Anesth Analg* 1995;80:242-248.

6. Indelli PF, Grant SA, Nielsen K, Vail TP: Regional anesthesia in hip surgery. *Clin Orthop Relat Res* 2005;441:250-255.

7. Vendittoli PA, Makinen P, Drolet P, et al: A multimodal analgesia protocol for total knee arthroplasty: A randomized, controlled study. *J Bone Joint Surg Am* 2006;88:282-289.

8. Watson MW, Mitra D, McLintock TC, Grant SA: Continuous versus single-injection lumbar plexus blocks: Comparison of the effects on morphine use and early recovery after total knee arthroplasty. *Reg Anesth Pain Med* 2005;30:541-547.

9. Horlocker TT, Wedel DJ, Benzon H, et al: Regional anesthesia in the anticoagulated patient: defining the risks (the second ASRA Consensus Conference on Neuraxial Anesthesia and Anticoagulation). *Reg Anesth Pain Med* 2003;28:172-197.

10. Lema MJ: Opioid effects and adverse effects. *Reg Anesth* 1996;21(Suppl):38-42.

11. Shoji H, Solomonow M, Yoshino S, D'Ambrosia R, Dabezies E: Factors affecting postoperative flexion in total knee arthroplasty. *Orthopedics* 1990;13:643-649.

12. Sinatra RS, Torres J, Bustos AM: Pain management after major orthopaedic surgery: Current strategies and new concepts. *J Am Acad Orthop Surg* 2002;10:117-129.

13. Bowrey S, Hamer J, Bowler I, Symonds C, Hall JE: A comparison of 0.2 and 0.5 mg intrathecal morphine for postoperative analgesia after total knee replacement. *Anaesthesia* 2005;60:449-452.

14. Horlocker TT, Wedel DJ, Benzon H, et al: Regional anesthesia and the anticoagulated patient: Defining the risks (The Second ASRA Consensus Conference on neuraxial anesthesia and anticoagulation). *Reg Anesth Pain Med* 2003;28:172-197.

15. Block BM, Liu SS, Rowlingson AJ, Cowan AR, Cowan JA Jr, Wu CL: Efficacy of postoperative epidural analgesia: A meta-analysis. *JAMA* 2003;290:2455-2463.

16. Kampe S, Weigand C, Kaufmann J, Klimek M, Konig DP, Lynch J: Postoperative analgesia with no motor block by continuous epidural infusion of ropivacaine 0.1% and sufentanil after total hip replacement. *Anesth Analg* 1999;89:395-398.

17. Kopacz DJ, Sharrock NE, Allen HW: A comparison of levobupivacaine 0.125%, fentanyl 4 microg/mL, or their combination for patient-controlled epidural analgesia after major orthopedic surgery. *Anesth Analg* 1999;89:1497-1503.

18. Wheatley RG, Schug SA, Watson D: Safety and efficacy of postoperative epidural analgesia. *Br J Anaesth* 2001;87:47-61.

19. Andersen G, Rasmussen H, Rosenstock C, et al: Postoperative pain control by epidural analgesia after transabdominal surgery: Efficacy and problems encountered in daily routine. *Acta Anaesthesiol Scand* 2000;44:296-301.

20. Ready LB: Acute pain: Lessons learned from 25,000 patients. *Reg Anesth Pain Med* 1999;24:499-505.

21. Coates MB: Combined subarachnoid and epidural techniques. *Anaesthesia* 1982;37:89-90.

22. Brownridge P: Central neural blockade and caesarian section: Part 1. Review and case series. *Anaesth Intensive Care* 1979;7:33-41.

23. Eldor J, Chaimsky G: Combined spinal-epidural needle (CSEN). *Can J Anaesth* 1988;35:537-539.

24. Cook TM: Combined spinal-epidural techniques. *Anaesthesia* 2000;55:42-64.

25. Herbstman CH, Jaffee JB, Tuman KJ, Newman LM: An in vivo evaluation of four spinal needles used for the combined spinal-epidural technique. *Anesth Analg* 1998;86:520-522.

26. Casati A, D'Ambrosio A, De NP, Fanelli G, Tagariello V, Tarantino F: A clinical comparison between needle-through-needle and double-segment techniques for combined spinal and epidural anesthesia. *Reg Anesth Pain Med* 1998;23:390-394.

27. Viscusi ER, Martin G, Hartrick CT, Singla N, Manvelian G: Forty-eight hours of postoperative pain relief after total hip arthroplasty with a novel, extended-release epidural morphine

formulation. *Anesthesiology* 2005;102:1014-1022.

28. Hartrick CT, Martin G, Kantor G, Koncelik J, Manvelian G: Evaluation of a single-dose, extended-release epidural morphine formulation for pain after knee arthroplasty. *J Bone Joint Surg Am* 2006;88:273-281.

29. Singelyn FJ, Deyaert M, Joris D, Pendeville E, Gouverneur JM: Effects of intravenous patient-controlled analgesia with morphine, continuous epidural analgesia, and continuous three-in-one block on postoperative pain and knee rehabilitation after unilateral total knee arthroplasty. *Anesth Analg* 1998;87:88-92.

30. Singelyn FJ, Gouverneur JM: Postoperative analgesia after total hip arthroplasty: IV PCA with morphine, patient-controlled epidural analgesia, or continuous "3-in-1" block? A prospective evaluation by our acute pain service in more than 1,300 patients. *J Clin Anesth* 1999;11:550-554.

31. Barrington MJ, Olive D, Low K, Scott DA, Brittain J, Choong P: Continuous femoral nerve blockade or epidural analgesia after total knee replacement: A prospective randomized controlled trial. *Anesth Analg* 2005;101:1824-1829.

32. YaDeau JT, Cahill JB, Zawadsky MW, et al: The effects of femoral nerve blockade in conjunction with epidural analgesia after total knee arthroplasty. *Anesth Analg* 2005;101:891-895.

33. Richman JM, Liu SS, Courpas G, et al: Does continuous peripheral nerve block provide superior pain control to opioids? A meta-analysis. *Anesth Analg* 2006;102:248-257.

34. Mollmann M: Continuous spinal anesthesia. [In German.] *Anaesthesist* 1997;46:616-621.

35. Macalou D, Trueck S, Meuret P, et al: Postoperative analgesia after total knee replacement: The effect of an obturator nerve block added to the femoral 3-in-1 nerve block. *Anesth Analg* 2004;99:251-254.

36. Hoek JA, Henny CP, Knipscheer HC, ten Cate H, Nurmohamed MT, ten Cate JW: The effect of different anaesthetic techniques on the incidence of thrombosis following total hip replacement. *Thromb Haemost* 1991;65:122-125.

37. Adam F, Jaziri S, Chauvin M: Psoas abscess complicating femoral nerve block catheter. *Anesthesiology* 2003;99:230-231.

38. Johr M: A complication of continuous blockade of the femoral nerve. [In German.] *Reg Anaesth* 1987;10:37-38.

39. Busch CA, Shore BJ, Bhandari R, et al: Efficacy of periarticular multimodal drug injection in total knee arthroplasty: A randomized trial. *J Bone Joint Surg Am* 2006;88:959-963.

40. Lombardi AV Jr, Berend KR, Mallory TH, Dodds KL, Adams JB: Soft tissue and intra-articular injection of bupivacaine, epinephrine, and morphine has a beneficial effect after total knee arthroplasty. *Clin Orthop Relat Res* 2004;428:125-130.

41. Rasmussen S, Kramhoft MU, Sperling KP, Pedersen JH: Increased flexion and reduced hospital stay with continuous intraarticular morphine and ropivacaine after primary total knee replacement: Open intervention study of efficacy and safety in 154 patients. *Acta Orthop Scand* 2004;75:606-609.

42. Vicente KJ, Kada-Bekhaled K, Hillel G, et al: Programming errors contribute to death from patient-controlled analgesia: Case report and estimate of probability. Can J Anaesth 2003;50:328-332.

43. Viscusi ER: Emerging techniques for postoperative analgesia in orthopedic surgery. *Am J Orthop* 2004;33(Suppl):13-16.

44. Sinatra R: The fentanyl HCl patient-controlled transdermal system (PCTS): an alternative to intravenous patient-controlled analgesia in the postoperative setting. *Clin Pharmacokinet* 2005;44(suppl 1):1-6.

45. Viscusi ER, Reynolds L, Tait S, Melson T, Atkinson LE: An iontophoretic fentanyl patient-activated analgesic delivery system for postoperative pain: A double-blind, placebo-controlled trial. *Anesth Analg* 2006;102:188-194.

46. Viscusi ER, Reynolds L, Chung F, Atkinson LE, Khanna S: Patient-controlled transdermal fentanyl hydrochloride vs intravenous morphine pump for postoperative pain: A randomized controlled trial. *JAMA* 2004;291:1333-1341.

Hip Resurfacing: Indications, Results, and Conclusions

Caroline Hing, BSc, MSc, MD, FRCS(Tr&Orth)
Diane Back, MBBS, FRCS Ed(Tr&Orth)
Andrew Shimmin, FAOrthA, FRACS, Dip Anat

Abstract

Hip resurfacing using metal-on-metal bearings has increased in popularity as a viable treatment option for young, active patients with osteoarthritis. Theoretic advantages of this procedure include preservation of bone stock, reduction in osteolysis, and a reduced risk of dislocation when compared with conventional hip arthroplasty with smaller diameter metal-on-polyethylene bearings. Concerns associated with the use of metal-on-metal bearings during hip resurfacing include the production of metal ions with unknown carcinogenic and immunologic effects. The long-term survival of the modern metal-on-metal hip resurfacing implant is also unknown. Hip resurfacing accounts for 7.5% of all hip replacements in Australia and has a 2.2% revision rate, with femoral fracture being the most common reason for revision. The cumulative survival rate at the authors' institution is 99.14% at 3-year follow-up.

Hip resurfacing arthroplasty has continued to increase in popularity over the past decade as a treatment option for young, active patients with osteoarthritis.[1-3] Metal-on-metal bearings of cobalt-chromium alloy may reduce the risk of particulate-related osteolysis when compared with metal-on-polyethylene bearings but may increase potential risks because of the systemic and local effects of metal ions.[4-7] Various designs of hip resurfacing implants have evolved over the years since their original inception in the 1960s. The Birmingham hip resurfacing implant (BHR, Smith & Nephew, Birmingham, England) in its present format has been in use since 1997, with an overall survival rate of 98% at 5-year follow-up reported by the center of its inception.[2,3] Radiostereophotogrammetric analysis to study the stability of resurfacing arthroplasty in the short term has also shown low values for cup migration and vertical and mediolateral migration of the implant head at 2-year follow-up. These results compared favorably with those for cemented components in conventional total hip replacements, confirming the favorable clinical and radiologic results of this implant in short-term use.[8]

Demographics of Hip Resurfacing in Australia

Metal-on-metal hip resurfacing has been performed in Australia since April 1999.[9] From September 1999 to December 2004, a total of 5,379 hip resurfacings were performed, accounting for 7.5% of all hip replacements. When compared with conventional total hip replacements, 2.2% of the hip resurfacings were revised as opposed to 1.9% of total hip replacements. Of the hip resurfacings, 86% used the BHR implant with a revision rate of 2%, and 14% used either the Cormet 2000 implant (Corin Medical, Cirencester, England), or the ASR (DePuy, Warsaw, IN) or Durom (Zimmer, Warsaw, IN) or Conserve Plus (Wright Medical Technology, Inc, Arlington, TN), with a revision rate of 3.6%.[9] The most common reason for revision was fracture of the femoral neck, with 59.3% of all resurfacing revisions performed for this reason; 84% of these fractures occurred within the first 6 months.[9]

When considering the 118 hip resurfacings that were revised, women had twice the risk of revision compared with men. Men older than 65 years had a higher percentage of revision compared with men younger than 65 years. For women, those 55 to 64 years of age had the highest risk of revision. Primary diagnosis also had an effect on the revision rate. Patients with osteoarthritis had the lowest number of early revisions (2%) compared with those with rheumatoid arthritis (8%), osteonecrosis (3.4%), and developmental dysplasia (3.2%).[9]

Conclusions from the Australian hip registry have confirmed that careful patient selection is important to ensure the longevity of a hip resurfacing implant, with the lowest number of revisions occurring in males younger than 65 years and in those with a primary diagnosis of osteoarthritis.

Indications for Hip Resurfacing

The ideal candidate for hip resurfacing is a man younger than 65 years with a primary diagnosis of osteoarthritis, good bone quality, and normal proximal femoral geometry.[3,9,10] Hip resurfacing cannot correct large limb-length inequality or change horizontal femoral offset.[10,11] Hence, patients with large limb-length inequality or significantly reduced horizontal offset are still best treated with conventional or extended offset stemmed implants.

Absolute contraindications to hip resurfacing include elderly and postmenopausal patients with osteoporosis, impaired renal function, and known metal hypersensitivity. Relative contraindications include inflammatory arthropathy, abnormal proximal femoral geometry, large femoral head geodes, and large areas of osteonecrosis.[1,10]

The proposed advantages of hip resurfacing as opposed to hip replacement are a lower dislocation rate, restoration of physiologic biomechanics, preservation of bone stock, and a return to a more active lifestyle.[1-3,11] Restoration of a normal femoral head size with preservation of hip biomechanics has contributed to a lower dislocation rate when compared with hip arthroplasty using a smaller femoral head.[1-3] A more physiologic pattern of femoral head loading following hip resurfacing is believed to produce compressive forces rather than hoop stresses, which may improve bone mineral density.[3] Favorable survivorship with a return to high-demand activities after hip resurfacing may be advantageous in younger patients who are actively employed in full-time positions.[1,3]

Early Results of Resurfacing at the Melbourne Orthopaedic Group

Between April 1999 and June 2001, 230 consecutive primary hip replacements using the BHR implant were performed by three surgeons at the Melbourne Orthopaedic Group. This series represented the first hip resurfacing performed using the BHR implant at this institution. All patients were available for follow-up. Patients were considered for the BHR implant rather than total hip replacement if they were active men younger than 75 years or active women younger than 60 years. Patients outside these age groups were considered on a case-by-case basis.[1] A clinical and radiologic review by an independent observer was performed at a mean follow-up of 3 years. Patients were assessed preoperatively using the Harris hip score,[12] the Medical Outcomes Study 12-Item Short Form Health Survey (SF-12),[13] and Charnley

grades.[14] Postoperatively, Oxford hip scores were also obtained.[15]

During radiologic review, radiolucent lines were recorded around the components in the zones described by Amstutz and associates[16] and DeLee and Charnley.[17] In addition, the preoperative femoral neck-shaft angle (A) was subtracted from the angle between the stem and the shaft (S) to determine varus or valgus implant positioning. If angle S was greater than angle A by more than 5°, the implant was considered to be valgus; if angle S was less than angle A by more than 5°, the implant was considered to be varus. The abduction angle of the acetabular component (C) was recorded, and the position of the stem relative to the femoral neck on the lateral radiograph was assessed[1] (Figure 1). The presence of heterotopic ossification was recorded using the classification of Brooker and associates.[18]

Demographics

Overall, 230 patients were included in the study (150 men and 80 women); 116 right hips and 114 left hips underwent resurfacing, and 17 patients underwent bilateral procedures. The mean age of patients at the time of surgery was 52 years (range, 18 to 82 years) (Figure 2). The mean patient height was 172.18 cm (standard deviation, 9.95 cm), the mean patient weight was 80.62 kg (standard deviation, 15.62 kg), and the mean body mass index was 27.02 kg/m^2 (standard deviation, 4.23 kg/m^2). The preoperative diagnoses are shown in Figure 3.

Results

At 3-year follow-up, one patient had died and one had undergone a revision to a total hip replacement because of a loose acetabular component. All surviving patients (228

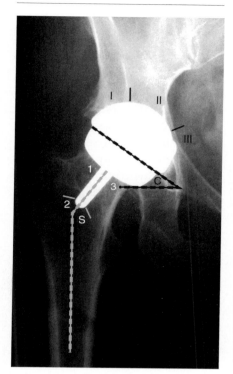

Figure 1 Postoperative radiographic measurements of implant position showing the zones of Amstutz (1, 2, and 3), the zones of DeLee and Charnley (I, II, and III), the stem shaft angle (S), and the cup angle (C).

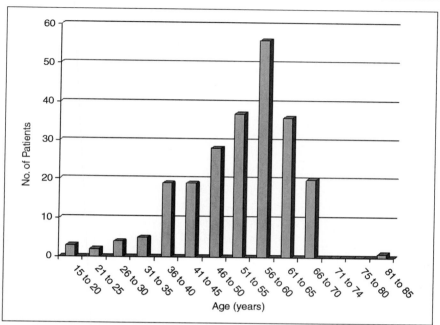

Figure 2 Graph showing age distribution of patients at the time of surgery.

hips) returned questionnaires, and 204 hips were available for clinical and radiologic review. The remaining 24 hips had been reviewed at a minimum 2-year follow-up. The cumulative survival rate was 99.14% at 3 years. The range of movement improved in all patients from a mean flexion of 92° (range, 25° to 130°) preoperatively to 110° (range, 80° to 130°) postoperatively. The mean postoperative Oxford hip score was 13.5 (range, 12 to 28). The Harris hip scores and SF-12 scores are summarized in Table 1.

Complications

Medical and surgical complications are summarized in Table 2. Patients also described clicking and squeaking. Fifty-three patients (22.9%) de-

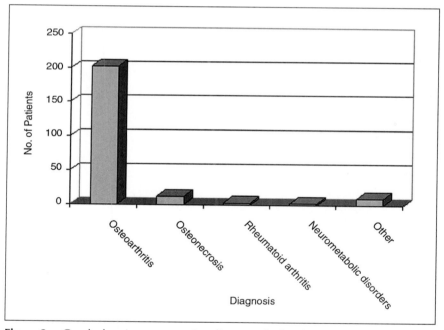

Figure 3 Graph showing preoperative diagnoses before hip resurfacing.

scribed painless clicking that was believed to be caused by the psoas tendon impinging on the anterior surface of the acetabular component. Nine patients (3.9%) described painless squeaking at ex-

treme flexion that was believed to be caused by a disruption in the fluid film between the bearing surfaces. One implant was revised to a total hip replacement 18 months after the original surgery because of

Table 1
Preoperative and 3-Year Harris Hip and SF-12 Scores After Hip Resurfacing

Charnley Category	No. of Arthroplasties	Harris Hip Score (range)	SF-12 Score (physical component)	SF-12 Score (mental component)
A				
Preoperative	162	63.9 (8 to 93)	31.1	58.6
3-year	162	97.7 (60 to 100)	54.1	56.9
B				
Preoperative	53	56.2 (18 to 82)	30.3	60.5
3-year	52	99.4 (90 to 100)	54.1	57.7
C				
Preoperative	15	64.8 (30 to 98)	31.5	52.2
3-year	14	85.5 (30 to 100)	48.2	55.9

Table 2
Number of Surgical and Medical Complications After Hip Resurfacing

Surgical Complications (No.)	Medical Complications (No.)
Superficial wound infection (11)	Hypotension (14)
Notched neck (5)	Deep venous thrombosis (11)
Acetabular introducer wire breakage (4)	Urinary tract infection (9)
Sciatic nerve palsy (2)	Sinus tachycardia (5)
Femoral nerve palsy (2)	Pressure sores (4)
Retained guidewires (2)	Pulmonary embolus (2)
Fracture, healed (1)	
Component mismatch (1)	
Common peroneal nerve palsy (1)	
Profunda femoris artery pseudoaneurysm (1)	
Femoral artery damage (1)	
Rectus femoris intramuscular hematoma (1)	

loosening of the BHR acetabular component.

Radiologic Results at 3-Year Follow-Up

No radiolucent lines were noted around either component. The mean abduction angle of the acetabular component was 45.8° (range, 37° to 65°). In eight patients, the initial postoperative radiographs showed that the acetabular component was inadequately seated; however, by 2-year follow-up, there was bony ingrowth in all instances. The femoral implant position was valgus in most patients (2.9°), with poor seating noted in 7 patients, and an anterior position noted in 115 patients. Six patients had notching of the femoral neck on the immediate postoperative radiographs, with one patient developing a femoral neck fracture 6 weeks after surgery that united with marked femoral neck narrowing after a 6-week period of not bearing weight. Four other patients presented with pain and a possible stress fracture of the femoral neck within 1 year of surgery. All pain resolved after a period of not bearing weight.

Heterotopic ossification was noted in 59.56% of patients (Brooker grade I in 38.26%, grade II in 13.48%, and grade III in 7.83%). This relatively high percentage of patients with heterotopic ossification may have been caused by several factors: the patient age group (young males often have hypertropic osteoarthritis); no routine use of prophylactic indomethacin in this high-risk group; and the surgical approach with the extensile exposure used in this procedure had a learning curve that could have resulted in more soft-tissue stripping. Three patients underwent excision of heterotopic ossification for pain and a reduced range of motion. Clinical review at 3-year follow-up showed no difference in outcome scores compared with those of patients who had undergone resurfacing but had not undergone additional surgery.

Results

This consecutive series of patients who underwent hip replacement using BHR implants had a cumulative survival rate of 99.14% at 3-year follow-up, which compares favorably with the results of resurfacings at other centers.[2,3,9,16] Radiologic review showed no evidence of osteolysis of either component at 3-year follow-up, although one acetabular component was revised at 18 months for loosening. Most of the femoral components were valgus, but the significance of femoral component position on survival is unknown at this stage. In this series, one femoral neck fracture occurred, which united with a period of not bearing weight, and six patients had evidence of notching that was treated with a period of protected weight bearing; none of these patients progressed to displaced femoral neck fracture. This series had a lower rate of femoral neck fracture than that reported in Australia (1.46%), possibly because patients with femoral neck notching and pain were identified early and treated with a period of protected weight bearing.[10,19] Further follow-up to determine the long-term outcomes of this cohort is ongoing.

Complications Associated With Hip Resurfacing Arthroplasty

Complications specific to hip resurfacing include femoral neck fracture, osteonecrosis, increased metal ion levels, and metal hypersensitivity.[1-4,10] Complications associated with hip arthroplasty that also apply to hip resurfacing include dislocation, heterotopic ossification, thromboembolic disease, nerve palsies, and vascular damage.

Careful patient selection is important in reducing the risk of complications, as is meticulous surgical technique and restoration of hip biomechanics.[10] Recent short-term reviews of hip resurfacing outcomes and hip registries have addressed some of the issues contributing to complications.[1,2,9]

Femoral Neck Fracture

In Australia, the most common reason for revision of a hip resurfacing has been a femoral neck fracture[9] (Figure 4). A recent survey of surgeons who had experienced a femoral neck fracture in their practice showed an overall fracture rate of 1.46% associated with the BHR implant.[19] The Australian national fracture rate for men undergoing resurfacing was 0.98% and for women was 1.91%. The absolute risk of femoral neck fracture is 0.0191 in women and 0.0098 in men. There is

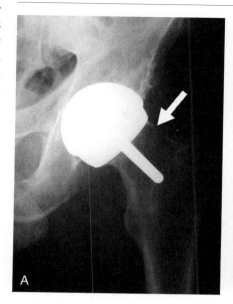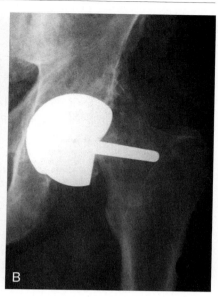

Figure 4   Radiographs showing a femoral neck stress fracture (*arrow*) (**A**) and propagation that occurred 6 weeks from hip resurfacing (**B**).

a statistically significant difference ($P < 0.001$) between men and women, with the relative risk for women versus men being 1.9496.[19] The mean time to fracture is 15 weeks from the time of initial surgery, with no significant difference between men and women.

Femoral neck notching and varus positioning have been implicated in increasing the risk of femoral neck fracture.[19-21] Finite element analysis using CT scans to reconstruct proximal femoral geometry and including the effect of muscle forces and hip loading in the boundary conditions has shown a change in bone mineral density up to 9 months from implantation. Bone resorption in this model was minimized by a valgus position of the femoral component, which may be the ideal alignment to prevent femoral neck fracture in the early postoperative period.[22] A cumulative effect of implant position and femoral neck bone density are likely to be important in the early postoperative period

for determining which patients are at risk of femoral neck fracture.

The effect of gender, age, and weight on the risk of femoral neck fracture and implant failure remains controversial. Obesity, which may contribute to poor surgical exposure, and osteoporosis in postmenopausal women may have osteoporosis, which may contribute to an increased risk of femoral neck fracture.[9,19] However, Beaulé and associates[23] have shown that weight less than 82 kg was significantly associated with a smaller femoral component size and a smaller fixation area and may result in adverse radiographic changes.

Femoral neck fracture has been shown to occur most commonly in the early postoperative period (mean time to fracture, 15 weeks); these fractures may be preceded by pain and limp that are not typically expected at that stage in the rehabilitation course.[19] Nondisplaced femoral neck fractures that are detected early may be successfully treated with a period of no weight bearing, which results in no compromise to clinical or radiologic outcomes.[24,25]

Osteonecrosis

Osteonecrosis as a result of femoral head resurfacing has been reported in the literature and may play a role in femoral neck fracture.[2,26] The true incidence of osteonecrosis with hip resurfacing is unknown because histologic studies have concentrated on failed retrieved resurfaced femoral heads.[26] Hip resurfacing has been shown to affect the oxygen concentration in the femoral head with an extended posterior approach, causing a mean 60% decrease in oxygen concentration; component insertion results in an additional 20% decrease.[27] Oxygen concentration does not improve significantly with wound closure, which raises concerns about the viability of the femoral head and neck after resurfacing. It can be postulated that osteonecrosis may be a cause of some femoral neck fractures if the interoperative reduction in oxygenation is permanent.[27]

Dual-energy x-ray absorptiometry (DEXA) can be used to measure changes in bone density around implants.[28] Most bone density changes occur within the first year after surgery. DEXA studies at 1 and 2 years postoperatively have shown that proximal femoral bone density is preserved, but the effect of implant position and notching on these measurements is unknown.[28] The findings from DEXA studies appear to concur with the finding of Freeman[21] that the vascular supply in the arthritic femoral head is mainly intraosseous, but do not concur with the findings of Steffen and associates[27] that femoral head oxygenation is reduced during surgery.[3]

Metal Ion Levels

Metal-on-metal bearing surfaces produce metal wear debris and corrode to produce metallic ions. The level of wear is dependent on metallurgy, implant design, and activity levels.[29] Theoretic risks of increased metal ion levels include local toxicity, osteolysis, and malignant change; however, the biologic long-term effects are unknown.[6,29,30] Various methods exist to measure serum chromium and serum cobalt, but the clinical relevance of raised metallic ions is uncertain.[10,29]

The BHR implant is made from a cobalt-chromium-molybdenum alloy, with a 4% carbide content that has been machine cast. A recent prospective longitudinal study of BHR implants found a peak in serum cobalt levels at 6 months postoperatively and a peak in serum chromium levels at 9 months postoperatively.[29] At 2-year follow-up, the mean serum ion levels were still higher than preoperative levels. No deterioration was found in renal function during the study period, and there was no radiographic evidence of lucency of either the femoral or acetabular components. Similar studies have also reported elevated cobalt and chromium levels with other bearing surface combinations, but it is difficult to compare these results because of differences in study designs and sampling. The local and systemic effects of elevated cobalt and chromium levels are still unknown.[7,29,31]

The mutagenic potential of metal ions is unknown because epidemiologic studies with these implants are of short duration. At present, orthopaedic implants are not classified based on carcinogenicity.[30] A recent in vitro study has demonstrated DNA damage in human cultured fibroblasts from synovial fluid of failed cobalt-chromium alloy prostheses, but this finding does not imply that DNA damage causes malignancy in humans.[6] Additional epidemiologic studies are needed to ascertain the malignant potential of metal ions in the context of hip resurfacing.

Dermal hypersensitivity to metal affects 10% to 15% of the population, with nickel being the most common sensitizer and cobalt-chromium being the second most common sensitizer.[32] Recent studies on metal hypersensitivity have shown a higher incidence in patients who have undergone arthroplasty than in the general population, but the relationship to osteolysis is unknown.[33] Patients with metal hypersensitivity may present with pain or an effusion. At a cellular level, free metal ions bind to native proteins to form allergens that activate a delayed cell-mediated immune response. Sensitized T-lymphocytes are activated and release cytokines with resultant macrophage activation. The histologic appearances of tissue samples from these patients are characterized by aseptic lymphocytic vasculitis associated lesions.[33] At present, no commercial hematologic tests are available for metal hypersensitivity, and the relevance of dermal hypersensitivity to metal in implant failure is yet to be defined.

Dislocation

Resurfacing the femoral head with a large femoral component and restoring the normal hip biomechanics may contribute to the low published dislocation rates of 0.75% at a mean of 3-year follow-up compared with conventional arthroplasty, which has a reported dislocation rate of up to 10%.[1,2,11,34] Smaller diameter metal-on-metal bearings have also been shown to exhibit suction

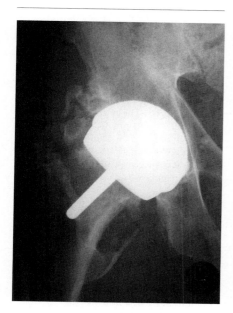

Figure 5 Radiograph showing heterotopic ossification (Brooker grade III) that occurred after hip resurfacing.

fit, which may contribute to stability. However, larger diameter metal-on-metal bearings have a greater diametric clearance and suction fit is less likely in the context of resurfacing.[35]

Heterotopic Ossification

Formation of heterotopic bone after hip resurfacing has been reported in 28% to 60% of patients[1,2,16] (Figure 5). Predisposition to formation of heterotopic bone is associated with male gender, bilateral simultaneous hip resurfacing, previous heterotopic bone formation, and extensive soft-tissue stripping.[36] Although the effect on clinical outcome scores is minimal, heterotopic ossification may reduce range of motion.[1,2,16] Indomethacin prophylaxis has been shown to reduce the risk of heterotopic bone formation.[33] Indications for the use of indomethacin vary from selective in high-risk patients to routine in all patients.[16,36]

Other Complications

Neurovascular injuries and thromboembolic disease have also been reported as complications of hip resurfacing, but these complications occur at rates comparable to those for conventional hip arthroplasty.[1,2,16]

Learning Curve

Implantation of the BHR using a posterior approach has an associated learning curve. A prospective study of two orthopaedic surgeons in the same unit, using the same approach and standard instrumentation, showed a significant improvement ($P < 0.001$) in surgical time and implant position, but no difference in clinical outcome when comparing the first to the second cohort of 50 patients who underwent implantation.[37] Because a significant learning curve is associated with hip resurfacing, this factor should be considered on initial introduction of this implant into clinical practice.

Summary

Hip resurfacing appears to provide a viable treatment option in the short term for young patients with degenerative arthritis. Careful patient selection is needed, with the best results obtained in young men with good bone stock. There is a learning curve associated with the procedure, and although short-term results are favorable, the long-term clinical and radiographic outcomes are still unknown. Concerns with hip resurfacing include the risk of femoral neck fracture in the early postoperative period, which is associated with varus implantation and intraoperative femoral neck notching. In addition, hip resurfacing is not ideal if the patient requires increased limb length or horizontal offset. The long-term effects of increased se-

rum metal ion levels is unknown. Serum cobalt levels appear to peak at 6 months postoperatively, whereas serum chromium levels appear to peak at 9 months postoperatively. Metal sensitivity has been implicated as a cause of groin pain in patients who have undergone hip resurfacing, but the relationship to osteolysis and whether it causes implant failure is unknown. Long-term independent studies of survivorship and complications are needed to determine ideal patient selection and reduce the risk of complications.

References

1. Back DL, Dalziel R, Young D, Shimmin A: Early results of primary Birmingham hip resurfacings. *J Bone Joint Surg Br* 2005;87:324-329.

2. Treacy RC, McBryde CW, Pynsent PB: Birmingham hip resurfacing arthroplasty. *J Bone Joint Surg Br* 2005;87:167-170.

3. Daniel J, Pynsent PB, McMinn DJ: Metal-on-metal resurfacing of the hip in patients under the age of 55 years with osteoarthritis. *J Bone Joint Surg Br* 2004;86:177-184.

4. MacDonald SJ: Metal-on-metal total hip arthroplasty: The concerns. *Clin Orthop Relat Res* 2004;429:86-93.

5. Dumbleton JH, Manley MT: Metal-on-metal total hip replacement: What does the literature say? *J Arthroplasty* 2005;20:174-188.

6. Davies AP, Sood A, Lewis AC, Newson R, Learmonth ID, Case CP: Metal-specific differences in levels of DNA damage caused by synovial fluid recovered at revision arthroplasty. *J Bone Joint Surg Br* 2005;87:1439-1444.

7. Jacobs JJ, Skipor AK, Doorn PF, et al: Cobalt and chromium concentrations in patients with metal on metal hip replacements. *Clin Orthop Relat Res* 1996;329(suppl):S256-263.

8. Itayem R, Arndt A, Nistor L, McMinn D, Lundberg A: Stability of the Birmingham hip resurfacing arthroplasty at two years. *J Bone Joint Surg Br* 2005;87:158-162.

9. Australian Orthopaedic Association: *National Joint Replacement Registry Annual*

Report. 2005, pp 29-63. Available at: www.dmac.adelaide.edu.au/aoanjrr/documents/corrigenda_2005.pdf. Accessed August 3, 2006.

10. Shimmin AJ, Bare J, Back DL: Complications associated with hip resurfacing arthroplasty. *Orthop Clin North Am* 2005;36-A:187-193.

11. Silva M, Haeng Lee K, Heisel C, Dela Rosa M, Schmalzried TP: The biomechanical results of total hip resurfacing arthroplasty. *J Bone Joint Surg Am* 2004;86-A:40-46.

12. Harris WH: Traumatic arthritis of the hip after dislocation and acetabular fractures: Treatment by mold arthroplasty: An end result study using a new method of result evaluation. *J Bone Joint Surg Am* 1969;51:737-755.

13. Dawson J, Fitzpatrick R, Murray D, Carr A: Comparison of measures to assess outcomes in total hip replacements. *Qual Health Care* 1996;5:81-88.

14. Charnley J: The long-term results of low-friction arthroplasty of the hip performed as a primary intervention. *J Bone Joint Surg Br* 1972;54:61-76.

15. Dawson J, Fitzpatrick R, Carr A, Murray D: Questionnaire on the perceptions of patients about total hip replacement. *J Bone Joint Surg Br* 1996;78:185-190.

16. Amstutz HC, Beaulé PE, Dorey FJ, Le Duff MJ, Campbell PA, Gruen TA: Metal-on-metal hybrid surface arthroplasty: Two to six-year follow-up study. *J Bone Joint Surg Am* 2004;86-A:28-39.

17. DeLee JG, Charnley J: Radiological demarcation of cemented sockets in total hip replacement. *Clin Orthop Relat Res* 1976;121:20-32.

18. Brooker AF, Bowerman J, Robinson RA, Riley LH Jr: Ectopic ossification following total hip replacement: Incidence and a method of classification. *J Bone Joint Surg Am* 1973;55:1629-1632.

19. Shimmin AJ, Back DL: Femoral neck fractures associated with hip resurfacing: A national review of 50 cases. *J Bone Joint Surg Br* 2005;87:463-464.

20. Freeman MA, Cameron HU, Brown GC: Cemented double-cup arthroplasty of the hip: A 5 year experience with the ICLH prosthesis. *Clin Orthop Relat Res* 1978;134:45-52.

21. Freeman MA: Some anatomical and mechanical considerations relevant to the surface replacement of the femoral head. *Clin Orthop Relat Res* 1978;134:19-24.

22. Kohan L, Gillies M: Effect of femoral component alignment on femoral neck remodelling after hip resurfacing: A finite element analysis. *Proceedings of the 65th Annual Scientific Meeting.* Australian Orthopaedic Academy, 2005, p 69.

23. Beaulé PE, Dorey FJ, LeDuff ML, Gruen T, Amstutz HC: Risk factors affecting outcome of metal-on-metal surface arthroplasty of the hip. *Clin Orthop Relat Res* 2004;418:87-93.

24. Cumming D, Fordyce M: The non-operative management of a peri-prosthetic subcapital fracture after metal-on-metal Birmingham hip resurfacing: A case report. *J Bone Joint Surg Br* 2003;85:1055-1056.

25. Cossey AJ, Back DL, Shimmin A, Young D, Spriggins AJ: The non-operative management of peri-prosthetic fractures associated with the Birmingham hip resurfacing procedure. *J Arthroplasty* 2005;20:358-361.

26. Little CP, Ruiz AL, Harding IJ, et al: Osteonecrosis in retrieved femoral heads after failed resurfacing arthroplasty of the hip. *J Bone Joint Surg Br* 2005;87:320-330.

27. Steffen RT, Smith SR, Urban JP, et al: The effect of hip resurfacing on oxygen concentration in the femoral head. *J Bone Joint Surg Br* 2005;87:1468-1474.

28. Kishida Y, Sugano N, Nishii T, Miki H, Yamaguchi K, Yoshikawa H: Preservation of the bone mineral density of the femur

after surface replacement of the hip. *J Bone Joint Surg Br* 2004;86:185-189.

29. Back DL, Young DA, Shimmin AJ: How do serum cobalt and chromium levels change after metal-on-metal hip resurfacing? *Clin Orthop Relat Res* 2005;438:177-181.

30. McGregor D, Baan RA, Portensky C, Rice JM, Wilbourne JD: Evaluation of the carcinogenic risks to humans associated with surgical implants and other foreign bodies: A report of an IARC Monographs Programme Meeting. *Eur J Cancer* 2000;36:307-313.

31. Jacobs JJ, Skipor AK, Patterson LM, et al: Metal release in patients who have had a primary total hip arthroplasty: A prospective controlled longitudinal study. *J Bone Joint Surg Am* 1998;80:1447-1458.

32. Hallab N, Merritt K, Jacobs JJ: Metal sensitivity in patients with orthopaedic implants. *J Bone Joint Surg Am* 2001;83-A:428-436.

33. Willert HG, Buchhorn GH, Fayyazi A, et al: Metal-on-metal bearings and hypersensitivity in patients with artificial hip joints. *J Bone Joint Surg Am* 2005;87:28-36.

34. Kelley SS, Lachiewicz PF, Hickman JM, Paterno SM: Relationship of femoral head and acetabular size to the prevalence of dislocation. *Clin Orthop Relat Res* 1998;355:163-170.

35. Clarke MT, Lee PT, Arora A, Villar RN: Levels of metal ions after small- and large-diameter metal-on-metal hip arthroplasty. *J Bone Joint Surg Br* 2003;85:913-917.

36. Back DL, Dalziel R, Young D, Shimmin A: The incidence of heterotopic bone formation following hip resurfacing. *J Bone Joint Surg Br* 2005;87(suppl I):44.

37. Back DL, Shimmin AJ: Learning curve associated with hip resurfacing arthroplasty. *J Bone Joint Surg Br* 2005;87(suppl I):45.

Advances in Hip Arthroplasty in the Treatment of Osteonecrosis

Thorsten M. Seyler, MD
Quanjun Cui, MD, MS
William M. Mihalko, MD, PhD
Michael A. Mont, MD
Khaled J. Saleh, MD, MSc, FRCSC, FACS

Osteonecrosis of the femoral head is a devastating disease for which many patients will eventually require total hip arthroplasty. Standard total hip arthroplasties have historically had poor results in patients with osteonecrosis. More recently, reports have shown excellent results with second- and third-generation designs that incorporate advances in bearing technology. However, there are still certain subpopulations of patients (those with sickle cell disease, those with systemic lupus erythematosus, and those who have undergone renal transplantation) that have less than optimal results. Other hip arthroplasty alternatives include bipolar hemiarthroplasty, limited femoral resurfacing, and metal-on-metal resurfacing. Bipolar hemiarthroplasty historically and currently has consistently poor results in most studies and should be avoided in patients with osteonecrosis. In multiple reports, limited femoral arthroplasty has demonstrated reasonable midterm and long-term outcomes as a temporizing procedure, with results being less predictable than for standard total hip arthroplasty. Recently, ceramic-on-ceramic and metal-on-metal resurfacing hip arthroplasty has emerged as a viable option that has been used to treat patients with osteonecrosis of the femoral head, and several studies have shown promising short-term outcomes. Overall, however, recent studies have shown more optimal outcomes with hip arthroplasty than resurfacing hip arthroplasty, which makes standard hip replacements, as well as other arthroplasty alternatives, more attractive for young patients with this disease.

Osteonecrosis is a devastating disease that usually leads to destruction of the hip joint. It typically occurs in young patients who are in the second through fifth decades of life.[1,2] In the early stages of the disease, various treatment alternatives such as core decompression, rotational osteotomy, and vascularized or nonvascularized bone grafting can be used to delay or avoid the need for total hip arthroplasty. Unfortunately, many patients present with late-stage disease (postcollapse) and have few alternatives that allow them to preserve the femoral head. Once the femoral head collapses or arthritis occurs on the acetabular side, the treatment of choice is reconstructive hip replacement.[3] Various types of hip replacement procedures such as limited resurfacing, bipolar hemiarthroplasty, standard total hip arthroplasty, and total resurfacing arthroplasty have been used to treat this patient population.[4]

Historically, the results of standard total hip replacements in patients with osteonecrosis have not been optimal in young patients with other disorders such as rheumatoid arthritis or primary osteoarthritis.[5-8] The poorest results have been found after bipolar hemiarthroplasty, probably because of the use of thin polyethylene, which can lead to extensive wear and subsequent osteolysis.[6,9,10] In addition, various other types of arthroplasty devices

One or more of the authors or the departments with which they are affiliated have received something of value from a commercial or other party related directly or indirectly to the subject of this chapter.

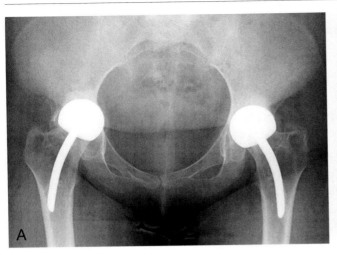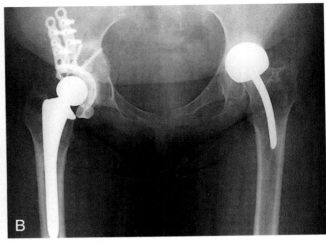

Figure 1 A, Preoperative AP radiograph shows bilateral limited resurfacing with protrusion on the right hip. **B,** Postoperative AP radiograph shows revision total hip arthroplasty has been performed on the right hip.

have been used. There is significant experience with the use of limited femoral resurfacing and renewed interest in metal-on-metal total joint prostheses, including metal-on-metal total resurfacings. Recent advances in prosthesis design, bearing surfaces, and bone ingrowth have led to improved results of reconstructive joint procedures. The selection and criteria for the use of these different devices, new technologies, or surgical techniques are discussed in this chapter.

It is important to make the appropriate choice of treatment for osteonecrosis of the femoral head because this patient population includes a large number of patients who will need to undergo a hip arthroplasty procedure. The true number of patients undergoing total hip arthroplasties annually for the treatment of osteonecrosis in the United States is unknown; however, recent data from both the Canadian Joint Arthroplasty Registry and the Australian National Joint Arthroplasty Registry have demonstrated that the diagnosis of osteonecrosis accounts for 5% of all primary total

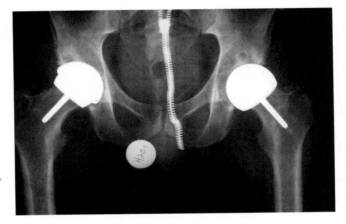

Figure 2 AP radiograph shows a metal-on-metal total hip resurfacing on the right side and a limited femoral resurfacing on the left side.

hip arthroplasties performed annually in those geographic areas.[11,12]

Limited Femoral Head Resurfacing

The high failure rate of total hip arthroplasty in young patients with osteonecrosis of the femoral head has historically made it an unfavorable treatment option (Figure 1). In advanced disease stages, procedures such as core decompression, rotational osteotomies, and nonvascularized and vascularized bone grafting do not have predictable results. In patients with large precollapse lesions and postcollapse disease, an-

other treatment option is femoral head resurfacing arthroplasty. Limited resurfacing (hemiresurfacing) of only the femoral side of the hip joint uses a cemented femoral head prosthesis that is matched in diameter with the native acetabulum (Figure 2). This procedure requires a pristine or relatively undamaged acetabular surface. The potential advantages of hemiresurfacing over total hip arthroplasty are removal of the damaged cartilage, bone stock preservation, lower dislocation rates, delay of a total hip arthroplasty, and easy conversion to hip arthroplasty if necessary.

Table 1
Literature Review of Limited Resurfacing for Osteonecrosis of the Femoral Head

Author(s)	Year	No. of Hips	Procedure	Average Follow-up (Range) [months]	Overall Clinical Success
Cuckler et al[17]	2004	59	Hemiresurfacing	54	68%
Beaulé et al[18]	2004	28	Hemiresurfacing	60 (28-100)	86%
Adili and Trousdale[16]	2003	29	Hemiresurfacing	34 (24-63)	94% (1-year follow-up)
Beaulé et al[14]	2001	37	Hemiresurfacing	78 (24-216)	76% (3-year follow-up) 79% (5-year follow-up) 59% (10-year follow-up) 45% (15-year follow-up)
Mont et al[13]	2001	30	Hemiresurfacing	84 (48-101)	90%
Siguier et al[19]	2001	37	Hemiresurfacing	49 (24-89)	85%
Nelson et al[15]	1997	21	Hemiresurfacing	> 60	82%
Grecula et al[20]	1995	10	Hemiresurfacing	96	70%
Tooke et al[21]	1987	12	Hemiresurfacing	39 (24-62)	92%
Langlais et al[22]	1979	86	Hemiresurfacing	78	85%
Hungerford et al[23]	1998	33	TARA	126 (48-168)	91%
Krackow et al[24]	1993	19	TARA	36 (24-72)	84%
Scott et al[25]	1987	25	TARA	37 (25-60)	88%

TARA = Total articular replacement arthroplasty.

Mont and associates[13] compared the outcome of hemiresurfacing to that of conventional total hip replacement for patients with postcollapse disease. At a mean 7-year follow-up for the hemiresurfacing group and a mean 8-year follow-up for the total hip arthroplasty group, they found that a higher percentage of patients who underwent hemiresurfacing were participating in sports (60% versus 27%). However, more patients who underwent hemiresurfacing had groin pain (20% versus 6%). Overall survivorship was similar in both groups: 90% for the hemiresurfacing group compared with 93% for the total hip arthroplasty group. Beaulé and associates[14] reported on a series of 37 hips followed for a mean of 6.5 years (range, 2 to 18 years) with conversion to total hip arthroplasty as the end point. The overall survival of hemiresurfacing in this study was 79% at 5-year follow-up, 59% at 10-

year follow-up, and 45% at 15-year follow-up. Nelson and associates[15] analyzed 21 hips treated with a custom-cemented titanium femoral component. At a mean follow-up of 6.2 years, the success rate was 82% (14 of 17 hips).

Recently, there have been a few reports detailing the less predictable outcomes and pain relief with resurfacing procedures. Adili and Trousdale[16] reviewed the clinical and radiographic results of 29 consecutive femoral head resurfacing procedures in 28 patients. They found that 17 patients (18 hips, 62%) reported feeling better than they did before surgery, with an overall survivorship of 75.9% at 3 years. At final follow-up, eight hips (27.6%) were converted to a total hip arthroplasty. Cuckler and associates[17] studied 59 hips for a mean follow-up of 4.5 years. They reported that in 16 patients (32%) the resurfacing procedure was considered a failure be-

cause of conversion to total hip arthroplasty or considerable groin pain requiring medication. Conversion of the failed implants to total hip arthroplasty was straightforward, confirming the conservative nature of the procedure. Both of these studies emphasized the unpredictable results obtained with resurfacing procedures.

On the basis of the previously cited reports and the results of the other studies[14-25] listed in Table 1, the following criteria are recommended for identifying appropriate candidates for limited femoral resurfacing: (1) young patients presenting with Ficat and Arlet stage III radiographic disease, (2) lesions with a combined necrotic angle greater than 200° or greater than 30% of femoral head involvement, (3) postcollapse lesions with greater than 2 mm of femoral head depression, and (4) no evidence of acetabular cartilage damage. With careful patient selection, hemiresurfacing is a viable option for the interim treatment of advanced disease stages.

Bipolar Hemiarthroplasty

Bipolar hemiarthroplasty has the same indications as hemiresurfacing. It has been designed to decrease the acetabular shear force through the use of an outer free acetabular cup that articulates with the prosthetic femoral head. Bipolar hemiarthroplasty has yielded variable success rates in patients with osteonecrosis of the femoral head, with many previous studies reporting less than optimal success. Although efforts have been made to improve results, hemiarthroplasty requires resection of the femoral neck and violation of the femoral canal, which may complicate future revisions. The most common complication associated with bipolar hemiarthroplasty is protrusio acetabuli.

In a series of 22 patients, Grevitt and Spencer[26] reported good or excellent results (full total hip arthroplasty was avoided) in 21 patients at a mean 40-month follow-up (range, 24 to 27 months). More recently, Chan and Shih[27] compared the outcomes of cementless total hip arthroplasty and hemiarthroplasty in a series of 28 patients with bilateral disease. At a mean 6.4-year follow-up (range, 4 to 12 years), a satisfactory outcome was found in 24 of 28 patients in the hemiarthroplasty group compared with 23 of 28 patients in the cementless total hip arthroplasty group.

Other reports have shown high complication rates in this patient population. Lachiewicz and Desman[9] analyzed 31 bipolar hip arthroplasties performed for osteonecrosis of the femoral head. At a mean 4.6-year follow-up, 48% of

the hips had excellent or good results. Sanjay and Moreau[28] reported 17 complications in 21 patients at a mean 4.6-year follow-up (range, 2.1 to 7.0 years). Ito and associates[29] reviewed 48 hips in 35 patients at a mean 11.4-year follow-up and found radiographic failure and/or acetabular degeneration in 42% of patients. Yamano and associates[30] reported the results of 29 cementless press-fit bipolar endoprostheses at a mean 12-year follow-up, with femoral loosening occurring in 6 hips (21%), acetabular protrusio occurring in 5 hips (17%), and osteolysis occurring in 11 hips (38%).

Because of these high failure and complication rates, there has been an overall decrease in the use of bipolar hemiarthroplasty for patients with osteonecrosis of the femoral head. In addition, osteolysis from polyethylene wear has been reported as a late complication in young, active patients probably because the polyethylene liner is often quite thin. Although bipolar hemiarthroplasty may be a reasonable treatment alternative for patients who have undergone renal transplant and have less activity in general,[31] it should not be used in this patient population. A summary of the results of using hemiarthroplasty to treat patients with osteonecrosis of the femoral head[6,9,10,26-35] appears in Table 2.

Standard Total Hip Arthroplasty

Standard total hip arthroplasty predictably provides excellent pain relief and a good functional outcome (Figure 3). However, it sacrifices more host bone and limits future surgical options. The most recent issue with regard to the results of total hip arthroplasty for the treatment of osteonecrosis is the longevity of the

prosthesis compared with the longevity reported for other diagnoses such as osteoarthritis and rheumatoid arthritis.[3-5,7,8] Factors that contribute to the high failure rates include relatively young age, long life expectancy, increased body weight, and poor quality of the femoral bone. Some authors have suggested that osteonecrosis of the femoral head itself is not a risk factor for failure of total hip arthroplasty. Historically, there have been poor results, with 30% to 50% failure rates reported with first-generation devices at short-term follow-up. Saito and associates[8] analyzed 29 hips treated with cemented total hip arthroplasty. At a mean 84-month follow-up, the clinical success rate was 52%. Similar results have been reported in studies by Dorr and associates[36] (45% failure rate), Cornell and associates[37] (39% failure rate), and Chandler and associates[7] (57% failure rate). More recently, improved results have been reported with the use of new bearing surfaces, cementing techniques, and new designs, but the results are still inferior to those reported for standard total hip arthroplasty performed for other diagnoses such as osteoarthritis or rheumatoid arthritis.

The results of using cemented standard total hip arthroplasty to treat patients with osteonecrosis of the femoral head vary. Early cementing techniques have had high failure rates, but studies assessing modern cementing methods have reported improved results. Kantor and associates[38] analyzed the results of 28 total hip arthroplasties with second-generation cementing techniques. At a mean 92-month follow-up, the survival rate was 86%. The authors concluded that despite the use of second-generation cementing techniques and improved results, the

Table 2
Literature Review of Bipolar Hemiarthroplasty for Osteonecrosis of the Femoral Head

Author(s)	Year	No. of Hips	Procedure	Average Follow-up (Range) [months]	Overall Clinical Success
Tsumura et al[32]	2005	32	Bipolar hemiarthroplasty	92 (60-180)	86%
Yamano et al[30]	2004	29	Bipolar hemiarthroplasty	144	62%
Lee et al[33]	2004	40	Bipolar hemiarthroplasty	96	95%
Nagai et al[34]	2002	12	Bipolar hemiarthroplasty	144-216	75%
Ito et al[29]	2000	48	Bipolar hemiarthroplasty	137 (84-216)	75%
Chan and Shih[27]	2000	28	Bipolar hemiarthroplasty	77 (48-144)	89%
Sanjay and Moreau[28]	1996	26	Bipolar hemiarthroplasty	55 (25-84)	57%
Grevitt and Spencer[26]	1995	22	Bipolar hemiarthroplasty	40 (24-71)	95%
Murzic and McCollum[31]	1994	32	Bipolar hemiarthroplasty	24-216	88%
Learmonth and Opitz[35]	1993	38	Bipolar hemiarthroplasty	56 (42-72)	87%
Takaoka et al[10]	1992	82	Bipolar hemiarthroplasty	66	86%
Cabanela[6]	1990	23	Bipolar hemiarthroplasty	110	59%
Lachiewicz and Desman[9]	1988	31	Bipolar hemiarthroplasty	55	48%

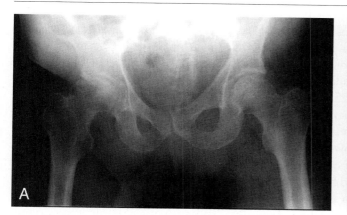

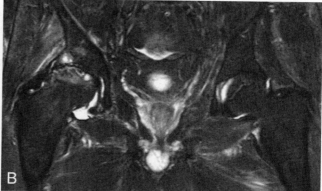

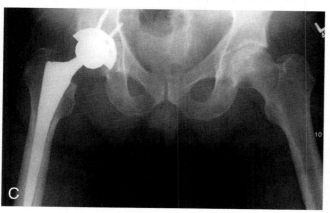

Figure 3 A, Preoperative AP radiograph shows collapse of the femoral head in a patient with osteonecrosis of the right femoral head. **B,** Preoperative MRI scan confirmed the diagnosis. **C,** Postoperative AP radiograph shows that metal-on-polyethylene total hip arthroplasty has been performed.

failure rate was still high. Garino and Steinberg[39] reviewed 123 cemented and hybrid total hip arthroplasties in patients with osteonecrosis. In their series, second-generation cementing techniques resulted in a 96% survival rate at a mean 54-month follow-up (range, 24 to 120 months). These results seem significantly better than previously reported. Recently, Kim and associates[40] prospectively studied the clinical and radiographic outcomes of total hip arthroplasty with so-called third-generation cementing and second-generation cementless total hip arthroplasties in 100 hips with osteonecrosis of the femoral head. At the final 122-month follow-up, they reported a survival rate of 98% in both groups. Radiographically, osteolysis of the femur occurred in 16% of the hips in the group treated with cement and in 24% of the hips in the group treated without cement.

Various reports have demonstrated improved implant fixation and implant longevity using newer designs of cementless total hip arthroplasties. Phillips and associates[41] reported on 20 cementless porous-coated primary total hip arthroplasties performed on 15 patients. At a minimum 24-month follow-up (mean, 62 months), no revisions were performed and one femoral component was loose. However, a high rate of acetabular component wear and osteolysis was radiographically noted and remained one of the major concerns for long-term outcome. Piston and associates[42] reviewed 35 cementless porous-coated total hip arthroplasties in 30 patients. At a mean 90-month follow-up (range, 60 to 120 months), the revision rate was 3% (1 of 30 hips) for the femoral side and 6% (2 of 30 hips) for the acetabular

side, which accounts for an overall failure rate of 6% (2 of 30 hips). All patients returned to a high level of activity postoperatively. Xenakis and associates[43] compared cementless total hip arthroplasties performed on 29 patients with osteonecrosis of the femoral head and on 29 patients with degenerative osteoarthritis. At a mean 7.6-year and 7.1-year follow-up, respectively, only one femoral implant failure occurred in the osteonecrosis group. With an overall survival rate of 96% for cementless total hip arthroplasty, this study demonstrated encouraging clinical results.

The underlying diagnosis associated with osteonecrosis of the femoral head appears to have an impact on implant longevity. Patients in certain subgroups such as those with osteonecrosis secondary to systemic lupus erythematosus, sickle cell disease, or renal transplantation have an increased risk for implant failure. Acurio and Friedman[44] retrospectively reviewed 25 total hip arthroplasties in 25 patients with sickle cell disease and osteonecrosis. At a mean 103-month follow-up (range, 24 to 216 months), 14 of 25 (40%) of the arthroplasties had been revised and 9 other hips (36%) were either radiographically and/or symptomatically loose. The overall complication rate was 49%, and the infection rate 20%. Lieberman and associates[45] reviewed 30 hips in patients with renal transplants and 16 hips in patients on chronic renal dialysis. Patients with renal transplants had generally satisfactory results that were comparable to the results of patients with osteonecrosis without underlying renal disease. However, patients undergoing hip arthroplasty while undergoing long-term renal dialysis demonstrated poor results (81% failure rate). Brinker and associates[5] re-

ported that patients who were younger than 35 years at the time of the total hip arthroplasty had a high failure rate, and the results varied by underlying diagnosis. Patients with systemic lupus erythematosus or an organ transplant had poorer results than those with idiopathic osteonecrosis of the femoral head. In contrast, Huo and associates[46] reported a 94.6% survival probability at 5 years and an 81.8% survival probability at 9 years for patients with osteonecrosis of the femoral head associated with systemic lupus erythematosus. Murzic and McCollum[31] compared cemented total hip arthroplasty, cementless bipolar hemiarthroplasty, and cementless total hip arthroplasty in 46 patients who underwent renal transplantation (77 hips) and had osteonecrosis of the femoral head. With a follow-up ranging from 24 to 216 months, loosening occurred in 46% of the hips treated with cemented total hip arthroplasty, 9% of the hips treated with bipolar hemiarthroplasty, and no hips treated with cementless total hip arthroplasty. The revision rates were 31%, 12.5%, and 0, respectively. Similar results have been reported by Zangger and associates.[47] These authors studied 19 patients with systemic lupus erythematosus and osteonecrosis of the femoral head who underwent 26 total hip arthroplasties. At a minimum follow-up of 24 months, one patient had developed a low-grade prosthetic infection and underwent successful revision, and there was one asymptomatic cup migration, accounting for an overall survival rate of 93%.

The use of ceramic alumina tribology in total hip arthroplasty is now well established (Figure 4). Retrieval studies have demonstrated that the wear rate in stable compo-

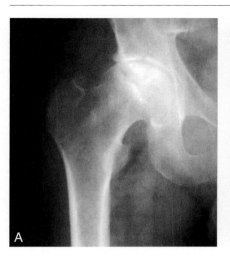
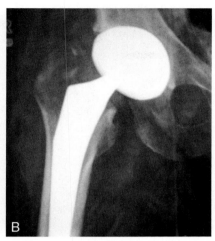

Figure 4   Preoperative **(A)** and postoperative **(B)** AP radiographs of a patient who underwent ceramic-on-ceramic total hip arthroplasty.

nents ranged from 0.025 μm to 2 μm per year. Nich and associates[48] recently reported the long-term results of ceramic-on-ceramic total hip arthroplasty in patients with osteonecrosis. Fifty-two ceramic-on-ceramic total hip arthroplasties were performed in 41 patients with osteonecrosis (mean age, 41 years; age range, 22 to 79 years). At an average 16-year follow-up (range, 11 to 24 years), no osteolysis was observed and no wear was detectable. With revision for aseptic loosening as the end point, the authors reported survival rates of 88.5% for the cup and 100% for the stem at 10-year follow-up. Fye and associates[49] analyzed 72 hips treated with either ceramic-on-ceramic or ceramic-on-polyethylene bearings. At a mean follow-up of 84 months (minimum follow-up, 48 months), the probability of survival for the entire series using revision as the end point was 97% at 11 years. The survival probability decreased to 89% when radiographic failures were included in the analysis. More recently, newer designs such as press-fit metal-backed alumina sockets have shown a better mid-

term outcome. However, long-term outcome studies are needed to further define the role of ceramic-on-ceramic total hip arthroplasty in patients with osteonecrosis of the femoral head.

Better implant designs, new technology, alternative bearings, and advanced surgical technique have shown promising long-term results that may minimize the negative impact of osteonecrosis on implant longevity. Even in patients who are at greater risk for implant failure, newer devices have demonstrated improved implant durability [8,31,39-45,47,49-70] (Table 3).

Metal-on-Metal Resurfacing
Metal-on-metal resurfacing was first introduced in the mid-1960s.[38] The early models of metal-on-metal resurfacing were abandoned because of component loosening and high failure rates.[71] Total hip resurfacing was used to replace both sides of the joint while preserving femoral bone stock. Additionally, the large diameter femoral head that is used permits an increased range of motion with less impingement and lower disloca-

tion rates.[72,73] Recently, there has been an advent in the use of metal-on-metal resurfacing with the development of new technology (Figure 5). Wear particle generation, osteolysis, and subsequent aseptic implant loosening is reduced by the advances in metal-on-metal bearing surfaces (Figure 6).[74-77] In addition, improved cemented fixation of femoral components has shown prolonged durability. The pain relief, function, and patient activity levels achieved using total resurfacing for patients with osteonecrosis are superior to those reported for hemiresurfacing and similar to the results for standard total hip arthroplasty. All these findings have led to an increase in metal-on-polyethylene total hip resurfacings, which have demonstrated low rates of long-term survivorship secondary to high rates of wear generation.

Despite all of the obvious advantages of total hip resurfacing, there are controversies concerning this procedure, including viability of the femoral head,[78] component loosening,[79] femoral neck fractures,[80] and metal ions.[81,82] The general concept that total hip resurfacing can induce femoral head osteonecrosis and subsequent implant failure was rebutted in various histologic studies analyzing the bone in retrieved femoral heads.[78,83-85] With the increasing number of metal-on-metal bearings used clinically, the concerns regarding the levels of metal in serum and urine have also increased.[81,82] Recent studies reported similar levels of cobalt and chromium ions in cohorts of metal-on-metal total hip resurfacings compared with conventional metal-on-metal total hip arthroplasties.[86] An initial peak in cobalt and chromium ion concentration has been detected with the use of newer metal-on-metal total

Table 3
Literature Review of Standard Total Hip Arthroplasty for Patients with Osteonecrosis of the Femoral Head

Author(s)	Year	No. of Hips	Procedure	Follow-up (Range) [months]	Overall Clinical Success
Berend et al[50]	2003	89	THA after failed Bone Grafting	110 (60-180)	82%
Al-Mousawi et al[51]	2002	35	Osteonecrosis secondary to SCD	114 (60-180)	80%
Zangger et al[47]	2000	26	Osteonecrosis secondary to SLE	55 (21-124)	93%
Chen et al[52]	1999	18	Osteonecrosis secondary to SLE	46 (24-85)	100%
Hickman and Lackiewicz[53]	1997	15	Osteonecrosis secondary to SCD	72 (24-144)	67%
Lieberman et al[45]	1995	46	Osteonecrosis and chronic renal failure	54	19%
Murzic and McCollum[31]	1994	77	Osteonecrosis after renal transplantation Cemented/Cementless THA	(24-216)	54%/100%
Moran et al[54]	1993	22	Osteonecrosis secondary to SCD	56	57%
Acurio and Friedman[44]	1992	25	Osteonecrosis secondary to SCD	103 (24-216)	60%
Clarke et al[55]	1989	27	Osteonecrosis secondary to SCD	66	41%
Hanker and Amstutz[56]	1988	8	Osteonecrosis secondary to SCD	78 (24-208)	38%
Schneider and Knahr[57]	2004	57	Cementless THA	(120-168)	82%
Kim et al[40]	2003	100	Cemented/Cementless THA	122	98%/ 98%
Xenakis et al[58]	2001	36	Cementless THA	136 (120-180)	93%
Taylor et al[59]	2001	70	Cementless THA	77	NA
Delank et al[60]	2001	66	Cementless THA	65 (58-94)	93%
Hartley et al[61]	2000	55	Cementless THA	117	79%
Fye et al[49]	1998	72	Cementless THA	84 (> 48)	97%/89%
Stulberg et al[62]	1997	98	Cementless THA	87 (31-134)	75%
Gonzalez et al[63]	1997	40	Cementless THA	58 (24-108)	80%
D'Antonio et al[64]	1997	53	Cementless THA	82 (60-96)	85%
Xenakis et al[43]	1997	29	Cementless THA	91	96%
Kim et al[65]	1995	78	Cementless THA	86 (72-108)	79%
Piston et al[42]	1994	35	Cementless THA	90 (60-120)	94%
Phillips et al[41]	1994	20	Cementless THA	64 (> 24)	95%
Lins et al[66]	1993	37	Cementless THA	48-72	81%
Katz et al[67]	1992	34	Cemented/Cementless THA	46 (24-84)	97%
Fyda et al[68]	2002	53	Cemented THA	> 120	83%
Ortiguera et al[69]	1999	188	Cemented THA	214 (120-304)	82%/50%
Wei et al[70]	1999	22	Revision THA	> 24	82%
Garino and Steinberg[39]	1997	123	Cemented THA	54 (24-120)	96%
Kantor et al[38]	1996	28	Cemented THA	92	86%
Saito et al[8]	1989	29	Cemented THA	84	52%

THA = total hip arthroplasty, SLE = systemic lupus erythematosus, SCD = sickle cell disease, NA=not available

hip resurfacing, followed by a gradual decline during the following 15 months. After a 2-year study period, the bearing has shown excellent wear properties, no radiolucency, and no adverse effects on renal function. There have been various other publications discussing elevated metal ion concentration in patients with metal-on-metal implants, but researchers have concluded that exposure to these elevated metal levels results in theoretic risks.[87,88] Additional studies are needed to elucidate the role of elevated metal ion levels in this patient population.

Grecula and associates[20] compared the outcome of patients younger than 50 years with osteonecrosis of the femoral head who were treated with one of four treatment modalities: standard cemented arthroplasty, total hip articular replacement by internal eccentric shells (THARIES), cementless total hip resurfacing, or cemented titanium femoral surface hemiarthroplasty. Similar degrees of clinical improvement were reported for the four treatments. The 96-month survivorship rates were 70% for cemented titanium femoral surface hemiresurfacing, 15% for cementless total hip resurfacing, 53% for THARIES, and 80% for standard cemented arthroplasty. Even better results have been reported with bone ingrowth total hip arthroplasty (Table 3). More recently, there have been several studies showing promising short-term results with newer devices. Beaulé and associates[18] compared the outcomes of 56 hips treated with metal-on-metal resurfacing arthroplasty with the outcomes of 28 hips treated with hemiresurfacing arthroplasty. The mean age of the patients was 41 years (age range, 16 to 56 years) for the metal-on-metal surface arthroplasty group and 36 years (age range, 22 to 51 years) for the hemiresurfacing group. At 55-month follow-up (range, 24 to 85 months) for the metal-on-metal surface arthroplasty group and 53-month follow-up (range, 25 to 96 months) for the hemiresurfacing group, University of California–Los Angeles hip

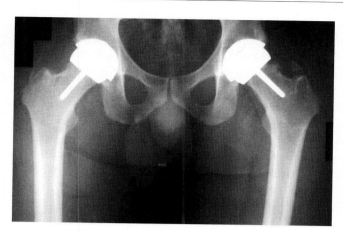

Figure 5
AP radiograph of a patient who underwent bilateral metal-on-metal total hip resurfacing arthroplasty.

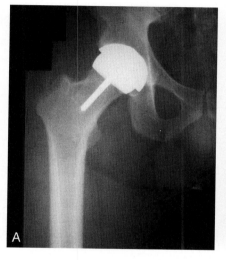
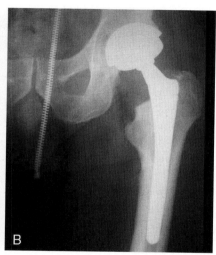

Figure 6 AP radiographs show a patient with a total hip resurfacing arthroplasty (A) and a patient with a standard total hip arthroplasty with a large femoral head (B).

Table 4
Literature Review of Metal-on-Metal Resurfacing for Osteonecrosis of the Femoral Head

Author(s)	Year	No. of Hips	Procedure	Average Follow-up (Range) [months]	Overall Clinical Success
Mont et al[91]	2005	41	Metal-on-metal	36 (24-48)	93%
Amstutz et al[89]	2004	36	Metal-on-metal	42 (26-74)	94%
Mohamad et al[90]	2004	12	Metal-on-metal	18 (17-46)	84%
Beaulé et al[18]	2004	56	Metal-on-metal	60 (28-100)	95%
Yoo[92]	2004	40	Metal-on-metal	36 (24-48)	93%
Grecula et al[20]	1995	19	Metal-on-metal	96	53%
Grecula et al[20]	1995	35	Metal-on-metal	96	15%
Dutton et al[93]	1982	42	Metal-on-metal	37	>76%

scores and Medical Outcome Studies 12-Item Short Form scores for the physical component were significantly better for the metal-on-metal surface arthroplasty group than the hemiresurfacing group. Two metal-on-metal surface replacements failed and were converted to total hip arthroplasties. Amstutz and associates[89] analyzed 400 metal-on-metal total hip arthroplasties done in 355 patients. This large series included 36 hips with osteonecrosis of the femoral head. All femoral head components were cemented. The patients had a mean age of 48 years (age range, 15 to 77 years). At a mean 42-month follow-up (range, 26 to 74 months), the overall survivorship was 94% and most patients had returned to a high level of activity. Twelve hips (3%) had been converted to a total hip arthroplasty, and 7 of those 12 hips (58%) were revised because of loosening of the femoral components. Three hips (25%) were revised for femoral neck fractures. The authors concluded that the most important risk factors for femoral component loosening were large femoral head cysts, low patient height, female gender, and smaller component size in male patients. Mohamad and associates[90] reported early experience with metal-on-metal total hip arthroplasty in 20 hips (19 patients). In this study, osteonecrosis of the femoral head was the diagnosis in 63% of the patients undergoing the procedure. The mean patient age was 43 years (age range, 25 to 58 years), and the mean follow-up was 18 months (range, 7 to 46 months). At final follow-up, 16 of 20 hips (84%) had good or excellent hip scores. Mont and associates[91] reported on 41 hips (37 patients) treated with metal-on-metal total hip arthroplasty for osteone-

crosis. At a mean follow-up of 36 months (range, 24 to 48 months), 38 of 41 hips (93%) had good or excellent results. There was no radiolucency and no component loosening, but heterotopic ossification was reported in three hips (7%).

Although total hip resurfacing may be a bone-preserving alternative for patients with advanced-stage disease and acetabular degeneration, most devices are still under investigation, and long-term outcome studies are necessary before the value of this treatment option can be truly determined. An overview of metal-on-metal studies for osteonecrosis of the femoral head[18,20,89-93] is provided in Table 4.

Summary
Treatment of the late stages of osteonecrosis of the femoral head has been challenging and controversial. There are multiple new devices and emerging new technology that are being proposed for use in patients with osteonecrosis. However, the goals of treatment remain the same and include pain relief, improving function and quality of life, and possibly preservation options for a lifelong treatment plan. Patient selection is important for the outcome, and treatment options depend on factors such as patient's age, underlying disease, and disease stage at presentation. Although hemiresurfacing and total resurfacing procedures are used for young patients with limited involvement of the femoral head, standard total hip arthroplasty may be more appropriate for older patients with significant involvement of the femoral head and acetabulum. The use of alternative bearing surfaces (metal-on-metal, ceramic-on-ceramic, and ceramic on ultra-high molecular weight polyethylene) and improved

surgical techniques provide a new promise for better long-term outcomes than those previously reported.

References
1. Mont MA, Hungerford DS: Nontraumatic avascular necrosis of the femoral head. *J Bone Joint Surg Am* 1995;77:459-474.
2. Assouline-Dayan Y, Chang C, Greenspan A, Shoenfeld Y, Gershwin ME: Pathogenesis and natural history of osteonecrosis. *Semin Arthritis Rheum* 2002;32:94-124.
3. Beaulé PE, Amstutz HC: Management of Ficat stage III and IV osteonecrosis of the hip. *J Am Acad Orthop Surg* 2004;12:96-105.
4. Lieberman JR, Berry DJ, Mont MA, et al: Osteonecrosis of the hip: Management in the 21st century. *Instr Course Lect* 2003;52:337-355.
5. Brinker MR, Rosenberg AG, Kull L, Galante JO: Primary total hip arthroplasty using noncemented porous-coated femoral components in patients with osteonecrosis of the femoral head. *J Arthroplasty* 1994;9:457-468.
6. Cabanela ME: Bipolar versus total hip arthroplasty for avascular necrosis of the femoral head: A comparison. *Clin Orthop Relat Res* 1990;261:59-62.
7. Chandler HP, Reineck FT, Wixson RL, McCarthy JC: Total hip replacement in patients younger than thirty years old: A five-year follow-up study. *J Bone Joint Surg Am* 1981;63:1426-1434.
8. Saito S, Saito M, Nishina T, Ohzono K, Ono K: Long-term results of total hip arthroplasty for osteonecrosis of the femoral head: A comparison with osteoarthritis. *Clin Orthop Relat Res* 1989;244:198-207.
9. Lachiewicz PF, Desman SM: The bipolar endoprosthesis in avascular necrosis of the femoral head. *J Arthroplasty* 1988;3:131-138.
10. Takaoka K, Nishina T, Ohzono K, et al: Bipolar prosthetic replacement for the treatment of avascular necrosis of the femoral head. *Clin Orthop Relat Res* 1992;277:121-127.
11. Canadian Institute for Health Information: *2005 Canadian Joint Replacement Registry Annual Report: Total Hip and Knee Replacements in Canada.*

Available at: http://secure.cihi.ca/cihiweb/dispPage.jsp?cw_page=AR_30_E. Accessed June 2, 2006.

12. Australian Orthopaedic Association National Joint Replacement Registry: 2004 Annual Report. Available at: http://www.dmac.adelaide.edu.au/aoanjrr/documents/aoanjrrreport_2004.pdf. Accessed June 2, 2006.

13. Mont MA, Rajadhyaksha AD, Hungerford DS: Outcomes of limited femoral resurfacing arthroplasty compared with total hip arthroplasty for osteonecrosis of the femoral head. *J Arthroplasty* 2001;16(suppl 1):134-139.

14. Beaule PE, Schmalzried TP, Campbell P, Dorey F, Amstutz HC: Duration of symptoms and outcome of hemiresurfacing for hip osteonecrosis. *Clin Orthop Relat Res* 2001;385:104-117.

15. Nelson CL, Walz BH, Gruenwald JM: Resurfacing of only the femoral head for osteonecrosis: Long-term follow-up study. *J Arthroplasty* 1997;12:736-740.

16. Adili A, Trousdale RT: Femoral head resurfacing for the treatment of osteonecrosis in the young patient. *Clin Orthop Relat Res* 2003;417:93-101.

17. Cuckler JM, Moore KD, Estrada L: Outcome of hemiresurfacing in osteonecrosis of the femoral head. *Clin Orthop Relat Res* 2004;429:146-150.

18. Beaulé PE, Amstutz HC, Le Duff M, Dorey F: Surface arthroplasty for osteonecrosis of the hip: Hemiresurfacing versus metal-on-metal hybrid resurfacing. *J Arthroplasty* 2004;19(suppl 3):54-58.

19. Siguier T, Siguier M, Judet T, Charnley G, Brumpt B: Partial resurfacing arthroplasty of the femoral head in avascular necrosis: Methods, indications, and results. *Clin Orthop Relat Res* 2001;386:85-92.

20. Grecula MJ, Grigoris P, Schmalzried TP, Dorey F, Campbell PA, Amstutz HC: Endoprostheses for osteonecrosis of the femoral head: A comparison of four models in young patients. *Int Orthop* 1995;19:137-143.

21. Tooke SM, Amstutz HC, Delaunay C: Hemiresurfacing for femoral head osteonecrosis. *J Arthroplasty* 1987;2:125-133.

22. Langlais F, Barthas J, Postel M: Adjusted cups for idiopathic necrosis: Radiological results. *Rev Chir Orthop Reparatrice Appar Mot* 1979;65:151-155.

23. Hungerford MW, Mont MA, Scott R, Fiore C, Hungerford DS, Krackow KA: Surface replacement hemiarthroplasty for

the treatment of osteonecrosis of the femoral head. *J Bone Joint Surg Am* 1998;80:1656-1664.

24. Krackow KA, Mont MA, Maar DC: Limited femoral endoprosthesis for avascular necrosis of the femoral head. *Orthop Rev* 1993;22:457-463.

25. Scott RD, Urse JS, Schmidt R, Bierbaum BE: Use of TARA hemiarthroplasty in advanced osteonecrosis. *J Arthroplasty* 1987;2:225-232.

26. Grevitt MP, Spencer JD: Avascular necrosis of the hip treated by hemiarthroplasty: Results in renal transplant recipients. *J Arthroplasty* 1995;10:205-211.

27. Chan YS, Shih CH: Bipolar versus total hip arthroplasty for hip osteonecrosis in the same patient. *Clin Orthop Relat Res* 2000;379:169-177.

28. Sanjay BK, Moreau PG: Bipolar hip replacement in sickle cell disease. *Int Orthop* 1996;20:222-226.

29. Ito H, Matsuno T, Kaneda K: Bipolar hemiarthroplasty for osteonecrosis of the femoral head: A 7- to 18-year followup. *Clin Orthop Relat Res* 2000;374:201-211.

30. Yamano K, Atsumi T, Kajwara T: Bipolar endoprosthesis for osteonecrosis of the femoral head: A 12-year follow-up of 29 hips. *ARCO Transactions,* 2004.

31. Murzic WJ, McCollum DE: Hip arthroplasty for osteonecrosis after renal transplantation. *Clin Orthop Relat Res* 1994;299:212-219.

32. Tsumura H, Torisu T, Kaku N, Higashi T: Five- to fifteen-year clinical results and the radiographic evaluation of acetabular changes after bipolar hip arthroplasty for femoral head osteonecrosis. *J Arthroplasty* 2005;20:892-897.

33. Lee SB, Sugano N, Nakata K, Matsui M, Ohzono K: Comparison between bipolar hemiarthroplasty and THA for osteonecrosis of the femoral head. *Clin Orthop Relat Res* 2004;424:161-165.

34. Nagai I, Takatori Y, Kuruta Y, et al: Nonself-centering Bateman bipolar endoprosthesis for nontraumatic osteonecrosis of the femoral head: A 12- to 18-year follow-up study. *J Orthop Sci* 2002;7:74-78.

35. Learmonth ID, Opitz M: Treatment of grade III osteonecrosis of the femoral head with a Charnley/Bicentric hemiarthroplasty. *J R Coll Surg Edinb* 1993;38:311-314.

36. Dorr LD, Takei GK, Conaty JP: Total hip arthroplasties in patients less than

forty-five years old. *J Bone Joint Surg Am* 1983;65:474-479.

37. Cornell CN, Salvati EA, Pellicci PM: Long-term follow-up of total hip replacement in patients with osteonecrosis. *Orthop Clin North Am* 1985;16:757-769.

38. Kantor SG, Huo MH, Huk OL, Salvati EA: Cemented total hip arthroplasty in patients with osteonecrosis: A 6-year minimum follow-up study of second-generation cement techniques. *J Arthroplasty* 1996;11:267-271.

39. Garino JP, Steinberg ME: Total hip arthroplasty in patients with avascular necrosis of the femoral head: A 2- to 10-year follow-up. *Clin Orthop Relat Res* 1997;334:108-115.

40. Kim YH, Oh SH, Kim JS, Koo KH: Contemporary total hip arthroplasty with and without cement in patients with osteonecrosis of the femoral head. *J Bone Joint Surg Am* 2003;85:675-681.

41. Phillips FM, Pottenger LA, Finn HA, Vandermolen J: Cementless total hip arthroplasty in patients with steroid-induced avascular necrosis of the hip: A 62-month follow-up study. *Clin Orthop Relat Res* 1994;303:147-154.

42. Piston RW, Engh CA, De Carvalho PI, Suthers K: Osteonecrosis of the femoral head treated with total hip arthroplasty without cement. *J Bone Joint Surg Am* 1994;76:202-214.

43. Xenakis TA, Beris AE, Malizos KK, Koukoubis T, Gelalis J, Soucacos PN: Total hip arthroplasty for avascular necrosis and degenerative osteoarthritis of the hip. *Clin Orthop Relat Res* 1997;341:62-68.

44. Acurio MT, Friedman RJ: Hip arthroplasty in patients with sickle-cell haemoglobinopathy. *J Bone Joint Surg Br* 1992;74:367-371.

45. Lieberman JR, Fuchs MD, Haas SB, et al: Hip arthroplasty in patients with chronic renal failure. *J Arthroplasty* 1995;10:191-195.

46. Huo MH, Salvati EA, Browne MG, Pellicci PM, Sculco TP, Johanson NA: Primary total hip arthroplasty in systemic lupus erythematosus. *J Arthroplasty* 1992;7:51-56.

47. Zangger P, Gladman DD, Urowitz MB, Bogoch ER: Outcome of total hip replacement for avascular necrosis in systemic lupus erythematosus. *J Rheumatol* 2000;27:919-923.

48. Nich C, Sariali el-H, Hannouche D, et al

Long-term results of alumina-on-alumina hip arthroplasty for osteonecrosis. *Clin Orthop Relat Res* 2003;417:102-111.

49. Fye MA, Huo MH, Zatorski LE, Keggi KJ: Total hip arthroplasty performed without cement in patients with femoral head osteonecrosis who are less than 50 years old. *J Arthroplasty* 1998;13:876-881.

50. Berend KR, Gunneson E, Urbaniak JR, Vail TP: Hip arthroplasty after failed free vascularized fibular grafting for osteonecrosis in young patients. *J Arthroplasty* 2003;18:411-419.

51. Al-Mousawi F, Malki A, Al-Aradi A, Al-Bagali M, Al-Sadadi A, Booz MM: Total hip replacement in sickle cell disease. *Int Orthop* 2002;26:157-161.

52. Chen YW, Chang JK, Huang KY, Lin GT, Lin SY, Huang CY: Hip arthroplasty for osteonecrosis in patients with systemic lupus erythematosus. *Kaohsiung J Med Sci* 1999;15:697-703.

53. Hickman JM, Lachiewicz PF: Results and complications of total hip arthroplasties in patients with sickle-cell hemoglobinopathies: Role of cementless components. *J Arthroplasty* 1997;12:420-425.

54. Moran MC, Huo MH, Garvin KL, Pellicci PM, Salvati EA: Total hip arthroplasty in sickle cell hemoglobinopathy. *Clin Orthop Relat Res* 1993;294:140-148.

55. Clarke HJ, Jinnah RH, Brooker AF, Michaelson JD: Total replacement of the hip for avascular necrosis in sickle cell disease. *J Bone Joint Surg Br* 1989;71:465-470.

56. Hanker GJ, Amstutz HC: Osteonecrosis of the hip in the sickle-cell diseases: Treatment and complications. *J Bone Joint Surg Am* 1988;70:499-506.

57. Schneider W, Knahr K: Total hip replacement in younger patients: Survival rate after avascular necrosis of the femoral head. *Acta Orthop Scand* 2004;75:142-146.

58. Xenakis TA, Gelalis J, Koukoubis TA, Zaharis KC, Soucacos PN: Cementless hip arthroplasty in the treatment of patients with femoral head necrosis. *Clin Orthop Relat Res* 2001;386:93-99.

59. Taylor AH, Shannon M, Whitehouse SL, Lee MB, Learmonth ID: Harris-Galante cementless acetabular replacement in avascular necrosis. *J Bone Joint Surg Br* 2001;83:177-182.

60. Delank KS, Drees P, Eckardt A, Heine J: Results of the uncemented total hip arthroplasty in avascular necrosis of the femoral head. *Z Orthop Ihre Grenzgeb*

2001;139:525-530.

61. Hartley WT, McAuley JP, Culpepper WJ, Engh CA Jr, Engh CA Sr: Osteonecrosis of the femoral head treated with cementless total hip arthroplasty. *J Bone Joint Surg Am* 2000;82:1408-1413.

62. Stulberg BN, Singer R, Goldner J, Stulberg J: Uncemented total hip arthroplasty in osteonecrosis: A 2- to 10-year evaluation. *Clin Orthop Relat Res* 1997;334:116-123.

63. Gonzalez MH, Ortinau ET, Buonanno W, Prieto J: Cementless total hip arthroplasty in patients with advanced avascular necrosis. *J South Orthop Assoc* 1997;6:162-168.

64. D'Antonio JA, Capello WN, Manley MT, Feinberg J: Hydroxyapatite coated implants: Total hip arthroplasty in the young patient and patients with avascular necrosis. *Clin Orthop Relat Res* 1997;344:124-138.

65. Kim YH, Oh JH, Oh SH: Cementless total hip arthroplasty in patients with osteonecrosis of the femoral head. *Clin Orthop Relat Res* 1995;320:73-84.

66. Lins RE, Barnes BC, Callaghan JJ, Mair SD, McCollum DE: Evaluation of uncemented total hip arthroplasty in patients with avascular necrosis of the femoral head. *Clin Orthop Relat Res* 1993;297:168-173.

67. Katz RL, Bourne RB, Rorabeck CH, McGee H: Total hip arthroplasty in patients with avascular necrosis of the hip: Follow-up observations on cementless and cemented operations Clin Orthop Relat Res 1992;281:145-151.

68. Fyda TM, Callaghan JJ, Olejniczak J, Johnston RC: Minimum ten-year follow-up of cemented total hip replacement in patients with osteonecrosis of the femoral head. *Iowa Orthop J* 2002;22-8-19

69. Ortiguera CJ, Pulliam IT, Cabanela ME: Total hip arthroplasty for osteonecrosis: Matched-pair analysis of 188 hips with long-term follow-up. *J Arthroplasty* 1999;14:21-28

70. Wei SY, Klimkiewicz JJ, Steinberg ME: Revision total hip arthroplasty in patients with avascular necrosis. *Orthopedics* 1999;22:747-757.

71. Amstutz HC, Grigoris P, Dorey FJ: Evolution and future of surface replacement of the hip. *J Orthop Sci* 1998;3:169-186.

72. Cuckler JM, Moore KD, Lombardi AV Jr, McPherson E, Emerson R: Large versus

small femoral heads in metal-on-metal total hip arthroplasty. *J Arthroplasty* 2004;19(suppl 3):41-44.

73. Crowninshield RD, Maloney WJ, Wentz DH, Humphrey SM, Blanchard CR: Biomechanics of large femoral heads: What they do and don't do. *Clin Orthop Relat Res* 2004;429:102-107.

74. Dorr LD, Long WT: Metal-on-metal: Articulations for the new millennium. *Instr Course Lect* 2005;54:177-182.

75. Schmalzried TP, Peters PC, Maurer BT, Bragdon CR, Harris WH: Long-duration metal-on-metal total hip arthroplasties with low wear of the articulating surfaces. *J Arthroplasty* 1996;11:322-331.

76. Sieber HP, Rieker CB, Kottig P: Analysis of 118 second-generation metal-on-metal retrieved hip implants. *J Bone Joint Surg Br* 1999;81:46-50.

77. Campbell P, Urban RM, Catelas I, Skipor AK, Schmalzried TP: Autopsy analysis thirty years after metal-on-metal total hip replacement: A case report. *J Bone Joint Surg Am* 2003;85:2218-2222.

78. Little CP, Ruiz AL, Harding IJ, et al: Osteonecrosis in retrieved femoral heads after failed resurfacing arthroplasty of the hip. *J Bone Joint Surg Br* 2005;87:320-323.

79. Beaule PE, Le Duff M, Campbell P, Dorey FJ, Park SH, Amstutz HC: Metal-on-metal surface arthroplasty with a cemented femoral component: A 7-10 year follow-up study. *J Arthroplasty* 2004;19(suppl 3):17-22.

80. Amstutz HC, Campbell PA, Le Duff MJ: Fracture of the neck of the femur after surface arthroplasty of the hip. *J Bone Joint Surg Am* 2004;86-A:1874-1877.

81. MacDonald SJ: Metal-on-metal total hip arthroplasty: The concerns. *Clin Orthop Relat Res* 2004;429:86-93.

82. Tharani R, Dorey FJ, Schmalzried TP: The risk of cancer following total hip or knee arthroplasty. *J Bone Joint Surg Am* 2001;83:774-780.

83. Campbell P, Mirra J, Amstutz HC: Viability of femoral heads treated with resurfacing arthroplasty. *J Arthroplasty* 2000;15:120-122.

84. Howie DW, Cornish BL, Vernon-Roberts B: The viability of the femoral head after resurfacing hip arthroplasty in humans. *Clin Orthop Relat Res* 1993;291:171-184.

85. Bradley GW, Freeman MA, Revell PA: Resurfacing arthroplasty: Femoral head viability. *Clin Orthop Relat Res* 1987;220:137-141.

86. Back DL, Young DA, Shimmin AJ: How

do serum cobalt and chromium levels change after metal-on-metal hip resurfacing? *Clin Orthop Relat Res* 2005;438:177-181.

87. MacDonald SJ: Can a safe level for metal ions in patients with metal-on-metal total hip arthroplasties be determined? *J Arthroplasty* 2004;19(suppl 3):71-77.

88. MacDonald SJ, Brodner W, Jacobs JJ: A consensus paper on metal ions in metal-on-metal hip arthroplasties. *J Arthroplasty* 2004;19(suppl 3):12-16.

89. Amstutz HC, Beaule PE, Dorey FJ, Le Duff MJ, Campbell PA, Gruen TA: Metal-on-metal hybrid surface arthroplasty: Two to six-year follow-up study. *J Bone Joint Surg Am* 2004;86:28-39.

90. Mohamad JA, Kwan MK, Merican AM, et al: Early results of metal on metal articulation total hip arthroplasty in young patients. *Med J Malaysia* 2004;59:3-7.

91. Mont MA, Ragland PS, Marulanda GA, Delanois RE, Seyler TM: Use of metal-on-metal resurfacing arthroplasty for avascular necrosis of the hip. *ARCO Transactions*, 2005.

92. Yoo TC: Results of metal-on-metal resurfacing for avascular necrosis of the femoral head. *ARCO Transactions*, 2005.

93. Dutton RO, Amstutz HC, Thomas BJ, Hedley AK: Tharies surface replacement for osteonecrosis of the femoral head. *J Bone Joint Surg Am* 1982;64:1225-1237.

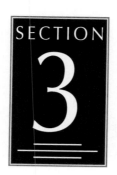

SECTION

3

Modern Management of Complications

Modern Management of Complications

Total hip arthroplasty (THA) has proved to predictably alleviate pain and restore function in patients with end-stage pathology of the hip joint. Its efficacy appears to apply to a wide range of diagnoses. The literature is continually populated with reports of favorable long-term results as it pertains not only to pain relief and restoration of function but also to implant survival. The articles in this section effectively emphasize the fact that very significant complications can occur following to THA. All surgeons performing THA must understand the incidence of these complications, the steps and methods required to avoid or minimize them, and perhaps most importantly the best ways to manage them when they occur.

Neurovascular injuries are not commonly encountered during or after THA. Barrack and Butler provide a comprehensive outline of all of the injuries that can occur in association with the procedure. As with many orthopaedic procedures, an informed understanding of the anatomy in the operative field is essential to avoid dramatic complications. The authors stress that avoiding structures at risk is the main way to minimize the incidence of injuries. Nerve injuries can be avoided by careful surgical exposure, cautious retractor placement, and strict attention to detail as it applies to restoration of limb length. Vascular injuries can be minimized by educated screw placement and screw length selection for acetabular components and cage constructs. Vascular injuries also can occur during implant removal, and the authors nicely define clinical scenarios that should cause the surgeon to be especially cautious and use exacting technique. The authors emphasize that a thorough knowledge of anatomy and understanding of surgical technique should be carried into the operative theater. A simple understanding of these principles should help minimize these dreaded injuries.

Dislocation following THA presents a significant challenge for the surgeon, and al-though all surgeons hope to be able to manage a dislocation without reoperation, the odds of success are against them. Two articles in this section focus on this relatively common complication; both define the patients and the circumstances that are of most concern and offer surgical solutions for prevention and management of this complication.

Mahoney and Pellici describe a robust anatomic repair of the posterior capsule and short external rotators to decrease the incidence of dislocation following THA performed via a posterior approach. Their results support the use of such a deliberate repair when using this approach.

Most hip surgeons would agree that the patient with recurrent dislocations is a real clinical challenge, particularly when the cause for dislocation is not evident. Daniel Berry offers a variety of surgical options for management of the trying patient with recurrent dislocations.

Both articles are extremely important and an excellent addition to this collection because they systematically define the patients that require the most care and that surgeons should be most concerned about. These patients must be readily identified so that appropriate preoperative planning, intraoperative decisions, and postoperative management plans can be formulated. Anticipation of the patient at risk for dislocation is critical because it allows the surgeon to make adjustments to surgical approach, implant selection, and postoperative rehabilitation.

Both articles reiterate that dislocation appears to be more common in the hands of the surgeon who does not perform THA regularly. This observation further underscores the importance of surgical technique and rigorous attention to detail as it pertains to implant placement, intraoperative stability assessment, and soft-tissue management. Dislocation inevitably occurs if a surgeon performs any reasonable number of hip arthroplasty procedures; understanding the material outlined in these two articles will help the surgeon weigh the advantages and disadvantages of nonsurgical and surgical management options, with an ultimate goal of minimizing the incidence of dislocation.

There is really no argument that hip surgeons are seeing more and more patients with periprosthetic fractures on the femoral side. Greidanus and associates provide an excellent review of this problem, including advice regarding prevention and management when it occurs. Emphasis is placed on awareness of differences in bone quality as it pertains to performing THA, differences in primary hip implant design, and the increased incidence of fracture in previously operated hips. This article appropriately stresses the importance of recognizing fractures intraoperatively in both the primary and revision settings. Surgical management of these fractures is technically demanding, and the authors provide a comprehensive management strategy for these patients. They also nicely describe the importance of issues such as implant selection, allograft supplementation, and postoperative rehabilitation, all of which must be considered and, in truth, mastered if a surgeon is going to attempt to manage these fractures.

THA, like any surgical procedure, has associated complications. As the field continues to evolve, however, we can only hope that the incidence of these complications will decrease. The numerous advances in technology keep us hopeful about the future. Intraoperative neurologic monitoring should eventually evolve to allow easy, cost-effective, real-time monitoring of the nerves exiting the hip during hip arthroplasty. We are hopeful that intraoperative CT and MRI someday can be mated to navigation not only to help avoid neurovascular structures but also to assist with placement of components in the ideal position, which could decrease the incidence of dislocation.

We continue to put hip stems in younger and younger patients and do not really know what problems we might be creating when placing a press-fit stem in a patient with a 50-or 60-year life expectancy. There is obviously great concern for periprosthetic femur fracture in this setting. There is some hope that hard-on-hard bearings (metal-on-metal and ceramic-on-ceramic) and perhaps hip resurfacing may allow for a more idealized outcome in these tough patients.

The implant manufacturers continue to provide us with more and more options in hip stems for the management of periprosthetic fractures. These newer modular stems are more forgiving than their fully porous-coated predecessors, and it is hoped that these new tools will enable us to manage these patients more effectively. We hope that the larger bearings, regardless of whether they are hard-on-hard or metal-on-highly cross-linked polyethylene, will help us reduce the incidence of dislocation, no matter what approach is used. Increased experience with and advances in instrumentation for the various approaches to the hip also are hoped to help us achieve this goal. It is essential to follow these new additions to our implant and surgical technique armamentarium prospectively to ensure that we are not creating new problems or making things worse are we move forward. The goal always should be to optimize patient outcomes and that will always require a special effort not only to minimize complications but also to perfect their management when they occur.

Michael P. Bolognesi, MD
Assistant Professor
Director, Adult Reconstruction
Division of Orthopaedic Surgery
Duke University Medical Center
Durham, North Carolina

Unstable Total Hip Arthroplasty: Detailed Overview

Daniel J. Berry, MD

Introduction

Dislocation is one of the most common complications of total hip arthroplasty (THA). Hip dislocation is a disturbing event for the patient and a frustrating problem for the surgeon and is associated with pain, morbidity,[1] and expense. Despite the increasing sophistication of THA implants and techniques, the problem of dislocation remains common, and although specific techniques may reduce the rate of dislocation, there is as yet no evidence that the overall prevalence has declined. Dislocation usually is treated nonsurgically initially, but recurrent dislocation usually requires surgical treatment. To date, most reports indicate that reoperation for recurrent instability carries with it a disconcertingly high chance of failure but, with better understanding of dislocation and improved technologies to treat dislocation, the success rate of surgical treatment probably can be improved. This chapter reviews the epidemiology of hip dislocation, measures that may be taken to avoid dislocation, and methods available to treat the dislocation.

Epidemiology

The prevalence of dislocation after THA varies widely, from 0.3% to 10% or more in different series.[2-6] In several large series the rate is 2% to 3%.[7-10] The rate in any specific series depends on many factors, including patient mix, the surgeon's experience,[11] and the surgical approach. It is clear that the reported prevalence of hip dislocation is higher if a specific program is in place at an institution to identify all patients who dislocate because many dislocations are not treated at the institution where the THA surgery was performed. Furthermore, the reported prevalence of dislocation is higher if patients are followed for longer periods of time, because first-time dislocations continue to occur for the life of the arthroplasty.

Risk Factors for Dislocation

Hip dislocation is well documented to be more common in specific demographic groups and is suspected to be more common in several others. Patient gender has an effect on the rate of dislocation: several series have shown women have a higher rate of dislocation than men.[9,10,12-15] Age at surgery appears to affect the risk of dislocation, with older patients at higher risk than younger patients, although the correlation between age and dislocation is not yet proven.[16-18] The reasons for a higher rate of dislocation in older patients may include a greater risk of falls, poorer soft tissues, and, perhaps, a greater incidence of confusion and noncompliance with dislocation precautions.

The underlying diagnosis leading to THA has an effect on dislocation risk. Patients treated with THA for a diagnosis of hip fracture are at high risk.[19-21] Advanced age, poorer or damaged muscles, greater propensity for falls, and altered proximal femoral anatomy probably all play a role in the increased risk of dislocation in these patients. The rate of dislocation in patients treated with THA for developmental dysplasia of the hip is elevated in some series.[21] In these patients, poorer muscle strength, bone deformity, and alterations from normal implant position may increase the risk.

Associated medical conditions and comorbidities also affect the risk of dislocation. Dislocation is more common in patients with neuromuscular conditions that lead to weakness in muscles around the hip or contractures around the hip.[4,22-25] Cognitive dysfunction increases the rate of hip dislocation, probably because impaired cognition leads to less compliance with hip dislocation precautions.[18,24]

Revision hip arthroplasty is associated with a considerably higher risk of dislocation than primary THA.[26] The main reasons for higher risk of dislocation after revision THA are compromised abductor muscles and bone loss that leads to compromises in implant location and orientation.

Chronology of Dislocation

Many authors[8,9,27,28] have reported that the majority of dislocations, on the order of 50% to 75%, occur in the first few months after THA. However, two studies[15,29] found that over 60% of dislocations occurred more than 4 to 5 weeks after surgery. Clearly, first-time dislocations continue indefinitely after a THA, and the longer patients are followed, the greater number that are identified late. Dislocations that occur in the first few months after THA, before the soft tissues have healed, are less likely to be recurrent than those that occur later according to most,[9,27] but not all,[29] authors. Late dislocation of a previously stable THA may be related to trauma or chronic changes around the hip (such as increased laxity of the pseudocapsule with time),[12] deteriorating muscle strength, or wear or deformation of the acetabular polyethylene.

Prevention of Dislocation

Measures to prevent dislocation can be divided into three main categories: preoperative measures, intraoperative measures, and postoperative measures.

Preoperative Measures

Some dislocation problems can be avoided by preoperatively identifying patients at high risk for dislocation and applying appropriate preventive measures. Knowledge of the epidemiologic factors discussed in the previous section helps the surgeon identify demographic groups at high risk for dislocation. Occasional patients may be at such high risk for dislocation that THA is considered contraindicated. Some patients with no preoperative abductor function, severe neuromuscular problems, or severe substance abuse or cognitive problems fall into this category. More commonly, patients will be recognized to be at increased risk for dislocation but nevertheless will be considered candidates for THA. Under these circumstances the surgeon may use a surgical exposure or implants that provide some protection against dislocation. For example, an elderly patient with Parkinson's disease, marked flexion contracture of the hip, and a diagnosis of subcapital hip fracture and little hip arthritis might be treated with an anterolateral approach rather than a posterolateral approach and a hemiarthroplasty rather than a THA.

Careful preoperative planning with implant templates helps prevent instability problems. Templating allows the surgeon to predict the optimal location and orientation of implants relative to bony landmarks of the pelvis and femur and predicts the proper level of femoral neck osteotomy. Importantly, preoperative templating allows the surgeon to choose implants that will restore leg length, femoral offset, and soft-tissue tension.

Intraoperative Measures

Approach Surgical approach affects the risk of dislocation. Multiple series have shown a higher risk of dislocation is associated with a posterior approach compared to an anterolateral approach.[2,14,15,30-35] The main reason for the difference is that in the posterior approach, the capsule and short external rotators that otherwise would provide posterior hip stability and act as a check rein to excessive hip internal rotation are taken down. There are also other reasons; inadequate acetabular component anteversion is more common with the posterior approach because the femur can interfere with socket insertion, leading to insufficient anteversion, and because when the patient is in the lateral position the pelvis tends to roll forward, creating the illusion of increased acetabular anteversion. Enhanced repair of the posterior soft tissues may reduce the risk associated with the posterior approach; recently a series in which preservation and meticulous repair of the posterior capsule and short external rotators was used demonstrated a low incidence of early postoperative dislocation.[36] Although the posterior approach has been associated with a higher dislocation rate, it also has advantages; the most important is that the abductor mechanism is not violated. The choice of exposure should be left to the surgeon's preference based on familiarity with each approach and the specifics of a given patient's situation. For patients at high risk for posterior dislocation, an anterolateral approach may reduce the risk.

Implant Orientation Implant orientation is one of the most important factors under the surgeon's control that strongly influences dislocation risk.[2-4,6,8,10,12,31,37-39]

Many series have demonstrated the importance of implant orientation for hip stability, and the orientation of both the acetabular component and femoral component are important. The classic article by Lewinnek and associates[39] showed that excess cup abduction or too little or too much cup forward flexion (hereafter called anteversion) increased the risk of hip instability. Barrack and associates (chapter 28) further refined the optimal cup position using a virtual reality computer model. They found the optimal cup position was approximately 45° of abduction and 20° of anteversion. Excessively abducted cups, that is, cups too vertical in orientation, lead to an increased risk of lateral hip dislocation with hip abduction. Insufficient abduction (that is, cups too horizontal in orientation) leads to less hip range of motion free of impingement in extension-external rotation and flexion-internal rotation. Insufficient anteversion increases the risk of posterior dislocation, whereas excessive anteversion increases the risk of anterior dislocation.

Femoral component orientation also plays a role in hip dislocation risk, but fewer studies have examined this factor because true femoral component version is difficult to measure radiographically without CT. One study showed femoral malposition to be a common source of hip instability.[7] The optimal femoral implant position appears to be about 15° of anteversion in most cases.

Acetabular and femoral component position have an additive influence on hip stability. Thus, modest additive malposition of both components may produce instability while modest malposition of one component may be partially compensated by the other.

Implant Location The location (as opposed to orientation) of the acetabular and femoral components affect hip stability. The location influences stability because it determines the likelihood of bony and soft tissue impingement, the efficiency of the abductor muscles, and the tension of the soft tissues. Marked socket medialization increases the likelihood of impingement of the femur against the pelvis, particularly in hip flexion and internal rotation, and can reduce the soft tissue tension in the hip unless a femoral stem with extra femoral offset is used. Markedly superior socket positioning increases the risk of impingement of the femur against the ischium in hip adduction, extension, and external rotation, and superior socket position also reduces the hip abductor tension if the leg is shortened. Thus, for primary hip replacements in the absence of bony deformity, hip stability can be optimized by avoiding excessively medial or superior placement of the socket.

Implant Choice Bipolar hemiarthroplasties appear to have a lower rate of dislocation than THA, probably because of the large outside diameter of the bipolar implant and the biarticular nature of the implant. These characteristics probably are the reason for a much lower reported hip instability risk for patients with femoral neck fractures treated with a bipolar arthroplasty when compared with THA.[40] For most patients with arthritic hips, however, resurfacing of the acetabulum with a fixed socket is preferred to optimize clinical results and pain relief.

A number of implant-related factors affect hip stability; these include femoral component offset, femoral component head-to-neck diameter ratio, femoral component neck geometry, and acetabular component design.[41,42] Although theoretically all these factors should affect hip stability, to date, proof in clinical series is lacking, probably because dislocation is a multifactorial problem and multiple confounding factors make it difficult to prove that a specific design factor affects hip stability. Nevertheless, if specific design features may improve hip stability, it is reasonable for the surgeon to consider using them, provided they have no major drawbacks.

Femoral offset is the horizontal distance from the center of the femoral canal to the center of the femoral head. The reproduction of femoral offset helps restore soft-tissue tension and reduces the hip-joint reactive force. Implants with increased femoral offset are an important recent design advance that for many patients better restore hip mechanics and, hopefully, will improve hip stability without excessive leg lengthening. The main drawback of higher offset femoral implants is increased torsional and bending stress on the femoral implant.

Increasing femoral component head diameter theoretically increases hip stability[41,43] by increasing the femoral head displacement necessary to cause dislocation. Increasing the femoral head-to-neck diameter ratio also should increase hip stability by increasing the arc of hip motion that can occur free of prosthetic impingement. Despite these theoretical advantages, clinical series have not shown a strong correlation between femoral head size and hip stability.[6,7,9,15,32,38,44] Large femoral head sizes do have a major disadvantage: increased volumetric polyethylene wear that can lead to increased periprosthetic osteolysis. Balancing the risks of instability and volumetric polyethylene wear, most surgeons prefer 28-, 26-, or 22-mm head sizes in most situations. However, the advantages of larger femoral head sizes may outweigh their disadvantages in specific patients at high risk for dislocation.

For a given femoral head size, the head-to-neck diameter ratio can be improved by reducing (within the constraints of material strength) the prosthetic femoral neck diameter. Neck geometries with a narrow anterior-posterior profile also help maintain implant strength while optimizing range of motion free of implant impingement. A better head-to-neck ratio is maintained by avoiding extra-long modular femoral heads that have reinforcing skirts on the

neck. Good preoperative planning will allow the surgeon to choose a sufficiently high femoral neck osteotomy level and an implant with sufficient neck length and offset to minimize the need for skirted modular femoral heads.

Elevated acetabular rim liners also affect hip stability, and different types of elevated rims are made by different manufacturers.[13] Some change the orientation of the face of the socket, while others provide an extended wall on one side of the socket. The two types of rim elevation are not identical; however, they both reorient the arc of hip stability but usually do not increase its magnitude.[45] Placement of an elevation posteriorly increases posterior stability at the expense of anterior stability, and placement of an elevation anteriorly increases anterior stability at the expense of posterior stability. Elevated rims can at times create prosthetic impingement and actually cause dislocation.[46] In one of the few clinical studies on the subject, Cobb and associates[47] found elevated liners provided a statistically significantly decreased likelihood of dislocation in patients treated with a primary THA using a posterior approach (but not an anterior approach) and in patients treated with revision THA.

Postoperative Measures
Postoperative patient education can help prevent dislocation. It is helpful for both the surgeon and physical therapists to emphasize the importance of hip dislocation precautions before the patient is discharged from the hospital after THA. Patients benefit from instruction on how to get in and out of chairs, bed, and automobiles, and how to put on shoes and socks safely. Prophylactic postoperative hip guide braces also can reduce the risk of dislocation in high-risk patients.

Treatment of Dislocation
The choice of surgical or nonsurgical treatment of hip dislocation depends on whether the dislocation is recurrent, the

chronology of the dislocation relative to the hip arthroplasty, and patient-specific factors.

Closed Reduction

Most dislocations that occur early after THA and most first or second dislocations are managed nonsurgically with closed reduction. Exceptions to this include dislocations associated with failed implants, dislocations associated with marked component malposition, and dislocations that cannot be reduced by closed means. During closed reduction, care needs to be taken to avoid implant dislodgment or modular implant disassembly.[48] Usually, some form of immobilization is used to reduce the risk of early redislocation; this immobilization can take the form of either a cast or a brace. Hip braces can minimize hip adduction and limit hip flexion. A hip spica cast provides even more constraint to motion, but, because it hinders ambulation and sitting, this treatment is reserved for very unstable hips.

The results of closed reduction followed by bracing or casting are available in a limited number of patients. Dorr and Wan[49] found 10 of 12 hips treated with a hip guide brace for 4 to 6 weeks became stable, and Clayton and Thirupathi[50] reported success in seven of nine patients treated with longer term bracing. Ritter[6] reported success in three of five hips treated with a hip spica cast. Bracing or casting are likely to be successful in treating first dislocations not associated with a clear-cut mechanical problem with the arthroplasty, but are less successful when the dislocation is recurrent. Stewart[51] found five of five first-time dislocations were treated successfully with a brace, but only three of eight recurrent dislocations were treated successfully.

The optimal duration of bracing or cast immobilization following dislocation is not known. For most patients 6 to 12 weeks after dislocation is a reasonable length of time that allows soft tissues disrupted by the dislocation to heal. Recur-

rent episodes of dislocation will usually require surgical treatment, although when strong medical or orthopaedic contraindications to surgery exist, prolonged nonsurgical treatment with bracing is an option.

Surgical Treatment

Surgical treatment of hip instability is estimated to be required after about 1% of THAs. This means that recurrent dislocation is probably the most frequent reason for early reoperation after THA. Although surgical treatment usually can solve a dislocation problem, the surgeon should not be complacent about this operation; in several of the largest series the redislocation rate after reoperation for hip instability was 20% to 40%.[52,53] These sobering statistics mean that historically, reoperation for instability has carried with it the highest likelihood of failure of any commonly performed reoperation after THA, including reoperation for infection. With improved understanding of hip dislocation, surgeons have become better at identifying the problems that lead to dislocation and solving them. Furthermore, powerful new technologies have become available to treat dislocation problems that once would not have been solvable. It is hoped that the rate of success now can be improved markedly.

When surgical management of dislocation is contemplated, an organized approach to analyzing the problem aids treatment. The surgeon first must understand the direction of dislocation: anterior, posterior, or directly lateral. When possible, this direction should be determined by a true lateral radiograph taken when the hip is dislocated. A detailed discussion about the hip position that led to dislocation also helps identify the direction of dislocation.

The surgeon should make every effort to understand the etiology of dislocation by considering the differential diagnosis of problems that lead to hip instability (Table 1). A discussion with the patient to determine cognitive or behavioral prob-

lems that contributed to dislocation, a careful physical examination aimed at determining leg length and abductor strength, and good-quality radiographs of the hip arthroplasty to determine implant stability and orientation[54,55] are all important parts of this evaluation. The etiology of a hip dislocation cannot always be identified, but, whenever possible, it is important, because understanding the cause leads to more directed and successful treatment.[11,52]

Component Malposition

When the main problem leading to hip instability is component malposition, the treatment is usually component reorientation (Fig. 1). Acetabular malposition is treated by reorienting the socket. Excess cup abduction, excess cup anteversion, or insufficient cup anteversion all can be treated by socket repositioning. Daly and Morrey[52] reported an 81% success rate (22 of 28 hips) when an unstable hip with insufficient acetabular component anteversion was revised by socket repositioning.

Elevated rim liners for modular sockets, or socket wall additions that are attached to nonmodular sockets with screws,[32,56-59] produce small adjustments in relative cup position. Placement of an elevated liner with the elevated hood laterally reduces the relative cup abduction; placement of an elevated rim posteriorly produces more cup anteversion; and placement anteriorly, less relative cup anteversion. The amount of reorientation of the safe zone of hip motion provided by elevated rim liners is modest, and they do not correct major abnormalities in acetabular component position. Fehring and associates[60] reported a high rate of failure when the only measure applied to treat recurrent instability was modular liner and modular head exchange. In a selected group of 29 patients treated in this manner, 16 (55%) had at least one redislocation in the study period.

Table 1
Differential diagnosis of hip dislocation after THA
Component malposition
Socket
Stem
Both socket and stem
Inadequate soft-tissue tension
Unrestored leg length/femoral offset
Excessively lax soft tissues
Impingement
Bone of femur against pelvis
Soft tissue or heterotopic bone interposed between femur and pelvis
Prosthetic femoral neck on acetabular component
Abductor mechanism deficiency
Abductor muscle deficiency due to poor healing, loss of substance, or superior gluteal nerve damage
Trochanteric osteotomy or fracture with proximal migration
Patient compliance problems
Cognitive
Behavioral
Substance abuse
Neuromuscular deficiency

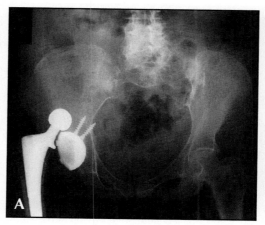 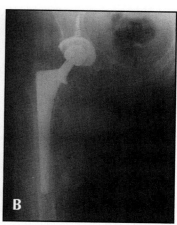

Fig. 1 A, AP pelvis radiograph of a patient with acetabular component malposition causing recurrent dislocation. **B,** AP hip radiograph after the acetabular component was revised to a less abducted position, thereby restoring hip stability.

Marked abnormalities in stem version can be treated with femoral component revision. However, revision of a well-fixed femoral component can be a major undertaking and can lead to substantial bone loss; thus, the surgeon must determine whether directed treatment of the problem (femoral component revision) is the best choice or whether the problem can be solved by compensating for the suboptimal femoral position in other ways.

Soft-Tissue Tension Insufficiency

The treatment of insufficient soft-tissue tension caused by lax but present soft tissues depends on its etiology and the implants in place. If the etiology is inadequate restoration of femoral offset or leg length, the soft tissues may be re-tensioned by increasing the femoral length or offset (by exchanging components). If modular implants are in place,

then a modular femoral head can be exchanged to a longer size. Modular "offset" or "lateralized" acetabular liners move the hip center of rotation laterally and inferiorly and increase the tension of the soft-tissue sleeve. If implants are not modular or if modular implants cannot provide a sufficient increase in soft-tissue tension, then the femoral component can be revised. Alternatively, trochanteric advancement can tension the abductor sleeve and thus improve hip stability. Ekelund[61] reported success with this technique in 19 of 21 patients, and Kaplan and associates[62] reported success with this technique in 17 of 21 patients. In both reports, a prerequisite for this form of treatment was satisfactory implant position. A disadvantage of trochanteric osteotomy is the risk that trochanteric nonunion, if it should occur, can cause an instability problem to worsen. Several factors determine the best method of restoring soft-tissue tension, including the desired leg length, whether the implants are modular, consideration of the pros and cons of long modular femoral heads with reinforcing skirts, and the suitability for advancement of the patient's trochanteric bone quality and abductors.

Impingement

Impingement can cause dislocation because the impingement source acts as a fulcrum levering the femoral head out of the socket. The impingement source can be the femur against the pelvis, interposed soft tissue, heterotopic bone, a migrated greater trochanter fragment, or the prosthetic neck against the prosthetic acetabulum. Impingement between the greater trochanter and pelvis with hip flexion and internal rotation may be treated either by excising some of the anterior greater trochanter or by removing hypertrophic soft tissues between the femur and pelvis in the region of the anterior capsule and the reflected head of the rectus femoris. Impingement between the femur and the ischium with the leg in extension, adduction, and external rotation can be treated by removing a small amount of prominent ischium or removing hypertrophic posterior inferior capsule or scar. Prosthetic impingement of the femoral neck against the acetabular component occurs with implant malposition, with a poor head-to-neck-diameter ratio, or when an acetabular component design has a very elevated rim. Prosthetic impingement is treated

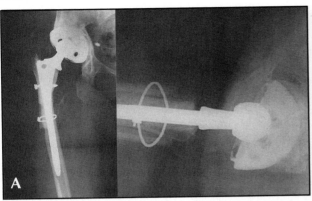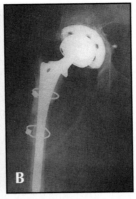

Fig. 2 A, AP and lateral hip radiographs of a patient with proximal femoral allograft, deficient abductors, and recurrent hip instability despite good implant position. **B,** AP hip radiograph after revision to a nonconstrained tripolar device using a custom, large-inside-diameter polyethylene liner.

by improving the implant position, optimizing the head-to-neck ratio, or removing an elevated acetabular rim liner.

Abductor Muscle Deficiency

The abductors normally contribute to hip stability by forming a dynamic sleeve around the hip. When the abductors are deficient or dysfunctional, the risk of hip instability is increased markedly. Abductor deficiency can be caused by trauma, failure of abductor or greater trochanteric healing after previous operations, or superior gluteal nerve dysfunction. Regardless of the etiology, abductor muscle insufficiency is one of the most difficult-to-solve causes of hip instability.

Fracture or nonunion of the greater trochanter with proximal migration leads to insufficiency of the abductor mechanism. Woo and Morrey[15] demonstrated that the dislocation rate increased from 2.8% to 17.6% when the trochanter failed to unite and migrated proximally. Reattachment of the greater trochanter can successfully restore continuity of the abductor mechanism and hip stability; however, trochanteric reattachment may not be possible when the trochanteric fragment is dysvascular or

small, or the trochanteric bed (the proximal lateral femur) is markedly deficient. Sometimes the greater trochanter can be advanced to healthy host bone by "pie crusting" tight scar and tendons of the abductor mechanism or by detaching the abductor mechanism from the proximal lateral ileum and advancing it distally on the superior gluteal neurovascular pedicle.

Abductor insufficiency also can result from the abductors failing to heal to the trochanter after an anterolateral approach to the hip. When the remaining abductors are of sufficient quality to allow reattachment, abductor repair sometimes can restore hip stability.[63] When the abductors cannot be repaired because of marked loss of abductor substance, severe scarring, or gluteal nerve damage, other measures to restore hip stability, such as constrained implants, must be considered.

Multifactorial Instability Problems

Many patients have some combination of implant malposition, impingement, or soft-tissue tension problems that together lead to instability. In these circumstances, combined measures aimed at solving in turn each of the contributing problems may be successful.

Conversion of THA to a Bipolar Femoral Head or Constrained Acetabular Component

The directed treatment methods discussed above are most effective when a specific problem leading to instability can be identified and solved. Unfortunately, the etiology of an instability problem cannot always be diagnosed, and, furthermore, some problems cannot be treated successfully by standard means. For such instability problems conversion to a bipolar femoral head or to a constrained acetabular component may be considered.

Conversion to Bipolar Femoral Head

Conversion of a conventional THA to a bipolar arthroplasty can restore hip stability.[64] Limited results of the technique have been reported. Zelicof and Scott[65] reported that all of 11 hips revised for instability were stabilized by conversion to a bipolar arrangement, and an 81% success rate (22 of 27 hips) in restoring hip stability was reported by Parvizi and Morrey.[66] The main disadvantage of conversion to a bipolar femoral head is that the mobile head articulates directly with acetabular bone and can cause pain and bone erosion; these problems are more likely when there is marked preexisting acetabular bone loss.

A bipolar or large-diameter monopolar head also can be articulated with a large inside diameter custom-made polyethylene liner of an acetabular component (Fig. 2). This approach gains the stability advantages of a bipolar head or very large head size while avoiding its main drawback—direct articulation of a mobile femoral head surface with bone. The technique requires a sufficiently large socket diameter to allow a custom-made large-inside-diameter polyethylene bearing surface to be inserted. Limited results of conversion to a tripolar arrangement (bipolar against a large-inside-diameter socket) have been reported. Grigoris and associates[67] reported that all of eight hips treated for instability with this method became stable.

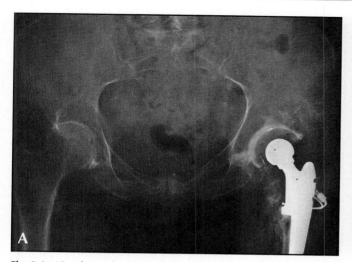
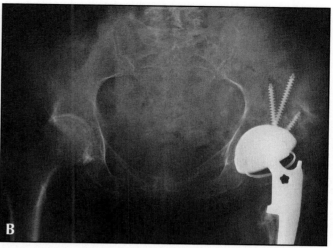

Fig. 3 A, AP pelvis radiograph of an elderly patient with recurrent hip instability after THA for an intertrochanteric hip fracture. The abductors were deficient. **B,** AP pelvis radiograph after the acetabular component was revised to a constrained tripolar component.

Constrained Implants These implants, which capture the femoral head, provide a powerful solution to manage many previously untreatable hip problems[30] (Figs. 3 and 4). These devices mostly have supplanted bipolar implants as a means of treating difficult instability problems. The advantages of these devices, however, come at a cost. Constrained implants have the potential to transmit high loads, which would otherwise lead to hip dislocation, to implant interfaces; these loads can lead to implant loosening (Fig. 5, *A*) or implant disassembly (Fig. 5, *B*). Most constrained liners provide less hip range of motion free of prosthetic impingement; repetitive impingement can lead to fatigue failure of the locking mechanism (Fig. 5, *C*). Constrained implants also have a risk of increased polyethylene wear and, potentially, osteolysis because of component impingement or multiple large-diameter metal-on-polyethylene articulating surfaces. Finally, if dislocation occurs when a constrained socket is in place, open reduction usually is required.

There is considerable variability in constrained implant designs. Different designs provide different levels of constraint and are subject to different modes

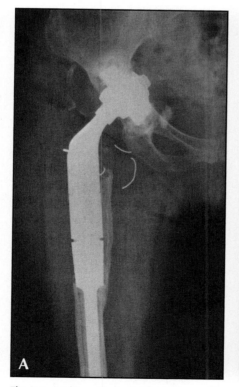
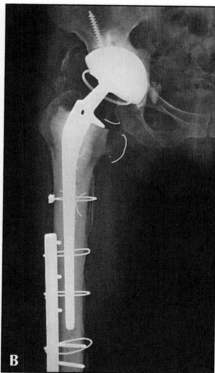

Fig. 4 A, AP hip radiograph of a patient with recurrent hip instability and failed tumor prosthesis. **B,** AP hip radiograph after revision to a constrained tripolar socket. The femur was revised to an allograft prosthetic composite.

of failure. The three main types of constrained implants are snap-fit sockets, sockets with constraint provided by a metal locking ring around the periphery of a polyethylene insert, and constrained tripolar devices. Snap-fit designs provide

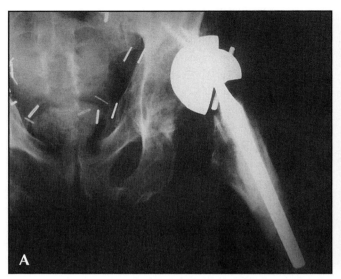
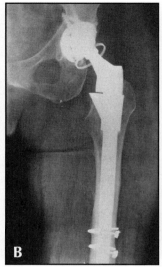
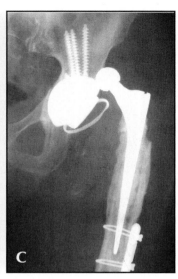

Fig. 5 A, AP hip radiograph demonstrating failure of a constrained uncemented socket at the implant-bone interface. **B**, AP hip radiograph demonstrating disassembly of the locking ring of a constrained socket. **C**, AP hip radiograph of a constrained socket that failed due to prosthetic impingement. The prosthetic femoral neck impinged on the locking ring (note deformation of the ring), leading to locking ring failure and dislocation.

less constraint than the other two design types. Constrained modular designs with locking rings can fail by disassembly of the locking ring,[68] dislocation of the head from the liner, or failure at the socket-bone, bone-cement, implant-cement, or polyethylene liner-shell interfaces. Failures can occur by acute overload or fatigue failure of the captured head locking mechanism. Anderson and associates[69] reported the results of 21 constrained S-ROM sockets (DePuy, Johnson & Johnson, Warsaw, IN); 18 of these were placed for recurrent instability. At a minimum of 2 years after surgery six had redislocated, and failures occurred at both the liner-shell interface and the head-liner interface. Lombardi and associates[70] reported 28 of 31 hips with previous instability treated with the same constrained socket were stable at a minimum of 2 years. Using a constrained tripolar device (Howmedica Osteonics, East Rutherford, NJ), Goetz and associates[71] reported a 96% (54 of 56 hips) success rate in 56 hips revised specifically for hip instability. In that

series, the constrained tripolar was used selectively for difficult instability problems in patients with a history of an average of six dislocations each. In 46 hips the tripolar component was placed without cement, and in 10 it was placed with cement (in four of which it was cemented into a well-fixed, porous-coated shell). One of the two failures occurred at the cement-metal interface of a constrained liner cemented into the metal-backed shell of another manufacturer, and the other failure occurred at the implant-bone interface of an uncemented socket.

The indications for use of constrained acetabular implants continue to evolve, and there are differing opinions about the indications for use of these devices. As a general rule, the threshold for using constrained implants is higher in younger than older patients because of the worrisome consequences of polyethylene wear and implant impingement in younger patients. Constrained implants are most helpful in the following situations: (1) patients who have failed

well-done attempts to solve an instability problem without constrained implants; (2) patients in whom the etiology of instability cannot be delineated, a situation in which the failure rate of other treatment methods is high; (3) patients with cognitive problems who cannot comply with reasonable dislocation precautions; (4) patients with deficient abductors (Figs. 4 and 5); (5) patients in whom the application of any other technique to gain stability carries a greater potential for problems or complications than would a constrained implant; and (6) some patients, particularly elderly or low-activity individuals, with reasonably well-positioned implants and a well-ingrown porous uncemented modular socket that is compatible with a constrained off-the-shelf or custom-made implant. (In this situation, constraint represents an expeditious, low-risk solution to a difficult problem. In the same patients, cementing a constrained liner into the well-fixed shell could be considered if a constrained liner were not available.)

Constrained implants should not be used when the bone quality is too poor for solid fixation of the implant to bone because constrained implants produce higher interface stresses. Constrained implants also should not be used to compensate for hopelessly malpositioned implants.

Summary

Hip dislocation is one of the most common complications of THA. Good preoperative planning, good postoperative patient education, accurate intraoperative component positioning, rigorous intraoperative testing of hip stability, and good repair of soft tissues during closure all help prevent dislocation. Early postoperative dislocations and first or second dislocations usually are treated with closed reduction and a hip guide brace or hip spica cast, but when dislocation becomes recurrent, surgical treatment usually is needed. When possible, surgical treatment is based on identifying and treating a specific problem leading to the dislocation, such as implant malposition, inadequate soft-tissue tension, or impingement. In selected circumstances, constrained implants or bipolar or tripolar implants provide powerful tools to restore hip stability.

References

1. Chandler RW, Dorr LD, Perry J: The functional cost of dislocation following total hip arthroplasty. Clin Orthop 1982;168:168-172.
2. Eftekhar NS: Dislocation and instability complicating low friction arthroplasty of the hip joint. Clin Orthop 1976;121:120-125.
3. Etienne A, Cupic Z, Charnley J: Postoperative dislocation after Charnley low-friction arthroplasty. Clin Orthop 1978;132:19-23.
4. Morrey BF: Instability after total hip arthroplasty. Orthop Clin North Am 1992;23:237-248.
5. Rao JP, Bronstein R: Dislocations following arthroplasties of the hip: Incidence, prevention, and treatment. Orthop Rev 1991;20:261-264.
6. Ritter MA: Dislocation and subluxation of the total hip replacement. Clin Orthop 1976;121:92-94.
7. Fackler CD, Poss R: Dislocation in total hip arthroplasties. Clin Orthop 1980;151:169-178.
8. Garcia-Cimbrelo E, Munuera L: Dislocation in low-friction arthroplasty. J Arthroplasty 1992;7:149-155.
9. Ali Khan MA, Brakenbury PH, Reynolds IS: Dislocation following total hip replacement. J Bone Joint Surg Br 1981;63:214-218.
10. Kristiansen B, Jorgensen L, Holmich P: Dislocation following total hip arthroplasty. Arch Orthop Trauma Surg 1985;103:375-377.
11. Hedlundh U, Ahnfelt L, Hybbinette CH, Weckstrom J, Fredin H: Surgical experience related to dislocations after total hip arthroplasty. J Bone Joint Surg Br 1996;78:206-209.
12. Coventry MB: Late dislocations in patients with Charnley total hip arthroplasty. J Bone Joint Surg Am 1985;67:832-841.
13. Nicholas RM, Orr JF, Mollan RA, Calderwood JW, Nixon JR, Watson P: Dislocation of total hip replacements: A comparative study of standard, long posterior wall and augmented acetabular components. J Bone Joint Surg Br 1990;72:418-422.
14. Turner RS: Postoperative total hip prosthetic femoral head dislocations: Incidence, etiologic factors, and management. Clin Orthop 1994;301:196-204.
15. Woo RY, Morrey BF: Dislocations after total hip arthroplasty. J Bone Joint Surg Am 1982;64:1295-1306.
16. Ekelund A, Rydell N, Nilsson OS: Total hip arthroplasty in patients 80 years of age and older. Clin Orthop 1992;281:101-106.
17. Newington DP, Bannister GC, Fordyce M: Primary total hip replacement in patients over 80 years of age. J Bone Joint Surg Br 1990;72:450-452.
18. Woolson ST, Rahimtoola ZO: Risk factors for dislocation during the first 3 months after primary total hip replacement. J Arthroplasty 1999;14:662-668.
19. Gregory RJ, Gibson MJ, Moran CG: Dislocation after primary arthroplasty for subcapital fracture of the hip: Wide range of movement is a risk factor. J Bone Joint Surg Br 1991;73:11-12.
20. Lee BP, Berry DJ, Harmsen WS, Sim FH: Total hip arthroplasty for the treatment of an acute fracture of the femoral neck: Long-term results. J Bone Joint Surg Am 1998;80:70-75.
21. Mallory TH, Lombardi AV Jr, Fada RA, Herrington SM, Eberle RW: Dislocation after total hip arthroplasty using the anterolateral abductor split approach. Clin Orthop 1999;358:166-172.
22. Hedlundh U, Fredin H: Patient characteristics in dislocations after primary total hip arthroplasty: 60 patients compared with a control group. Acta Orthop Scand 1995;66:225-228.
23. Hedlundh U, Karlsson M, Ringsberg K, Besjakov J, Fredin H: Muscular and neurologic function in patients with recurrent dislocation after total hip arthroplasty: A matched controlled study of 65 patients using dual-energy x-ray absorptiometry and postural stability tests. J Arthroplasty 1999;14:319-325.
24. Paterno SA, Lachiewicz PF, Kelley SS: The influence of patient-related factors and the position of the acetabular component on the rate of dislocation after total hip replacement. J Bone Joint Surg Am 1997;79:1202-1210.
25. Pierchon F, Pasquier G, Cotten A, Fontaine C, Clarisse J, Duquennoy A: Causes of dislocation of total hip arthroplasty: CT study of component alignment. J Bone Joint Surg Br 1994;76:45-48.
26. Berry, DJ: Dislocation, in Steinberg ME, Garino JP (eds): Revision Total Hip Arthroplasty. Philadelphia, PA, Lippincott-Williams & Wilkins, 1999, pp 463-481.
27. Lindberg HO, Carlsson AS, Gentz C-F, Pettersson H: Recurrent and non-recurrent dislocation following total hip arthroplasty. Acta Orthop Scand 1982;53:947-952.
28. Williams JF, Gottesman MJ, Mallory TH: Dislocation after total hip arthroplasty: Treatment with an above-knee hip spica cast. Clin Orthop 1982;171:53-58.
29. Joshi A, Lee CM, Markovic L, Vlatis G, Murphy JC: Prognosis of dislocation after total hip arthroplasty. J Arthroplasty 1998;13:17-21.
30. Browne AO, Sheehan JM: Trochanteric osteotomy in Charnley low-friction arthroplasty of the hip. Clin Orthop 1986;211:128-133.
31. Horwitz BR, Rockowitz NL, Goll SR, et al: A prospective randomized comparison of two surgical approaches to total hip arthroplasty. Clin Orthop 1993;291:154-163.
32. McCollum DE, Gray WJ: Dislocation after total hip arthroplasty: Causes and prevention. Clin Orthop 1990;261:159-170.
33. Roberts JM, Fu FH, McClain EJ, Ferguson AB Jr: A comparison of the posterolateral and anterolateral approaches to total hip arthroplasty. Clin Orthop 1984;187:205-210.
34. Unwin AJ, Thomas M: Dislocation after hemiarthroplasty of the hip: A comparison of the dislocation rate after posterior and lateral approaches to the hip. Ann R Coll Surg Engl 1994;76:327-329.
35. Vicar AJ, Coleman CR: A comparison of the anterolateral, transtrochanteric, and posterior surgical approaches in primary total hip arthroplasty. Clin Orthop 1984;188:152-159.
36. Pellicci PM, Bostrom M, Poss R: Posterior approach to total hip replacement using enhanced posterior soft tissue repair. Clin Orthop 1998;355:224-228.
37. Carlsson AS, Gentz CF: Postoperative dislocation in the Charnley and Brunswik total hip arthroplasty. Clin Orthop 1977;125:177-182.
38. Dorr LD, Wolf AW, Chandler R, Conaty JP: Classification and treatment of dislocations of total hip arthroplasty. Clin Orthop 1983;173:151-158.
39. Lewinnek GE, Lewis JL, Tarr R, Compere CL, Zimmerman JR: Dislocations after total hip-replacement arthroplasties. J Bone Joint Surg Am 1978;60:217-220.
40. Barnes CL, Berry DJ, Sledge CB: Dislocation after bipolar hemiarthroplasty of the hip. J Arthroplasty 1995;10:667-669.

Complications in Primary Total Hip Arthroplasty: Avoidance and Management of Dislocations

Craig R. Mahoney, MD
Paul M. Pellicci, MD

Abstract

Dislocation in primary total hip arthroplasty is common and problematic and is attributable to several factors, including previous hip surgery, neuromuscular disorders, cerebral dysfunction, psychosis, alcoholism, and female gender. Factors under the control of the surgeon include component orientation and restoration of soft-tissue tension. Prosthetic factors lowering the risk of dislocation include increasing the size of the prosthetic femoral head, keeping femoral neck circumference to a minimum, and optimizing the geometry of the acetabular component. Postoperatively, patients should be expected to comply with standard hip precautions.

Treatment is with immediate closed reduction. Multiple dislocations can be treated by advancing the trochanter in the presence of inadequate soft-tissue tension, revision arthroplasty in the presence of malpositioned components, or the use of a constrained cup when intraoperative instability persists.

Because the risk of redislocation is much higher than that for first-time dislocation, prevention is critical. An enhanced repair technique can be used to reconstruct the posterior soft-tissue sleeve during the posterior surgical approach. This technique has been successful in lowering the dislocation rate from 4% to 0% in a series of 395 consecutive patients.

Dislocation in primary total hip arthroplasty (THA) can be attributed to risk factors involving the patient, the surgeon, the prosthesis, and postoperative care.[1] This chapter focuses on these factors and nonsurgical and surgical treatment options. The senior author's current surgical technique for repairing the soft tissues will be presented as a possible means to avoid dislocation.

Epidemiology

Reports regarding dislocations document only true dislocation events; therefore, the incidence of instability is likely understated. Dislocation rates of less than 5% are often reported in the literature. Morrey[2] reviewed 16 studies between 1973 and 1987 that did not control for approach, type of prosthesis, or postoperative regimen. Of 35,000 procedures, a dislocation rate of 2.23% was found. Individual rates ranged from 0.7% to 7.0%.

Dislocations can occur in a posterior or anterior direction. Posterior dislocation is usually secondary to a combination of excessive flexion, adduction, and internal rotation and has been historically associated with the posterior surgical approach to the hip. An anterior dislocation occurs during excessive extension, adduction, and external rotation. Anterior dislocations have been associated more frequently with anterior surgical approaches to the hip but may occur with posterior approaches as well.

Risk Factors
Patient Factors

A preoperative assessment should be done to look for any possible factor that may predispose the patient to dislocation. Previous studies have focused on the diagnosis prior to THA, previous hip surgery, comorbid states, gender, age, and body habitus as predisposing factors.[3-7]

Diagnosis Higher dislocation rates have occurred when THA is done in the presence of hip fracture.[3] Soft-tissue and bony trauma alter surgical landmarks and affect stability. Woo and Morrey[4] compared other preoperative diagnoses, including osteoarthritis, rheumatoid arthritis, osteonecrosis, and developmental dysplasia of the hip as possible predisposing factors for dislocation and found no association.

Prior Hip Surgery One of the most significant patient factors predisposing to dislocation is THA in a previously operated hip. Woo and Morrey[4] reviewed over 10,000 THAs and noted that the dislocation rate doubled with revision surgery when compared with primary surgery. Many other studies have substantiated this finding with dislocation rates as high as 20% reported by some authors.[5-7] Trauma to the soft tissues, including the external rotators and abductors of the hip, and postoperative capsular laxity are thought to contribute to the problem. Lower rates of dislocation after primary procedures have been reported when more complete methods of closure are used.[8]

Comorbid Diagnosis Neuromuscular disorders have long been implicated as contributing to dislocation. Hedlundh and Fredin[9] performed a matched controlled study and postural and stability tests for 65 patients. Balance and vibration sense were impaired in the patients with dislocations when compared with those with no dislocations.

An increased incidence of dislocations in patients with cerebral dysfunction, psychosis, and alcoholism has been reported. Woolson and Rahimtoola[10] defined cerebral dysfunction as a state of mental confusion occurring during the hospital stay, a history of dementia, or a history of consumption of six or more alcoholic beverages per day. The dislocation rate in this group was significantly higher than for control patients. Other studies have further implicated alcoholism as a risk factor for dislocation after revision.[11]

Gender Female gender has also been recognized as a contributing factor; female to male ratios of 2:1 to 3:1 have been reported in the literature.[4,5,9,12] This factor may be secondary to decreased muscle tone or increased flexibility in females; however, further research is needed to determine the cause.

Age and Body Habitus Several studies have looked at age as a risk factor for dislocation; no statistical significance has been shown to date. Woolson and Rahimtoola[10] reported a slight trend for increased age of the patient as a risk factor, but statistical significance was not reached.

There is limited data on body habitus and the rate of dislocation. Paterno and associates[11] reviewed 380 primary procedures, comparing dislocation rates in obese patients (body mass index > 30 kg/m^2) and nonobese patients, with dislocation rates of 3% and 5%, respectively. Again, no statistical significance was shown.

Surgical Factors

The surgeon's experience level, surgical approach, orientation of the components, and restoration of soft-tissue tension of the hip all play a role in maintaining stability of the hip. The surgeon has direct control of all of these factors.

Surgeon Experience Kreder and associates[13] reviewed the records of more than 8,000 THAs and found that for surgeons performing two or fewer procedures per year, there are significantly higher rates for mortality, infections, revision, and more serious complications during their patients' index hospitalization.

Hedlundh and associates[14] reviewed 4,230 primary THAs done using a posterior approach. The overall rate of dislocation was 3%. However, an inexperienced surgeon, defined as having done fewer than 15 THAs, had double the number of dislocations when compared with more experienced colleagues. The frequency of dislocation diminished with increasing surgeon experience and remained fairly constant after approximately 30 THAs had been performed. For every 10 hips replaced per year, the risk of dislocation was reduced by 50%.

Approach The posterior approach to the hip has long been thought to play a role in dislocation. Many authors have reported dislocation rates two to three times higher than those reported for the anterior approach.[4,15,16] Woo and Morrey[4] reported dislocation rates of 2.3% for the anterior approach and 5.8% for the posterior approach. Differences in dislocation rates may be because of insufficient anteversion of the acetabular component during the posterior approach. Orientation and size of capsular defects that exist after surgery and the soft-tissue trauma inherent with each approach are factors that may also account for the different rates. Many other studies have had similar findings, leading to the conclusion that the posterior approach has a higher dislocation rate.[15,16]

The lack of well-controlled studies of both approaches make comparison of dislocation rates difficult. Many studies included more than one surgeon, different prostheses, and included changes in surgical technique as the studies progressed. In addition, one of the largest series, encompassing more than 6,000 THAs, found no evidence of surgical approach as a risk factor for dislocation.[5]

Recently, an enhanced repair technique following the posterior approach in which the capsule, short external rotators, and the quadratus femoris are reattached to their original anatomic positions has been extremely successful in reducing dislocation.[8] A consecutive series of nearly 800 patients were compared; the first 395 did not use the repair and the second 395 did. There were 16 dislocations in the first group and no dislocations in the second group. Notably, in this study, the same surgeon using the same prosthesis changed only the method by which the closure was completed when comparing dislocation rates.

Orientation of Components Component position has long been known to be critical to stability when performing a THA. The acetabulum has received the most attention in the literature secondary to the difficulty experienced in accurately placing the component. Prior to beginning the procedure, secure and consistent positioning of the patient is vital to avoid incorrect estimates of pelvic orientation.

Lewinnek and associates,[17] using plain radiographs, took measurements postoperatively in order to define abduction and anteversion of the acetabular components. The dislocation rate for the cups in anteversion of 15° ± 10° and abduction of 40° ± 10° was 1.5%. Cups falling outside this range had a dislocation rate of 6.1%.

D'Lima and associates,[18] in a computer model, determined the effects of the positions of the acetabular and femoral components and of varying head-neck ratios on impingement and range of motion. Acetabular abduction angles of less than 45° decreased flexion and abduction of the hip, whereas higher angles decreased adduction and rotation. Femoral and acetabular anteversion increased flexion but decreased extension. Acetabular abduction angles of between 45° and 55° permitted a better overall range of motion and stability when combined with appropriate acetabular and femoral anteversion. Other studies support the contention that acetabular malposition predisposes to dislocation.[5,19]

Rotation of the femoral component has also been implicated in dislocation; however, accurate measurement of component rotation is difficult to assess.[20] Herrlin and associates[21] analyzed total hip replacements with and without dislocation and found that decreased femoral anteversion was linked to a reduction in range of motion resulting from impingement and was present in the group of patients with dislocations. They recommended inserting the femoral component in 10° to 20° of anteversion. Fackler and Poss[6] found dislocation to be frequently associated with component malposition not noted at the time of surgery. The most common orientation error in their series was excessive femoral anteversion.

Soft-Tissue Tension Reestablishing the tension of the soft tissues surrounding the hip joint is very important in decreasing the risk of dislocation after THA. Several structures assist in stabilizing the femoral head within the acetabulum of the normal hip joint. During THA, some of these structures are violated or are surgically removed to facilitate surgical exposure. This surgical trauma is known to negatively affect the stability of the hip.

Dennis and associates[22] examined 20 subjects (5 normal hip joints, 10 nonconstrained clinically normal THAs, and 5 constrained THAs) fluoroscopically while performing active hip abduction. Fluo-

roscopic videos of the normal hips were used to measure the distance between the femoral head and acetabulum, looking specifically for separation between these two structures. No separation was observed in normal hips or those subjects implanted with constrained THA, while 100% of patients with unconstrained THA demonstrated femoral head separation averaging 3.3 mm. The authors hypothesized that the soft-tissue supports create a passive, resistant force at the hip, preventing femoral head separation from the acetabulum. This study highlights the role that the soft-tissue structures play in overall hip stability.

Previous studies have indicated that reestablishing soft-tissue tension is important in maintaining a stable hip postoperatively. Fackler and Poss[6] hypothesized that changes in their surgical technique, specifically foregoing trochanteric osteotomy and placing the stems in more valgus, may have reduced the tension of the hip abductors and possibly led to increased dislocation rates in their series. Woo and Morrey[4] equated myofascial tension with limb length or changes in limb length. Although they did not believe that myofascial tension had a strong influence on the risk of instability in their study, matching preoperative and postoperative limb length has become the most popular way to reestablish soft-tissue tension around the hip.

Complete soft-tissue repair has been discussed more frequently as part of the posterior approach in an effort to reestablish soft-tissue tension around the hip.[10] The goals of the repair are to provide a more stable soft-tissue cuff during the immediate postoperative period and a biologic scaffold to support the formation of a pseudocapsule. During the posterior approach, an anterior pseudocapsule often forms after surgery and can actually act as a source of impingement in the absence of a posterior repair. In this situation, the presence of a posterior soft-tissue sleeve becomes even more important.

Component Factors
Component geometry and its relationship to stability in THA has been the topic of numerous studies. The geometry of the femoral head and neck, the ratio between the size of the head and neck, and the geometry and size of the acetabular component have received the most attention.

Head Size Reports of increasing dislocation rates in THA during the 1970s led some surgeons to increase femoral head size from 22 mm to larger diameters ranging from 26 mm to 32 mm,[19] with the belief that stability would improve by increasing the distance necessary to fully displace the femoral head from the acetabulum. A larger head would also increase soft-tissue tension prior to dislocation by the same mechanism. Most retrospective studies looking at head size as a factor in dislocation have not supported this assertion, however, as most could find no correlation between size and dislocation rate.[4,5,19]

Bartz and associates[23] used a dynamic cadaver model of THA to examine the influence of the size of the head of the femoral component on range of motion prior to impingement and posterior dislocation following total hip replacement. Significant associations were noted between the femoral head size and the degree of flexion at dislocation. Increasing the femoral head size from 22 to 28 mm increased the range of flexion prior to impingement and posterior dislocation. Increasing the head size from 28 to 32 mm did not lead to more significant improvement in the range of joint motion. The site of impingement prior to dislocation varied with the size of the femoral head. The authors concluded that increasing the diameter of the femoral head component increased the range of motion prior to impingement and dislocation.

Kelley and associates,[24] in a prospectively randomized study, demonstrated a decrease in dislocation rates when a 28-mm head (no dislocation) was substituted for a 22-mm head (36% dislocations). Along with head size, the authors believed that the use of large uncemented acetabular components, along with subtle differences in the geometry of the neck (specifically the absence of a recessed neck in their study) led to the increased rate of dislocation compared with historic controls.

Acetabular Component Acetabular component modularity has increased the variation in geometry available to the surgeon. Changes in design have included elevating the posterior wall, changing the geometry of the articulating surface, or creating a constrained polyethylene component to prevent dislocation.

Polyethylene modifications of wall height are designed to increase the relative depth on one side of the acetabulum. This forces the femoral head to travel an increased distance before dislocation, much like increasing femoral head size. Significant reductions in dislocation rates have been shown using elevated-rim acetabular liners.[25] The advantage of this liner is counterbalanced by an overall decrease in the range of motion allowed by the components. Impingement will occur earlier in the motion cycle when motion is directed toward the elevated rim. This so-called rim impingement of the femoral neck on the acetabulum has also been associated with an accelerated rate of polyethylene wear.[26]

Constrained acetabular components consist of a polyethylene insert that locks the femoral head into the acetabulum. They have been used in both primary and revision THA as prophylaxis for patients predisposed to dislocation.[27,28] Anderson and associates[27] reported a redislocation rate of 29% in 21 patients using the S-ROM (DePuy, Warsaw, IN) constrained acetabular socket. In 18 patients, the device was placed to treat a chronically dislocating THA; in three patients, intraoperative instability during revision THA necessitated its use. No dislocations occurred in the three patients with

instability. Goetz and associates[28] reviewed 101 constrained acetabular components in 98 patients. The indications included intraoperative instability in 38 patients and neurologic impairment in seven patients. Four patients experienced recurrent dislocation or component failure (4%), two of which occurred in patients without previous dislocation. Dissociation of modular acetabular components in THA has been reported.[29] This has led many authors to recommend judicious use of this component for desperate cases of hip instability during THA.[27,28]

Although long-term concerns involved in using constrained liners have been recognized, it is our opinion that constrained sockets can be considered in patients who exhibit instability intraoperatively. There is a lack of early radiographic or clinical evidence of loosening in the literature.[27,28] We also believe that constrained sockets can be considered for patients who have other factors, such as the presence of previous hip surgery, neuromuscular disorders, or poor abductor musculature that would predispose them to dislocation.

Cup Size Recently, a relationship between the outer diameter of the acetabular component and the rate of dislocation has been shown. Kelley and associates[24] compared dislocation rates in hips with acetabular components larger than 56 mm to those with cups 54 mm and smaller. There was a significantly reduced rate of dislocation in the group with smaller cup size. Prior to this study, there was limited information regarding hip stability as a function of acetabular diameter.

In the same study, a mismatch between head and cup diameter, specifically small femoral heads and large acetabular diameters, was found to be highly predictive of dislocation. The authors believed this could be the result of a mismatch of the femoral head component of the THA compared with the size of the patient's anatomic femoral head. The pseudocapsule attachment, which would be moved

farther away from the femoral head when using a large acetabular component, and prosthetic impingement resulting from the increased width of the acetabulum available to impinge against the femoral component, could also contribute to instability.

Neck Diameter/Head-Neck Ratio Neck diameter is known to cause a restricted range of motion before impingement and dislocation can occur. D'Lima and associates,[18] using a computer model, determined the effects of varying head-neck ratios on impingement and range of motion. They found that lower head-neck ratios decreased the range of motion that was possible without prosthetic impingement. The addition of a modular sleeve that increased the diameter of the femoral neck by 2 mm decreased the range of motion by 1.5° to 8.5°, depending on the direction of motion that was studied. Kelley and associates[24] believed that subtle differences in the geometry of the neck, specifically the absence of a recessed neck in their study, led to an increased rate of dislocation.

Postoperative Factors

Most dislocation events take place relatively soon after surgery, usually within the first 3 months.[4-6,17,30] According to results from a study by Fackler and Poss,[6] 68% of dislocations had occurred by 1 month postoperatively, with over half of the patients in the study experiencing a dislocation prior to discharge from the hospital. Ali Khan and associates[5] reported that most of the dislocations in their study occurred within 5 weeks postoperatively.

Physical therapy and the patient's ability to comply with therapy recommendations are postoperative factors that also play a large role in dislocation.

Physical Therapy/Rehabilitation In the rehabilitation setting, dislocation is devastating because it is potentially preventable. Many patients are now discharged to a rehabilitation center after their acute hospitalization to assist in their recovery. There are few studies that focus on incidence of hip dislocation after THA and the role of physical therapy.

Krotenberg and associates[31] studied the differences in dislocation rates between patients in rehabilitation centers and those in acute hospital settings. The rate of hip dislocation among total hip replacement patients in rehabilitation hospitals was not significantly higher than that in acute settings. Among bipolar hemiarthroplasty patients, however, the dislocation rate was markedly and significantly lower in rehabilitation than in acute settings. The authors hypothesized that a lower rate may be secondary to subconscious shifting of forces acting on the hip; however, further research is needed.

Compliance As previously noted, there has been an increased incidence of dislocations in patients with cerebral dysfunction, psychosis, and the propensity to abuse alcohol.[10] Patients with altered mental status have difficulty complying with postoperative hip precautions. Krotenberg and associates[31] noted that at least 50% of the dislocations in their series were secondary to compliance issues.

Redislocation

Once a dislocation has occurred, the risk of redislocation is high, with a reported incidence of approximately 33%.[4] The time of dislocation has been implicated as an important factor. Ali Khan and associates[5] reported a 60% recurrence rate after late dislocation and a 40% recurrence rate after dislocations occurring within 5 weeks of surgery.

Treatment
Nonsurgical
Historically, in the absence of obvious component malposition, most dislocations are treated with closed reduction and some form of immobilization, such as bracing, for up to 12 weeks. In addition, in cases where comorbid states increased the likelihood of postoperative instability, postoperative bracing has been

used to reduce the risk of dislocation or redislocation.[32,33] There is little information in the literature to support specific external treatment modalities other than bracing or casting. Bracing is easy to apply and use, can be applied during the immediate postoperative period, and is economically advantageous because of the reduced number of dislocation events postoperatively.[34] Detractors of bracing contend they are expensive, poorly tolerated by patients, and ineffective.[35]

Clayton and Thirupathi[32] used a hip abduction brace in nine patients in whom the position of components was satisfactory and who had postoperative dislocations; the brace was placed as a prophylactic measure in one patient who had a spastic muscle disorder. No further dislocations occurred in the nine patients after 6 to 9 months of brace treatment.

A hip cast brace was used prophylactically by Mallory and associates[33] on patients with revision and primary THAs whose hips were thought to be unstable at the completion of surgery or who had a neurologic diagnosis predisposing them to dislocation. Dislocation occurred in three patients who had undergone previous revision THA. Of these three patients, one dislocation occurred while the cast brace was worn. In the patients with primary THAs, the average time in the cast brace was 15 days and no dislocations occurred.

Surgical
A precise determination of the cause of the instability made preoperatively will optimize the results of the surgery postoperatively.[36] Recurrent dislocations caused by malpositioned components should be treated by revision arthroplasty. In the absence of component malposition, when the patient has had repeated dislocations not amenable to nonsurgical modalities, surgical intervention can be considered.

Trochanteric Advancement As stated previously, reestablishing the tension of the soft tissues surrounding the hip joint is

very important in decreasing risk of dislocation after THA.[37] When soft-issue tension is inadequate and suspected of contributing to chronic hip instability, some surgeons have advocated distal and lateral transfer of the greater trochanter.[38,39]

Fraser and Wroblewski[38] reported on the revision of 21 Charnley low-friction arthroplasties for recurrent or irreducible dislocation. Specific indications for revision included trochanteric detachment, iatrogenic shortening of the limb, and malorientation of the components. Sixteen patients had no further complications after revision.

Kaplan and associates[39] reported on 21 patients who underwent trochanteric advancement for multiple dislocations. The trochanter was advanced an average of 16 mm. Four patients with rheumatoid arthritis had trochanteric migration greater than 1 cm. Seventeen of the 21 hips had no further dislocations at a mean follow-up of 2.7 years. The authors stated that trochanteric advancement is an effective and safe procedure for prevention of recurrent dislocations after THA in patients without component malposition.

Nonunion is one complication associated with transfer of the trochanter. Gottschalk and associates[40] found that the original reduction of the greater trochanter influenced the rate of union. Fixation of the trochanter in a tilted position led to a delay in union and in nine cases led to a nonunion.

Constrained Cup Certain constrained acetabular components have been shown to be effective in treating recurrent dislocation after THA.[27,28] Anderson and associates[27] had a redislocation rate of 29% using the S-ROM constrained acetabular socket insert in treating chronically dislocating THAs. Patients who redislocated had a significantly increased acetabular abduction angle of the metallic acetabular cup, averaging 70°. No evidence of loosening in the acetabular components was observed. Goetz and associates[28] reviewed 101 Osteonics constrained acetabular

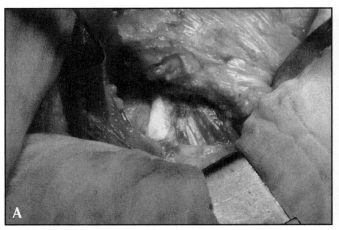
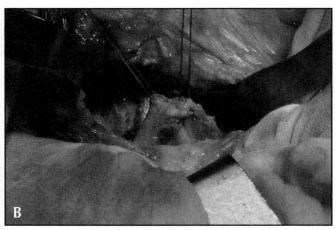

Fig. 1 A, Retractors placed superior to the piriformis and superior to the quadratus femoris, isolating the short external rotators and posterior capsule. **B,** The piriformis and the conjoined tendons are tagged using nonabsorbable suture.

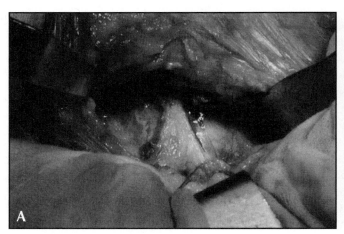
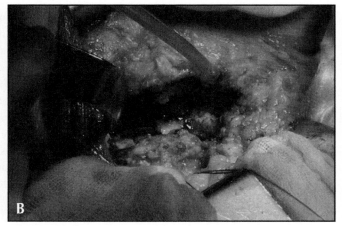

Fig. 2 A, The posterior hip capsule is fully exposed, after the inferior retractor is replaced just inferior to the capsule, and the superior retractor is placed under the gluteus minimus. **B,** The posterior capsule and quadratus are detached in a large flap-like fashion. A small cuff of the quadratus is retained on the femur for subsequent repair.

components (Osteonics, Mahwah, NJ) implanted into 98 patients. A 4% incidence of recurrent dislocation or component failure was reported, and no evidence of an increased femoral or acetabular component loosening was found radiographically.

Prevention of Dislocation

Dissatisfaction with existing rates of dislocation led the senior author to revise his method of repair of the soft tissues during the posterior approach to the hip. The goal of the enhanced repair is to reconstruct, as completely as possible, the posterior soft-tissue sleeve, which includes the tendinous short external rotators, the posterior capsule, the quadratus femoris, and the tendinous insertion of the gluteus maximus.

During the exposure, after the fascia of the gluteus maximus and the fascia lata have been divided, the insertion of the gluteus maximus is partially divided using electrocautery. A retractor is placed superior to the piriformis and superior to the quadratus femoris (Fig. 1, A). The piriformis and the conjoined tendons are isolated as a unit and divided and tagged using nonabsorbable suture (Fig. 1, B). After the conjoined tendon is released, the inferior retractor is replaced just inferior to the capsule. The gluteus minimus is lifted from the superior hip capsule, and the superior retractor is placed under the gluteus minimus (Fig 2, A). The posterior capsule, now isolated, is detached in a large flap-like fashion. The quadratus is then released, retaining a small cuff of tissue on the femur for subsequent repair (Fig 2, B). After the acetabular and femoral components have been implant-

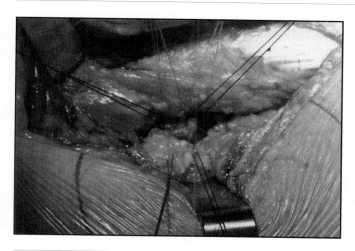

Fig. 3 Sutures are passed through two drill holes in the posterior aspect of the greater trochanter, and the posterior capsule is tagged with two permanent sutures at the locations closest to the drill holes in the femur.

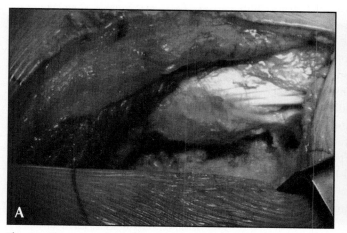
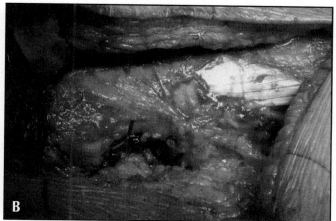

Fig. 4 A, The sutures from the superior capsule and the piriformis are tied over the greater trochanter to the corresponding inferior capsular and conjoined tendon. **B,** The quadratus is repaired back to its insertion using absorbable suture.

ed, two drill holes are made in the posterior aspect of the greater trochanter. Sutures are passed through the holes using free needles with a looped end left on the medial surface of the femur. After the hip is reduced, the posterior capsule is tagged with two permanent sutures at the locations closest to the drill holes in the femur (Fig. 3). The permanent sutures from the superior capsule and the piriformis are pulled through the looped ends. The looped ends are pulled back through the drill holes, drawing the permanent sutures out with them. The sutures from the superior capsule and the piriformis are tied to the corresponding inferior capsular and conjoined tendon

(Fig. 4, A). The quadratus is then repaired back to its insertion using absorbable suture. The leading edge of the muscle typically has a small amount of myofascia that will hold the sutures for the repair (Fig. 4, B).

The senior author used the enhanced repair method on 395 consecutive primary THAs over a 22-month period.[8] At a minimum follow-up of 1 year, there were no dislocations. Before the enhanced posterior repair was done, there were 16 dislocations (4%). The enhanced posterior repair was not used to treat any of the 16 patients with a dislocation. The difference in dislocation rates is significant with a P value of less than 0.0001. There

were no significant differences in the demographics of the two consecutive groups of patients. The prosthesis used was identical in both groups (Omnifit stems [class II], Osteonics, Allendale, NJ; HGP/Trilogy sockets [class II], Zimmer, Warsaw, IN), except for 32 consecutive patients in the second group who received a different but similar femoral component (Spectron [class II], Smith & Nephew, Memphis, TN).

A second surgeon used the enhanced repair in 124 consecutive primary total hip replacements between January of 1994 and October of 1996. At 6-month follow-up, there was one dislocation (0.8%). Prior to using the enhanced repair, in a consecutive series of 160 primary total hip replacements performed between January 1991 and December 1993, there were 10 dislocations (6.2%). The difference in dislocation rate is significant with a *P* value of 0.014. There were no significant differences in the demographics of the two groups. Although the prostheses used in the two groups were made by different manufacturers, a comparison reveals they have similar head-neck angles and similar offsets, and the acetabular components in both groups are of a hemispherical design and allow similar prosthetic ranges of motion. In the group without the enhanced repair, 76% of the stems were either Omnifit (Osteonics) or Anatomic (class II) (Zimmer). Duraloc (class II) (DePuy) was used for 97% of the acetabular components. In 38 hips, modular combinations that included risk factors for dislocation were used because of decreased prosthetic range of motion: 26 modular femoral heads with a skirt, and 12 acetabular polyethylene liners that used an elevated rim. Of the 10 dislocations, 80% were in patients who had either an Omnifit or Anatomic stem, two of the patients had long femoral necks (with skirt); there were no elevated rim liners in this group.

In the group with enhanced repair, 98% of the stems were Zimmer or Omnifit stems, while 73% of the acetabular components were Reflection (class II) (Smith & Nephew) or Trilogy (Zimmer) acetabular components. The single patient who sustained a posterior dislocation had an anatomic stem with a Reflection (Smith & Nephew Richards) acetabulum, a 7-mm neck with a short skirt, and a neutral (not elevated) acetabular liner. In both groups, 98% of the patients had either 26- or 28-mm femoral head diameters. All patients who dislocated in both groups had 28-mm head diameters.

The demographics of the two groups were not significantly different. In the group without the enhanced repair, the majority had Omnifit stems and Duraloc cups. In the group with enhanced repair, the majority had anatomic stems and Reflection or Trilogy sockets.

Summary

Dislocation remains a common and problematic complication. Although there are several risk factors that predispose patients to dislocation, other factors under the surgeon's control can reduce the risk of dislocation.

If dislocation does occur, the patient should be treated immediately with closed reduction. Multiple dislocations can be treated by trochanteric advancement in the presence of inadequate soft-tissue tension, revision arthroplasty in the presence of malpositioned components, or the use of a constrained cup when intraoperative instability persists.

Prevention is critical because the risk of redislocation is much higher than first time dislocation. The enhanced repair technique presented herein can be used to reconstruct, as completely as possible, the posterior soft-tissue sleeve during the posterior approach. The dislocation rate reported by the senior author in a consecutive series of 395 patients was zero using this technique.

References

1. Berry DJ: Unstable total hip arthroplasty: Detailed overview. *Instr Course Lect* 2001;50: 265-274.

2. Morrey BF: Dislocation, in Morrey BF, An KN (eds): *Reconstructive Surgery of the Joints*, ed 2. New York, NY, Churchill Livingstone, 1996, vol 2, pp 1247-1260.

3. Lee BP, Berry DJ, Harmsen WS, Sim FH: Total hip arthroplasty for the treatment of an acute fracture of the femoral neck: Long-term results. *J Bone Joint Surg Am* 1998;80:70-75.

4. Woo RY, Morrey BF: Dislocations after total hip arthroplasty. *J Bone Joint Surg Am* 1982;64:1295-1306.

5. Ali Khan MA, Brakenbury PH, Reynolds IS: Dislocation following total hip replacement. *J Bone Joint Surg Br* 1981;63:214-218.

6. Fackler CD, Poss R: Dislocation in total hip arthroplasties. *Clin Orthop* 1980;151:169-178.

7. Williams JF, Gottesman MJ, Mallory TH: Dislocation after total hip arthroplasty: Treatment with an above-knee hip spica cast. *Clin Orthop* 1982;171:53-58.

8. Pellicci PM, Bostrom M, Poss R: Posterior approach to total hip replacement using enhanced posterior soft tissue repair. *Clin Orthop* 1998;355:224-228.

9. Hedlundh U, Fredin H: Patient characteristics in dislocations after primary total hip arthroplasty: 60 patients compared with a control group. *Acta Orthop Scand* 1995;66:225-228.

10. Woolson ST, Rahimtoola ZO: Risk factors for dislocation during the first 3 months after primary total hip replacement. *J Arthroplasty* 1999;14:662-668.

11. Paterno SA, Lachiewicz PF, Kelley SS: The influence of patient-related factors and the position of the acetabular component on the rate of dislocation after total hip replacement. *J Bone Joint Surg Am* 1997;79:1202-1210.

12. Coventry MB: Late dislocations in patients with Charnley total hip arthroplasty. *J Bone Joint Surg Am* 1985;67:832-841.

13. Kreder HJ, Deyo RA, Koepsell T, Swiontkowski MF, Kreuter W: Relationship between the volume of total hip replacements performed by providers and the rates of postoperative complications in the state of Washington. *J Bone Joint Surg Am* 1997;79:485-494.

14. Hedlundh U, Ahnfelt L, Hybbinette CH, Weckstrom J, Fredin H: Surgical experience related to dislocations after total hip arthroplasty. *J Bone Joint Surg Br* 1996;78:206-209.

15. Morrey BF: Difficult complications after hip joint replacement: Dislocation. *Clin Orthop* 1997;344:179-187.

16. Roberts JM, Fu FH, McClain EJ, Ferguson AB Jr: A comparison of the posterolateral and anterolateral approaches to total hip arthroplasty. *Clin Orthop* 1984;187:205-210.

17. Lewinnek GE, Lewis JL, Tarr R, Compere CL, Zimmerman JR: Dislocations after total hip-replacement arthroplasties. *J Bone Joint Surg Am* 1978;60:217-220.

18. D'Lima DD, Urquhart AG, Buehler KO, Walker RH, Colwell CW Jr: The effect of the orientation of the acetabular and femoral components on the range of motion of the hip at different head-neck ratios. *J Bone Joint Surg Am* 2000;82:315-321.

19. Ritter MA: Dislocation and subluxation of the total hip replacement. *Clin Orthop* 1976;121: 92-94.

20. Herrlin K, Selvik G, Pettersson H, Kesek P, Onnerfalt R, Ohlin A: Position, orientation and component interaction in dislocation of the total hip prosthesis. *Acta Radiol* 1988;29:441-444.

21. Herrlin K, Pettersson H, Selvik G, Lidgren L: Femoral anteversion and restricted range of motion in total hip prostheses. *Acta Radiol* 1988;29:551-553.

22. Dennis DA, Komistek RD, Northcut EJ, Ochoa JA, Ritchie A: In vivo determination of hip joint separation and the forces generated due to impact loading conditions. *J Biomech* 2001;34:623-629.

23. Bartz RL, Nobel PC, Kadakia NR, Tullos HS: The effect of femoral component head size on posterior dislocation of the artificial hip joint. *J Bone Joint Surg Am* 2000;82:1300-1307.

24. Kelley SS, Lachiewicz PF, Hickman JM, Paterno SM: Relationship of femoral head and acetabular size to the prevalence of dislocation. *Clin Orthop* 1998;355:163-170.

25. Cobb TK, Morrey BF, Ilstrup DM: The elevated-rim acetabular liner in total hip arthroplasty: Relationship to postoperative dislocation. *J Bone Joint Surg Am* 1996;78:80-86.

26. Urquhart AG, D'Lima DD, Venn-Watson E, Colwell CW Jr, Walker RH: Polyethylene wear after total hip arthroplasty: The effect of a modular femoral head with an extended flange-reinforced neck. *J Bone Joint Surg Am* 1998;80: 1641-1647.

27. Anderson MJ, Murray WR, Skinner HB: Constrained acetabular components. *J Arthroplasty* 1994;9:17-23.

28. Goetz DD, Capello WN, Callaghan JJ, Brown TD, Johnston RC: Salvage of total hip instability with a constrained acetabular component. *Clin Orthop* 1998;355:171-181.

29. Fisher DA, Kiley K: Constrained acetabular cup disassembly. *J Arthroplasty* 1994;9:325-329.

30. Dorr LD, Wolf AW, Chandler R, Conaty JP: Classification and treatment of dislocations of total hip arthroplasty. *Clin Orthop* 1983;173: 151-158.

31. Krotenberg R, Stitik T, Johnston MV: Incidence of dislocation following hip arthroplasty for patients in the rehabilitation setting. *Am J Phys Med Rehabil* 1995;74:444-447.

32. Clayton ML, Thirupathi RG: Dislocation following total hip arthroplasty: Management by special brace in selected patients. *Clin Orthop* 1983;177:154-159.

33. Mallory TH, Vaughn BK, Lombardi AV Jr, Kraus TJ: Prophylactic use of a hip cast-brace following primary and revision total hip arthroplasty. *Orthop Rev* 1988;17:178-183.

34. Dorr LD: Bracing after revision THA: Essential, expedient, and economical. *Orthopedics* 2001;24:228.

35. Cameron H: Bracing after revision THA: Unnecessary, expensive, and cruel. *Orthopedics* 2001;24:230.

36. Daly PJ, Morrey BF: Operative correction of an unstable total hip arthroplasty. *J Bone Joint Surg Am* 1992;74:1334-1343.

37. Eftekhar NS: Dislocation and instability complicating low friction arthroplasty of the hip joint. *Clin Orthop* 1976;121:120-125.

38. Fraser GA, Wroblewski BM: Revision of the Charnley low-friction arthroplasty for recurrent or irreducible dislocation. *J Bone Joint Surg Br* 1981;63:552-555.

39. Kaplan SJ, Thomas WH, Poss R: Trochanteric advancement for recurrent dislocation after total hip arthroplasty. *J Arthroplasty* 1987;2:119-124.

40. Gottschalk FA, Morein G, Weber F: Effect of the position of the greater trochanter on the rate of union after trochanteric osteotomy for total hip arthroplasty. *J Arthroplasty* 1988;3:235-240.

Avoidance and Management of Neurovascular Injuries in Total Hip Arthroplasty

Robert L. Barrack, MD
R. Allen Butler, MD

Abstract

Neural injuries that occur after total hip arthroplasty (THA) can be classified as involving either the central nervous system or peripheral nerves. Central nervous system changes after THA may be attributed to increased appreciation of fat embolism syndrome associated with THA. Certain maneuvers such as impacting the acetabulum, femoral reaming, and cement pressurization can force marrow fat into the venous system. When there is an associated right to left shunt, paradoxical embolization can occur, which may account for previously unexplained cases of confusion and mental status changes after surgery. Peripheral nerve injuries are rare and can involve either distant sites or nerves in the immediate vicinity of the hip joint. Upper extremity nerve injuries are usually associated with patient positioning. Sciatic nerve injury is the most common nerve injury following THA. In comparison, femoral nerve injury is much less common and is associated with an anterior approach. Diagnosis is often delayed, and the prognosis is generally better than with sciatic nerve injury. The superior gluteal nerve is at risk during the direct lateral approach. Obturator nerve injury is the least common type of injury and has the least functional consequence. It can present as groin or inguinal pain. Vascular injuries are less common but more immediately life threatening. The mechanisms of vascular injury include occlusion associated with preexisting peripheral vascular disease and vascular injury during removal of cement during screw fixation of acetabular components, cages, or structural grafts. Perioperative assessment should include vascular evaluation of patients with absent pulses, previous vascular bypass surgery, or dysvascular limbs. A CT scan should be considered when cement or components extend medially into the pelvis.

Major neurovascular injury is the least common but most distressing complication of total hip arthroplasty (THA). Vascular injury is the most immediate life-threatening intraoperative event associated with THA. The incidence of vascular injury may, in fact, be increasing because of two potential reasons: a higher volume of increasingly complex revision procedures being performed in recent years, and the increased use of screws in the pelvis because of the popularity of techniques using jumbo or large acetabular components requiring adjunctive screw fixation, the use of structural grafts, and the more widespread use of antiprotrusio cages.

The incidence of peripheral nerve injury remains static and may actually be decreasing. This decrease may be related to surgeons' increased experience with arthroplasty and the awareness of risk factors and relevant anatomy associated with these injuries. Persistent nerve palsy usually results in patient dissatisfaction.[1] Neurovascular injury is traumatic to both the patient and the surgeon, as well as being a common cause of litigation.

Peripheral nerve injuries are the complications most apt to cause litigation across all surgical specialties. Injuries to nerves of the pelvis and leg have been listed as the number four cause of claims and the ninth leading reason for indemnity payout, according to one study.[2] Peripheral nerve injuries cannot be entirely eliminated but can be minimized by preoperative assessment of risks, informed consent, knowledge of relevant anatomy, and early recognition coupled with appropriate treatment.

Neural injuries can be classified as involving either the central nervous system or peripheral nerves. Peripheral nerve injures can be further classified into those involving a distant site or the contralateral limb and those involving nerves in the vicinity of the operated hip. Involvement of the sciatic nerve is the most common by far, followed by that of the femoral, superior gluteal, and obturator nerves.

Central Nervous System Injury

In recent years, there has been increasing awareness of central nervous system changes following THA and total knee arthroplasty. This is partially the result of more extensive use of transesophageal echocardiography, which has confirmed the presence of significant embolic phenomena associated with the insertion of total hip components, particularly at the time of femoral stem insertion.[3,4] This technology has also confirmed a higher

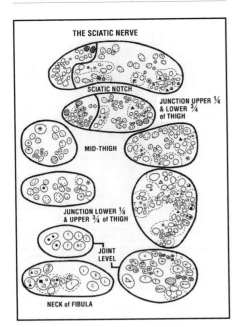

Fig. 1 Cross-sectional analysis of the sciatic nerve and its divisions at different levels demonstrate that at the level of the hip joint the peroneal division has a higher density of nerve fibers with less interstitial tissue, making it more vulnerable to compression neuropathy. (Reproduced with permission from Schmalzried TP, Noordin S, Amstutz HC: Update on nerve palsy associated with total hip replacement. *Clin Orthop* 1997;344: 188-206.)

incidence of cardiac conditions such as patent foramen ovale, which can lead to right to left shunting. The clinical results of embolization at the time of THA include pulmonary shunting, desaturation, adult respiratory distress syndrome, and cerebrovascular injury. Paradoxical embolization occurs in 10% to 20% of adults, a much higher incidence than previously thought, and may cause neurologic deficits and mental status changes postoperatively. The surgical maneuvers most commonly associated with embolization include impacting the acetabular component, femoral reaming, and, most particularly, femoral cement pressurization.[4] The risk of embolic phenomena can be minimized by obtaining a preoperative echocardiogram in high-risk patients, such as those with cardiovascular disease. Pulsatile lavage of fat and marrow elements prior to cementing is also likely to decrease the risk of fat embolization. In patients with signs of pulmonary shunting or cardiovascular lability, surgeons should consider minimizing cement pressurization or possibly using press-fit components. Evidence shows that venting of the femur decreases the risk of embolization.[5]

Nerve Injury at Distant Sites

Peripheral nerve injury distant from the operated hip, such as in the upper extremities or the contralateral limb, is relatively infrequent and usually related to patient positioning. Patients with rheumatoid arthritis are likely at higher risk for distant nerve injuries probably because many of them are thin with less soft-tissue padding, which increases the risk of nerve damage from extrinsic compression. Patients with ankylosed hips, which often require excessive retraction, are also at increased risk. Nercessian and associates[6] described peripheral neuropathies distant from the surgical site following THA. Eleven of 45 nerve injuries distant from the hip occurred in the upper extremity, which represented only 11 of 7,133 overall peripheral nerve injuries (0.15%) and included 5 ulnar nerve injuries and 4 brachial plexus injuries. Nine of the 11 injuries resolved; the 2 injuries that did not resolve were in patients with rheumatoid arthritis.

Peripheral nerve injuries in the contralateral limb were described by Smith and associates.[7] In their study, transient nerve deficits in the contralateral limb occurred in 5 of 919 cases. Factors associated with injury included the lateral decubitus position, trochanteric osteotomy with lateral dislocation of the hip, and long surgical times in which there was prolonged pressure on the contralateral femoral triangle. If a trochanteric osteotomy is performed in the lateral decubitus position and the operated limb is brought across the table so that it is placing pressure on the contralateral limb, attention should be focused on relieving pressure periodically and adequate padding of the contralateral limb.

Sciatic Nerve Injury

Peripheral nerve injuries in the vicinity of the operated hip are much more common, with an overall incidence of 1% to 2% following THA. The known risk factors include female gender, hip dysplasia, and revision THA. The sciatic nerve is most commonly affected. One review of 28 studies that comprised over 25,000 cases showed that the sciatic nerve was involved in 79% of injuries, followed by the femoral nerve in 13.2%, sciatic and femoral nerves in 5.8%, and obturator nerve in 1.6%. The etiology of the nerve injury was undetermined in 47% of cases and caused by traction in 20%, contusion in 18.5%, hematoma in 11.2%, dislocation in 2.3%, and laceration in 1.2%.[1,8] Lengthening of the surgical side, although generally accepted as a risk factor for development of sciatic nerve palsy, remains somewhat controversial. In one study, Johanson and associates[9] reported nerve palsy in 13 of 46 hips (28%) in which lengthening of more than 4 cm occurred. In comparison, in 54 hips in which lengthening of less than 4 cm occurred, nerve palsy did not occur. Conversely, Nercessian and associates[10] reported that of 1,287 THAs, 66 had lengthening of more than 2 cm. The single sciatic nerve palsy in this group was caused by intraoperative transsection.

The peroneal division of the sciatic nerve is involved much more frequently than the tibial portion. At the level of the hip joint, the peroneal division is in much closer proximity to retractors used to expose the hip and is therefore more vulnerable to compression. At this level, the peroneal division also has a much higher density of nerve fibers, making it more susceptible to compression neuropathy (Fig. 1). Other risk factors for development of sciatic or peroneal palsy include ipsilateral peripheral neuropathy and lumbar disk disease. Both conditions should be assessed and treated preoperatively if possible. In these cases, special attempts should be made to minimize traction on the nerve. If nerve palsy does occur in patients with these risk factors, the prognosis is not as good as that of the general population.

Perioperative Considerations

Surgical maneuvers that can minimize the risk of nerve palsy at the time of THA include palpation of the nerve and continuous protection with soft tissue and retractors that minimize the tension on the soft tissue adjacent to the nerve. It is also advisable to routinely note in the surgical report that the nerve was identified, palpated, and protected throughout the case. In addition, flexing the knee decreases the tension on the nerve. Studies using somatosensory evoked potentials (SSEP) have established that positions that change the potential and therefore place pressure on the nerve include retracting the femur anteriorly during acetabular reaming and retracting the femur laterally at the time of canal instrumentation. It is therefore advisable to relax traction on the femur in longer cases. Excessive rotation of the femur during trochanteric osteotomy has also been shown to place direct pressure on the nerve. The sciatic nerve is in the surgical field and potentially more vulnerable during a posterior approach. In spite of this, the type of surgical approach has not been associated with a higher incidence of nerve palsy. Intraoperative risk factors include previous trauma (especially open reduction and internal fixation), excision of heterotopic ossification, and absence of the posterior acetabular wall. In these cases, the sciatic nerve is frequently trapped in scar tissue immediately adjacent to the posterior rim of the acetabulum. If there is hardware in place that must be removed and heterotopic ossification that must be excised in the

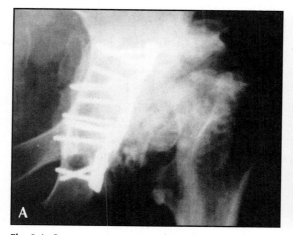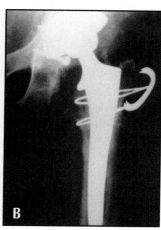

Fig. 2 A, Severe posttraumatic arthritis following open reduction and internal fixation of posterior column fracture. **B,** Plate removal and excision of heterotopic ossification was associated with peroneal nerve palsy following total hip replacement.

same vicinity, the sciatic nerve is particularly vulnerable to injury (Fig. 2). Therefore, careful preoperative assessment of sensation and motor function should be performed. If clinical examination reveals abnormality, an electromyogram (EMG) and nerve conduction velocity study and/or SSEP should be considered preoperatively. If the patient is at high risk because of dysplasia with anticipated lengthening of more than 2 cm, an extensive revision with anticipated lengthening, or posterior plating or structural grafting, it is important to document informed consent because of the increased potential for nerve injury. In exceptionally high-risk cases, SSEP can be considered although there is no compelling evidence that this will lower the incidence of nerve injury. A final intraoperative consideration is protection of the sciatic nerve during wire passage, as there are documented cases of nerve injury during this maneuver.

The role of SSEP remains controversial, and this technique is certainly not justified in routine cases. Studies have identified a surprising high incidence of changes in potential of the SSEP during various maneuvers involved in THA.[11-14] The overall incidence of nerve injury,

however, has not been found to be different in monitored versus unmonitored cases.[12] The SSEP does have some notable disadvantages including increasing surgical time, equipment expense, specific anesthetic requirements (such as nitrous/narcotic technique), and operator dependence.

Effective treatment of nerve palsy begins with early recognition. The neurovascular status of the extremity should be documented both preoperatively and in the recovery room postoperatively. The method of assessing peroneal function is important. The patient should not be asked to just "wiggle the toes." This maneuver can elicit active toe flexion with passive extension that may give the false impression of extensor hallucis longus or toe extensor function. The patient should be asked to actively extend the great toe and the ankle against resistance and should be tested for light touch compared with the other foot. These findings should be documented in order to be compared with any subsequent findings. If a change in neurovascular function is found, the patient and family should be counseled immediately. If there is loss of active extension against gravity, early bracing and physical therapy including passive stretching should be instituted to prevent heel cord contracture. If there is substantial loss of sensation, attention must be directed toward skin care to prevent skin ulceration. EMGs are advisable at 4 to 6 weeks to document the level and degree of the injury. Patients who have painful dyesthesia should be considered for a number of alternative medical treatments, including tricyclic antidepressants.

Etiology

After a diagnosis is made, it is important to attempt to determine whether an etiology can be found. A potential etiology to be considered for early nerve palsy is leg lengthening. If the operated leg was substantially lengthened, a split mattress technique may be considered, which allows flexion of the knee to relieve tension on the sciatic nerve. If a long modular head has been placed, a shorter head may be considered. In one study, acute shortening with a modular head has been associated with early return of an acute nerve deficit.[15] However, this may lead to instability and soft-tissue laxity and may require trochanteric advancement.

Another etiology of early nerve palsy is impingement on bone graft, screws, or components. Radiographs should be scrutinized for potential areas of impingement; Judet views or a CT scan may be considered if this appears to be a possibility. The fibular head is another source of potential impingement and would lead to a more distal nerve palsy that should be distinguishable on EMG. Patients who have had epidural anesthesia are at higher risk for this type of injury because of lack of sensation or motor control for several hours after surgery during which time the nerve can be compressed against the fibular head either by a Velcro strap of an abduction pillow or through direct pressure on a traction splint.

Hematoma is a common cause of late palsies that further emphasizes the importance of early diagnosis and docu-mentation. If a late palsy does occur, it is important to check for signs of an expanding hematoma in the thigh or buttock. The thigh circumference can be measured and documented. In addition, the hematocrit level should be checked and coagulation studies done to ensure that excessive anticoagulation has not occurred. A CT scan or ultrasound can be obtained to try to document the presence of a hematoma.

Surgical evacuation of the hematoma should be performed as soon as safely feasible. In cases of definite overlengthening with profound palsy, a shortening should be considered in the early postoperative period. Definite impingement on a component or screw should be corrected as soon as possible. Surgical transection also should be repaired early when possible. However, most patients are treated nonsurgically and fortunately, most achieve some return of function.

The role of exploration and neurolysis during the original surgical procedure is somewhat controversial. It is advisable to palpate the nerve routinely and to perform a limited neurolysis when there is abnormal anatomy, scarring around the nerve, and the presence of preoperative symptoms. It is also advisable to check the tension on the nerve initially and after reduction to ensure that there is not excessive tension with the components in place and reduced.

Outcome

The expected outcome of sciatic or peroneal palsy is variable. In one review of 21 studies encompassing over 23,000 cases in which 228 palsies were identified, 41% were asymptomatic at final follow-up, 44% were left with a mild deficit, and 15% were left with a major deficit.[8] The vast majority of those with a major deficit were classified as having a poor result. Good prognostic signs for recovery following nerve injury include early return of motor function within the first 2 weeks postoperatively and the presence of partial motor or sensory function. Poor prognostic signs included the presence of painful dyesthesia and complete motor and sensory loss with no return within the first 2 weeks.[1,8,12]

Femoral Nerve Injury

Femoral nerve injury is much less common than sciatic palsy following THA and is generally associated with an anterior surgical approach. The most common etiology is direct compression from either retractors, cement, or screws. Anatomically, the femoral nerve is located just medial to the rectus tendon level of the hip joint and lies lateral to the artery and vein (Fig. 3). A retractor must be placed under the rectus tendon for it to be safely protected from the femoral nerve. A retractor that is placed in soft tissue and lies anterior to the rectus tendon is at risk for direct compression of the femoral nerve. Risk factors for femoral nerve palsy include a prior anterior surgical approach, an absent or released psoas tendon, and anterior bone deficiency. Diagnosis of femoral nerve palsy is often delayed because testing for femoral nerve function is somewhat more subtle and less familiar to many practitioners. One helpful trick is for the examiner to place a hand beneath the popliteal space and ask the patient to press the leg down against the examiner's hand, which allows observation of the quadriceps muscles for contraction. The prognosis is generally better for femoral nerve injuries than for sciatic or peroneal injuries. Observation is normally undertaken routinely unless there is definite evidence of impingement by cement, screws, bone graft, or hematoma. When there is profound muscle weakness, temporary bracing may be necessary with an orthotic device such as a long leg drop-lock brace.

Superior Gluteal Nerve Injury

Superior gluteal nerve injury has become more clinically relevant with the increased popularity of transgluteal surgical approaches such as the direct lateral or Hardinge approach.[13,16] The superior gluteal nerve exits the sciatic notch above the piriformis and can be found at the posterior border of the gluteus medius proximally. It innervates the gluteus medius, gluteus minimus, and tensor fascia lata. The safe zone has been described as an area 5 cm above the greater trochanter; however, it may lie as close as 3 cm anteriorly. The safe zone is more difficult to delineate in the revision situation, in which case there may be substantial proximal migration of the femur, making the safe zone markedly diminished.

Numerous studies have identified electrical evidence of damage to the superior gluteal nerve during THA with estimates of from 14% to 77% based on EMG changes.[11,13,16] The clinical relevance of the injury is much less well documented. Clinical evidence of damage has only been found in 11% to 40% of cases.[13,16] With denervation of the gluteus medius and minimus, a marked Trendelenburg gait may be observed. It may be difficult to distinguish superior gluteal nerve damage from partial avulsion of a portion of the gluteus medius and minimus. The transgluteal approaches partially detach the abductor insertions, and subsequent dehiscence may clinically mimic a superior gluteal nerve injury. An EMG may be useful in making this distinction. One recent study compared the direct lateral and the transtrochanteric approaches and found that perioperative injury was more common than previously appreciated.[13] Even more common, however, was preoperative evidence of nerve injury. The nerve injuries were not related to the presence of a Trendelenburg gait and were not particularly related to the surgical approach used.

Obturator Nerve Injury
Obturator nerve palsy is the least commonly documented nerve injury following THA and is of the least functional consequence. It is generally caused by

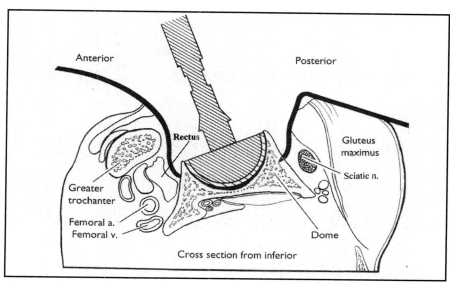

Fig. 3 Anterior anatomy of the hip with a retractor placed under the rectus tendon. Retractors placed over these tendons present a risk to the femoral neurovascular bundle. (Adapted with permission from Pellicci PM, Padget DE: Acetabular exposure and reaming, in *Atlas of Total Hip Replacement*. Philadelphia, PA, Churchill Livingstone, 1995, p 45.)

medial protrusion of cement, screws, or components. It may present late, with the clinical presentation usually being that of groin pain or inguinal pain. Local nerve block can confirm the diagnosis. If there is a screw or cement in the vicinity that is accessible, surgical removal may be indicated.[17] Obturator neurectomy is also an option to relieve persistent symptoms if an obturator block is successful.[18]

Vascular Injuries
Vascular injuries are uncommon but are associated with the most dramatic complication of THA. Vascular injuries can occur through different mechanisms and at different stages of performing a THA. Occlusion or embolization can occur during the course of a THA, particularly in patients with peripheral vascular disease. Other major types of vascular injury are associated with the surgical approach, component removal, and component insertion, particularly the increasingly common use of screws in recent years.

Preoperative assessment is a crucial first step in minimizing the risk of vascular complications. Patients with a dysvascular limb, absent or markedly diminished pedal pulses, and/or prior vascular bypass surgery should undergo preoperative vascular evaluation. Patients who have significant arteriosclerotic cardiovascular disease or who have had prior vascular bypass surgery are at risk for plaque embolization and occlusion of distal vessels. These conditions can occur during positioning or during the surgical approach when the hip is dislocated, which can cause kinking of the vessels or grafts. In such cases, consideration can be given to modifying the surgical approach in an attempt to minimize the amount of time spent in positions that place the graft at risk for occlusion. In addition, careful preoperative and postoperative assessment of the vascular status of the extremity should be performed in such cases.

Intrapelvic cement or components should also be carefully assessed preoperatively. Cement that was present inside the pelvis immediately postoperatively poses a greater risk to vascular structures than cement that has migrated into the

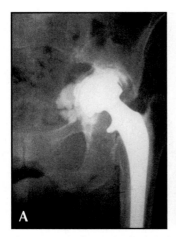
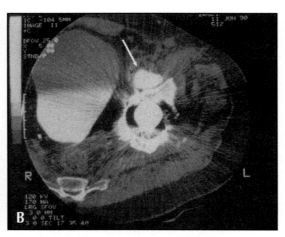

Fig. 4 A, AP radiograph of a failed cemented acetabular component with intrapelvic cement. **B,** CT scan demonstrates that the medial cement is immediately adjacent to and displacing the iliac vessels (*arrow*).

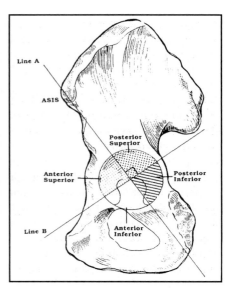

Fig. 5 Depiction of the quadrant system for safe placement of acetabular screws during THA. (Reproduced with permission from Wasielewski RC, Cooperstein LA, Kruger MP, Rubash HE: Acetabular anatomy and the transacetabular fixation of screws in total hip arthroplasty. *J Bone Joint Surg Am* 1990;72:501-508.)

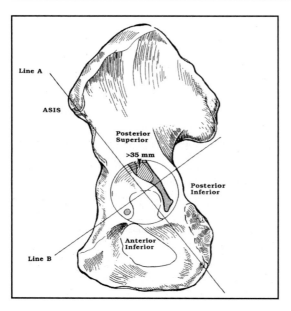

Fig. 6 Areas of the quadrant that are safest for placement of longer screws. Longest depths are most consistently available on the posterior superior quadrant. (Reproduced with permission from Wasielewski RC, Cooperstein LA, Kruger MP, Rubash HE: Acetabular anatomy and the transacetabular fixation of screws in total hip arthroplasty. *J Bone Joint Surg Am* 1990;72: 501-508.)

pelvis over time. Polymerizing methacryclate can adhere to vessel walls, and removing cement in this case is much more likely to lead to a vascular complication than cement that has migrated into the pelvis and displaced vessels long after the polymerization process. When cement is visible medial to Köhler's line, a CT scan to determine the proximity of the cement to major vascular structures should be considered (Fig. 4). Components that are immediately adjacent to

major vessels may be more safely removed through a retroperitoneal intrapelvic approach.

The popularity of cementless acetabular fixation with adjunctive screws increases the risk of major vascular injury by intrapelvic screw placement. This risk can be minimized by understanding the relevant anatomy. Wasielewski and associates[19,20] described the quadrant system for the safe screw placement through an acetabular component. Line A connects

the anterior superior iliac spine and the center of the acetabular component and divides the acetabulum into two equal halves. Line B is drawn perpendicular to line A at the acetabular midpoint. The anterior superior quadrant places the external iliac artery and vein at greatest risk (Fig. 5). The anterior inferior quadrant places the obturator nerve, artery, and vein at risk for injury. The posterior superior quadrant is the safest. The longest screws can be placed in this orientation. Depths of greater than 35 mm are only obtained on a routine basis in the posterior superior quadrant (Fig. 6). Excessively long screws, however, can jeopardize the sciatic nerve or superior gluteal artery when placed in this orientation. The posterior inferior quadrant is the next safest quadrant; however, shorter screws must be used in this quadrant.

Details of surgical technique can also minimize the risk of vascular complications. Most importantly, only superior and posterior screw placement should be selected whenever possible, particularly avoiding orientation of screws anterior to line A of the quadrant system (Fig. 7). Engagement of only one cortex is necessary. Bicortical drilling should be avoided except in safe quadrants posteriorly. Bicortical fixation does impart greater strength; however, it is not necessary and should be undertaken with care when using screws that are not assured of being in a safe quadrant. Constant pressure should be maintained on the drill, and if there is not firm, secure resistance, further drilling should not be undertaken. A firm end point should be felt with a depth gauge prior to determining screw placement. Screws longer than 25 mm are not necessary unless there is assurance on drilling and depth gauge placement that the screws are either within bone or that the end point of the second cortex is not in doubt. An uncontrolled plunge with the drill should be a cause of concern. Pulsatile bleeding from a screw hole, along with unexplained hypotension and tachycardia immediately following drilling or screw placement and abdominal or thigh distension following screw placement are also cause for concern.

Management of bleeding following acetabular screw placement is an uncommon problem but should be familiar to surgeons who use screws in the pelvis. If the patient is hemodynamically stable, then immediate volume and blood replacement should be undertaken and close observation should follow. If the patient is hemodynamically unstable or pulsatile bleeding persists, immediate laparotomy should be performed with an approach to the iliac vessels. If there is continued blood loss following blood and volume replacement, then postoperative angiography with transcatheter embolization should be considered[21] (Fig 8).

With increased use of acetabular cages, screws are placed further proximal in the ilium as well as inferiorly in the ischium, placing different structures at

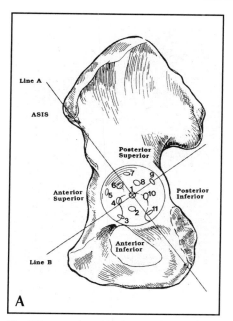
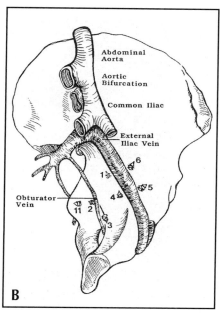

Fig. 7 Screws placed in the anterior quadrant (1, 4, 5, and 6) (**A**) are particularly dangerous because they exit immediately adjacent to the iliac vessels inside the pelvis (**B**). (Reproduced with permission from Wasielewski RC, Cooperstein LA, Kruger MP, Rubash HE: Acetabular anatomy and the transacetabular fixation of screws in total hip arthroplasty. *J Bone Joint Surg Am* 1990;72:501-508.)

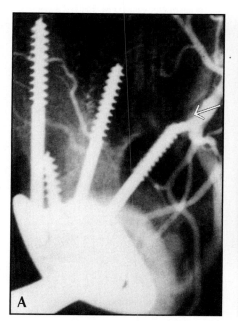
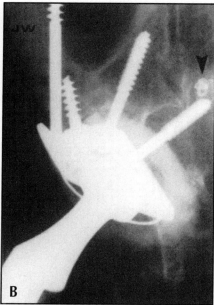

Fig. 8 A, Postoperative angiogram demonstrating interruption of the superior gluteal artery by an errant long screw (*white arrow*). **B,** Bleeding was controlled with a transcatheter embolization (*black arrowhead*). (Reproduced with permission from Rothman RH, Hozack WJ: *Complications of Total Hip Arthroplasty.* Philadelphia, PA, WB Saunders, 1997, pp 14-30.)

risk. A study by Lavernia and associates[22] defined the location of screws and the associated structures at risk when inserting an antiprotrusio cage. Posterior rim screws through an acetabular cage can endanger the iliac vessels. Ischial screws come in close proximity to the pudendal neurovasclar bundle. The iliac extensions of many cages extend proximally, and screws greater than 20 mm in length can endanger the bowel if they extend more than a few millimeters medial to the inner table. Placement of acetabular screws during revision THA when there has been proximal migration leading to a high hip center also increases the risk of neurovascular complications as reported by Meldrum and associates.[23] When a high hip center is used in revision surgery the anterior half of the posterior superior quadrant was found to be unsafe in some cases.

Summary

Neurovascular injuries are fortunately an uncommon complication of THA. Knowledge of the relevant anatomy and predisposing factors allows surgeons to identify patients at risk for these complications. This enables surgeons to obtain informed consent from patients so that they are more aware of and have a greater understanding of potential complications. More careful preoperative planning is necessary in order to minimize risk.

References

1. Schmalzried TP, Amstutz HC, Dorey FJ: Nerve palsy associated with total hip replacement: Risk factors and prognosis. *J Bone Joint Surg Am* 1991;73:1074-1080.

2. Hofmann AA, Skrzynski MC: Leg-length inequality and nerve palsy in total hip arthroplasty: A lawyer awaits! *Orthopedics* 2000;23:943-944.

3. Ereth MH, Weber JG, Abel MD, et al: Cemented versus noncemented total hip arthroplasty: Embolism, hemodynamics, and intrapulmonary shunting. *Mayo Clin Proc* 1992;67:1066-1074.

4. Woo R, Minster GJ, Fitzgerald RH Jr, Mason LD, Lucas DR, Smith FE: Pulmonary fat embolism in revision hip arthroplasty. *Clin Orthop* 1995;319:41-53.

5. Engesaeter LB, Strand T, Raugstad TS, Husebo S, Langeland N: Effects of a distal venting hole in the femur during total hip replacement. *Arch Orthop Trauma Surg* 1984;103:328-331.

6. Nercessian OA, Macaulay W, Stinchfield FE: Peripheral neuropathies following total hip arthroplasty. *J Arthroplasty* 1994;9:645-651.

7. Smith JW, Pellicci PM, Sharrock N, Mineo R, Wilson PD Jr: Complications after total hip replacement: The contralateral limb. *J Bone Joint Surg Am* 1989;71:528-535.

8. Schmalzried TP, Noordin S, Amstutz HC: Update on nerve palsy associated with total hip replacement. *Clin Orthop* 1997;344:188-206.

9. Johanson NA, Pellicci PM, Tsairis P, Salvati EA: Nerve injury in total hip arthroplasty. *Clin Orthop* 1983;179:214-222.

10. Nercessian OA, Piccoluga F, Eftekhar NS: Postoperative sciatic and femoral nerve palsy with reference to leg lengthening and medialization/lateralization of the hip joint following total hip arthroplasty. *Clin Orthop* 1994;304:165-171.

11. Abitbol JJ, Gendron D, Laurin CA, Beaulieu MA: Gluteal nerve damage following total hip arthroplasty: A prospective analysis. *J Arthroplasty* 1990;5:319-322.

12. Lewallen DG: Neurovascular injuries associated with hip arthroplasty. *J Bone Joint Surg Am* 1997;79:1870-1880.

13. Kenny P, O'Brien CP, Synnott K, Walsh MG: Damage to the superior gluteal nerve after two different approaches to the hip. *J Bone Joint Surg Br* 1999;81:979-981.

14. Pereles TR, Stuchin SA, Kastenbaum DM, Beric A, Lacagnino G, Kabir H: Surgical maneuvers placing the sciatic nerve at risk during total hip arthroplasty as assessed by somatosensory evoked potential monitoring. *J Arthroplasty* 1996;11:438-444.

15. Silbey MB, Callaghan JJ: Sciatic nerve palsy after total hip arthroplasty: Treatment by modular neck shortening. *Orthopedics* 1991;14:351-352.

16. Ramesh M, O'Byrne JM, McCarthy N, Jarvis A, Mahalingham K, Cashman WF: Damage to the superior gluteal nerve after the Hardinge approach to the hip. *J Bone Joint Surg Br* 1996;78:903-906.

17. Pecina M, Lucijanic I, Rosic D: Surgical treatment of obturator nerve palsy resulting from extrapelvic extrusion of cement during total hip arthroplasty. *J Arthroplasty* 2001;16:515-517.

18. Siliski JM, Scott RD: Obturator nerve palsy resulting from intrapelvic extrusion of cement during total hip replacement: Report of four cases. *J Bone Joint Surg Am* 1985;67:1225-1228.

19. Wasielewski RC, Cooperstein LA, Kruger MP, Rubash HE: Acetabular anatomy and the transacetabular fixation of screws in total hip arthroplasty. *J Bone Joint Surg Am* 1990;72:501-508.

20. Wasielewski RC, Crossett LS, Rubash HE: Neural and vascular injury in total hip arthroplasty. *Orthop Clin North Am* 1992;23:219-235.

21. Thomas CD, Asumu T, Chalmers N, Hirst P: Therapeutic embolization for sustained hemorrhage following total hip replacement in a patient with hemophilia A. *Orthopedics* 2000;23:849-850.

22. Lavernia CJ, Cooke C, Hernandez RA: Abstract: Anatomic consequences of screw placement in acetabular reconstruction cages. *J Arthroplasty* 2000;15:254-255.

23. Meldrum RD, Johansen RL: Abstract: Safe screw placement in acetabular revision surgery. *67th Annual Meeting Proceedings*. Rosemont, IL, American Academy of Orthopaedic Surgeons, 2000, pp 327-328.

Principles of Management and Results of Treating the Fractured Femur During and After Total Hip Arthroplasty

Nelson V. Greidanus, MD, MPH, FRCSC
Philip A. Mitchell, MD, FRCS (Tr and Orth)
Bassam A. Masri, MD, FRCSC
Donald S. Garbuz, MD, FRCSC
Clive P. Duncan, MD, FRCSC

Abstract

The management of fractures of the femur during and after total hip arthroplasty can be difficult, and treatment can be fraught with complications. The ideal scenario would be one in which these fractures are prevented. It is important that the surgeon has a thorough understanding of the principles of managing these fractures and has access to a variety of fixation and prosthetic devices and allograft bone when necessary in order to provide the best treatment. Because periprosthetic fractures range from the very simple (requiring no surgical intervention) to the complex (requiring major revision), a classification system of these fractures aids in understanding both the principles of management and results of treatment.

A discussion of the etiology, classification, treatment options, and historical results is important in order to optimize current management of intraoperative and postoperative periprosthetic fractures. Whether surgical or nonsurgical treatment is used depends on various factors.

Intraoperative Fractures
Epidemiology
Berry[1] reported a detected intraoperative periprosthetic fracture rate of 1.0% of primary hip arthroplasties (238 of 23,980) and 7.8% of revision hip arthroplasties (497 of 6,349) on review of the Mayo Clinic Joint Registry. The higher prevalence of intraoperative femoral fracture in revision total hip arthroplasty (THA) has

also been reported by other authors.[2,3] Khan and O'Driscoll[4] reported a similar rate of intraoperative fracture, 1.0% (17 of 1,751) prevalence in primary and revision arthroplasties. Johansson and associates[5] describe 23 intraoperative periprosthetic fractures at their institution, all of which occurred during revision THA. These fractures are more common when the femoral component is inserted without cement at the time of primary hip replacement, with a prevalence of 5.4% (170 of 3,121) compared with a prevalence of 0.3% (68 of 20,859) when the femoral component is inserted with cement.[1] A fracture rate of 1.2% (7 of 605) has been reported when cement is used[6] compared with a fracture rate of

3.0% (39 of 1,318) when cement is not used for femoral fixation.[7]

A similar increased prevalence of fracture with cementless femoral stems is seen in the revision setting. Berry[1] reported a fracture rate of 21.0% in cementless revision procedures (322 of 1,536) in comparison with 3.6% in cemented revision procedures (175 of 4,813). Although the series did not stratify the analysis on the basis of stem length, stem geometry, or bone defect classification, this difference is understood to be a result of the technical nuances of obtaining a tight press-fit within a femur of potentially compromised bone stock.

Classification
Intraoperative fractures may include cortical perforations, longitudinal cracks, or displaced fractures with or without comminution (Fig. 1). Many are not recognized at the time of surgery and are only later detected on postoperative radiographs.[5,7] Successful treatment requires that the implant remain stable and is dictated by fracture location and configuration.

Several fracture classification systems have been reported in the literature.

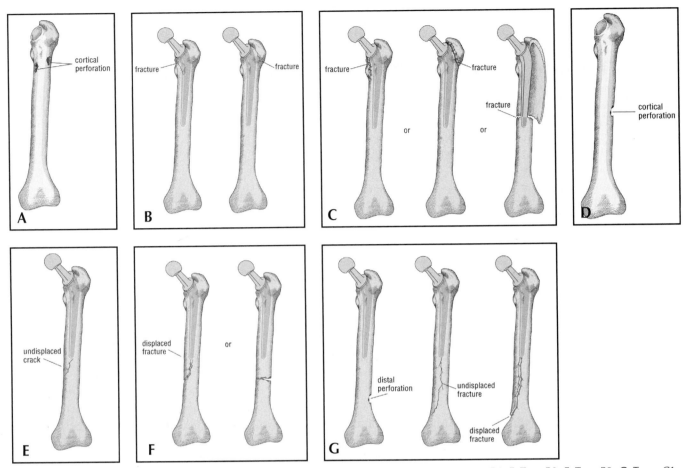

Fig. 1 Intraoperative periprosthetic fractures of the femur. **A**, Type A1. **B**, Type A2. **C**, Type A3. **D**, Type B1. **E**, Type B2. **F**, Type B3. **G**, Types C1, C2, and C3.

Johansson and associates[5] described type 1 fractures proximal to the tip of the prosthesis, type 2 fractures at the distal tip of the prosthesis, and type 3 fractures beyond the tip of the prosthesis. Mallory and associates[8] describe type 1 fractures as occurring in the most proximal portion of the femur, type 2 around the stem, and type 3 at the tip of the prosthesis. Schwartz and associates[7] classify fractures as proximal to the tip of the stem or distal to the tip of the stem with further subclassification identifying them as complete or incomplete. Stuchin[9] describes type 1 fractures as proximal fractures, type 2 as long spiral fractures originating at the tip of the prosthesis, type 3 as originating from a stress riser in the femur, and

type 4 as not otherwise classifiable. Kavanagh[10] describes type 1 as occurring down to the level of the lesser trochanter, type 2 as proximal to the isthmus, and type 3 at or below the isthmus, with all types subclassified as A or B according to displacement of the fracture. These classification systems are in agreement in that each suggests an increasing level of complexity among fractures with greater degrees of distal host-bone involvement.

Vancouver Classification Because different configurations of intraoperative fracture can occur, the Vancouver classification of periprosthetic fractures has been modified for the intraoperative scenario to describe and help in the management of these fractures[11] (Fig. 2). This

new classification system depends on the location, configuration, and stability of the fracture. The femur is divided into three zones, each representing a major type of fracture. Type A fractures would be classified as proximal metaphyseal, not extending into the diaphysis; type B fractures would be diaphyseal, not extending into the distal diaphysis and therefore not precluding diaphyseal long-stem fixation; and type C fractures would be distal fractures extending beyond the longest extent of the longest revision stem and can include the distal metaphysis. Each type is then subclassified into either subtype 1, representing a simple cortical perforation; subtype 2, representing an undisplaced linear crack; or subtype 3, representing a displaced or unstable fracture.[12-15] These subtypes are described in Table 1.

Treatment and Results

Several studies in the literature discuss the results of femoral fracture occurring at the time of THA. Khan and O'Driscoll[4] studied 17 intraoperative fractures in 1,751 arthroplasties. Their suggestions for management included standard implants for short, oblique fractures, open reduction and fixation of long, oblique fractures, and traction for fractures distal to the tip of the stem. Taylor and associates[6] studied 11 intraoperative fractures in 605 arthroplasty procedures (1.8% of cases). The majority of fractures were in the proximal femur and did not compromise final integrity of the arthroplasty; however, they were associated with prolonged convalescence and greater morbidity. Johansson and associates[5] describe 6 of 23 cases of femoral fracture proximal to the tip of the prosthesis that were managed with either nonsurgical or surgical intervention. Only two of these cases had a satisfactory outcome, and both were treated with early surgical intervention and managed with internal fixation and prolonged immobilization or long stem revision and early mobilization. The other four cases had unsatisfactory results arising from prosthetic loosening or infection. Fifteen additional cases of femoral fracture occurring at the distal tip of the femoral prosthesis were managed with surgical treatment. Eight of these cases had a satisfactory result with internal fixation or long stem fixation, and the remaining seven cases had unsatisfactory results caused by malunion, loosening, or heterotopic ossification. Two additional cases were reported with fractures distal to the tip of the prosthesis, both of which had unsatisfactory results caused by refracture or loosening of the prosthesis.

More favorable outcomes for intraoperative fractures have been reported.

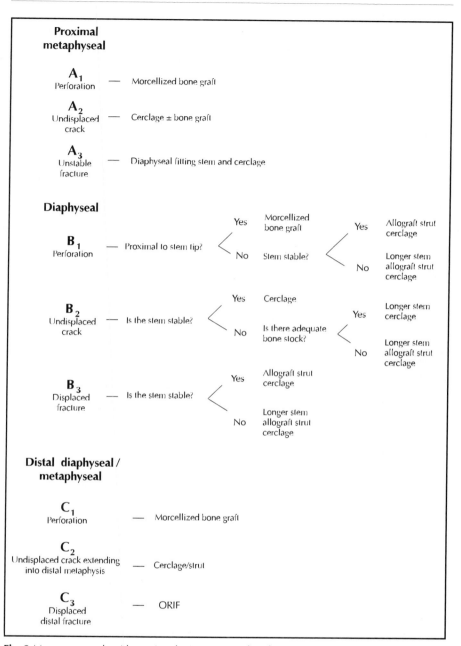

Fig. 2 Management algorithm using the Vancouver classification system for intraoperative periprosthetic fractures. ORIF = open reduction and internal fixation.

Fitzgerald and associates[2] reported an intraoperative fracture rate of 6.3% (40 of 630 cementless femoral stems). All 40 fractures were satisfactorily treated with Parham bands or cerclage wires and, in most cases, bone grafts. One fracture beyond the distal tip that was diagnosed postoperatively was treated successfully with a spica cast. All patients were treated with protected weight bearing for 2 to 4 months. Christensen and associates[16] described 10 patients with intraoperative fractures during 159 revision procedures (6.3%), all of which were treated with open reduction and internal fixation. Although all fractures united, only 6 of

Table 1
Adaptation of the Vancouver Classification

Fracture Subtype	Description	Treatment
A1	Cortical perforation	Simple bone grafting from locally harvested bone
A2	Undisplaced linear crack (occurring at the time of proximal broaching or stem insertion	Cerclage wire fixation
A3	Displaced or unstable fracture of the proximal femur or greater trochanter (occurring at the time of a proximally coated femoral stem)	Diaphyseal-fitting, cementless femoral stem; wires, cables, or a trochanteric fixation claw and cables
B1	Diaphyseal cortical perforation (occurs from cement removal devices or reamers during canal preparation)	Bypass with a cortical strut; bone grafting at the time of strut insertion and fixation
B2	Undisplaced linear crack (usually occurs during broaching or implant insertion)	Protected weight bearing for 6 weeks to 3 months; cerclage wire fixation and bypass of the fracture; cortical struts in patients with poor bone structure
B3	Displaced fracture of the midfemur (occurs at the time of dislocation of the femur through an area of weak bone or at the time of femoral cement removal or femoral preparation)	Reduction and fixation with cerclage wires (spiral or oblique fractures) or one or two cortical struts (transverse fractures); extramedullary and strut and cable augmentation in fractures with well-impacted femoral stems
C1	Cortical perforation (occurs during cement removal or canal preparation)	Bone grafting and bypass of the fracture with a cortical strut
C2	Undisplaced linear crack extending just above the knee joint	Cerclage wires and/or an onlay cortical strut allograft
C3	Displaced fracture of the distal femur that cannot be bypassed by a femoral stem	Open reduction and internal fixation

these 10 patients regained satisfactory function.

Mallory and associates[8] evaluated 56 fractures occurring at the time of cementless arthroplasty that united without major complication or morbidity and compared them with a THA cohort without fractures. Successful union occurred in 45 fractures (80%) of the proximal femur only, 9 fractures (16%) involving the length of the prosthesis, and 2 fractures (4%) located at the tip of the stem. Schwartz and associates[7] reported excellent results in their study of 39 intraoperative fractures diagnosed in 1,318 cases of consecutive THAs. Approximately half of the fractures were diagnosed intraoperatively. The majority of fractures were incomplete and stable; however, those that were complete, unstable, and com-

promised the implant were treated with a fully coated or four-fifths coated stem to provide distal fixation. Adjuvant cerclage wiring was used when needed. Intraoperative fractures that were diagnosed postoperatively were treated with spica casts and protected weight bearing if the fracture was incomplete and did not violate the posterior femoral cortex; however, complete fractures were best treated with open reduction and internal fixation. All fractures in this study united successfully with no long-term consequences or complications. Stuchin[9] obtained good results in his study of 12 intraoperative fractures in 79 press-fit femoral component arthroplasties, with the majority occurring during a revision procedure. All fractures united without compromising patient function when

treated with techniques that were determined by the exact location of the fracture.

Other studies of revision cementless femoral fixation describe intraoperative fracture rates ranging from 8.8% to 46%.[17-20] Paprosky and associates[20] report an intraoperative fracture rate of 8.8% (15 of 170 fractures) and an intraoperative cortical perforation rate of 5.9% (10 of 170) in their long-term review of cementless femoral revision arthroplasty procedures. A review of 87 second-generation cementless (tapered distal tip, bowed options) revision stems revealed only one significant intraoperative fracture, which was successfully treated with a longer femoral stem that bypassed the fracture.[21] The majority of these fractures are diagnosed intraoperatively and treated appropriately without adversely affecting the outcome of the revision procedure. The increasing use of extensile osteotomies in revision arthroplasty may help minimize the rate of stem-tip fractures during femoral revision; however, they also have been associated with an increased incidence of proximal femoral fractures related to the creation of the osteotomy fragment.[22] These proximal femoral fractures have been successfully treated with cerclage wire fixation with or without cortical strut allograft, without compromising the outcome of the revision procedure.[22]

Intraoperative Fractures Diagnosed in the Immediate Postoperative Period

Occasionally, an intraoperative periprosthetic fracture is diagnosed in the immediate postoperative period. These fractures should be fully evaluated with radiographic imaging to determine the extent of the fracture. Many of these fractures are stable, minimally displaced, do not compromise the fixation of the revision prosthesis, and will unite successfully without complication.[7] An effort should be made to attempt to treat these stable

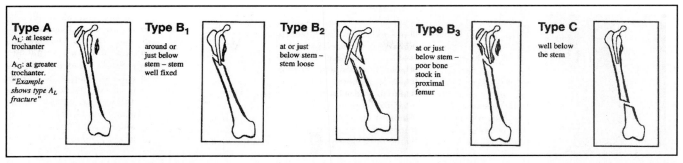

Fig. 3 Vancouver classification of postoperative periprosthetic fractures of the femur. Type A fractures are located in the trochanteric region; the type A fracture shown is located at the lesser trochanter. Type B is located around or just distal to the stem; type B1 is prosthesis stable; type B2 is prosthesis unstable; type B3 is bone stock inadequate. Type C fractures are located well below the stem. (Reproduced from Duncan CP, Masri BA: Fractures of the femur after hip replacement. *Instr Course Lect* 1995;44:293-304.)

fractures with nonsurgical methods, including protected weight bearing and possible use of spica casts or braces, until union is complete. Complex, unstable fractures are rarely diagnosed during the immediate postoperative period because the majority will have been detected intraoperatively. However, they should be treated as early as is appropriate for their fracture configuration.

The literature suggests that the intraoperative periprosthetic fracture can be successfully treated without adversely affecting the function of the prosthetic reconstruction if care is taken to stabilize the fracture, prevent fracture propagation, and maintain prosthetic alignment and stability until union occurs.

Postoperative Fractures
Epidemiology
Studies suggest that the prevalence of postoperative periprosthetic fractures ranges from 0.1% to 2.1%.[1,23-32] The largest study identified to date is from the Mayo Clinic Joint Registry, in which fractures were identified after 1.0% of primary THAs (238 of 23,980) and after 4.0% of revision hip arthroplasties (252 of 6,349).[1]

Etiology
The most frequent cited cause of periprosthetic fracture of the femur is a

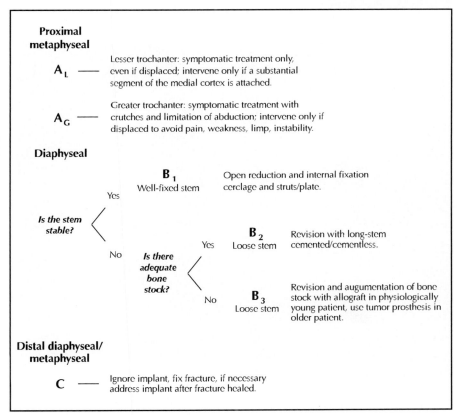

Fig. 4 Management algorithm using the Vancouver classification system for postoperative fractures.

minor episode of trauma. In studies by Adolphson and associates[23] and Beal and Tower,[33] fractures were caused by minor trauma in 88% (28 of 32) and 84% (72 of 86), respectively. Major trauma appears to account for approximately 8% (6 of 75) of reported cases.[34] Undiagnosed osteolytic defects are another risk factor. Lewallen and associates[35] reported that up to 50% of their patients presented with insidious pain and fracture with no history of fall or trauma preceding the fracture event.

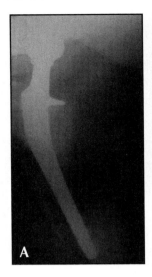
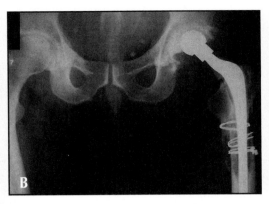
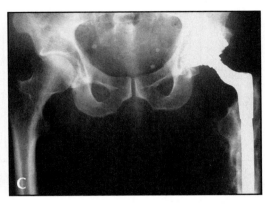

Fig. 5 A, Fracture around infected prosthesis with infection diagnosed on aspiration prior to surgery. **B,** The same fracture treated with PROSTALAC. **C,** The same fracture after stage 2 revision to long-stem insertion, which took place once the infection was eradicated and the fracture united.

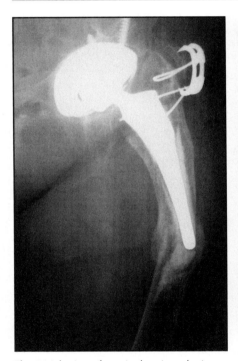
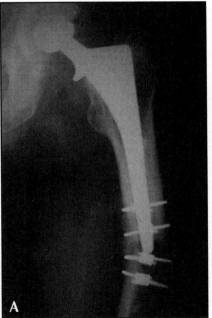
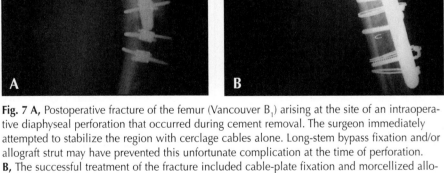

Fig. 6 Malunion of a united periprosthetic fracture resulting from nonsurgical treatment of a Vancouver B_2 fracture.

Fig. 7 A, Postoperative fracture of the femur (Vancouver B_1) arising at the site of an intraoperative diaphyseal perforation that occurred during cement removal. The surgeon immediately attempted to stabilize the region with cerclage cables alone. Long-stem bypass fixation and/or allograft strut may have prevented this unfortunate complication at the time of perforation. **B,** The successful treatment of the fracture included cable-plate fixation and morcellized allograft because the stem was well osseointegrated.

Classification

Periprosthetic fracture treatment decisions depend on five important factors: fracture location, stability of the implant and fracture, quality of host bone stock, patient physiology and age, and surgeon experience.[33] These factors can be determined through a series of questions, the answers to which can be used to formulate a treatment algorithm.[36] For a classification system to be useful as a guide to management, it should incorporate these factors so that similar fractures can be compared.

Several periprosthetic fracture classification systems have been described.[5,24,33,34,37] Most of these classification systems are simply based on the location of the fracture, with the exception of the classification system of Roffman and Mendes,[37] which takes the stability of the implant into consideration.

Vancouver Classification The Vancouver classification of periprosthetic fractures (Fig. 3) was developed to consolidate the three most important factors for treatment decision making: site of the fracture, stability of the implant, and quality of surrounding bone stock.[11,38,39] This classification has been demonstrated to be both reliable and valid and can provide the surgeon with a useful treatment algorithm.[39] To the best of our knowledge, this is the only such classification system that has been subjected to reliability and validity testing.

As with its modification for intraoperative fractures, the Vancouver classification system divides fractures into the following three major types, depending on the location of the fracture: type A, denoting the trochanteric region; type B, denoting a fracture around or just distal to the femoral stem; and type C, denoting fractures that are so far below the femoral stem that their treatment is independent of the presence of a hip replacement in situ. Types A and B are then subdivided according to the stability of the implant and remaining bone stock (Fig. 4). Type A fractures are further identified as either fractures of the greater trochanter, type A_G, which tend to be stable and are often related to osteolysis in the greater trochanter; or fractures of the lesser trochanter, type A_L, which may lead to implant instability as the medial buttress is lost. Type B fractures are further identified according to the stability of the femoral implant and the remaining bone stock as follows: Type B_1, in which the femoral implant is solidly fixed; type B_2, in which the femoral implant is loose but the remaining bone stock is good; or type B_3, in which there is severe bone stock loss (osteopenia, osteolysis, or comminution) in the presence of a loose implant.

Type C fractures are well away from the stem and can be treated independently of the arthroplasty using standard techniques of fracture reduction and stabilization.

Treatment and Results

Whenever a periprosthetic fracture is encountered for which a revision THA is contemplated, infection is a possibility. Unfortunately, serologic markers such as erythrocyte sedimentation rate and C-reactive protein level are not useful in the presence of a fracture, unlike failed THA without a fracture.[40] Therefore, routine aspiration biopsy can be used to rule out infection in these cases. If the aspiration biopsy suggests infection at the site of the THA, the patient can be treated in two stages using the PROSTALAC system (DePuy, Warsaw, IN) as an interim spacer that allows healing of the fracture while the infection is being eradicated[41,42] (Fig. 5).

Historical management options have included protected weight bearing,[43] traction[5,12,23,33,44] casts and braces,[12] internal fixation with plates and screws,[12,33] internal fixation with modified cable-plate devices,[45-51] or revision arthroplasty with or without allograft.[11,23,33,52-54]

The trend over the past 20 years has been a move from nonsurgical management toward surgical management. Several factors, including early failures with nonsurgical management and improved surgical techniques and prosthetic options, contribute to this trend. The quality of the published reports remains poor in that most studies span large periods and are compilations of cases managed by different surgeons using different techniques. However, distinct trends of success and failure document the historical management of these fractures.

Nonsurgical Treatment Several studies describe the results of various methods of nonsurgical treatment. In one study of 37 periprosthetic femoral fractures, 14 occurred postoperatively, 8 had associated complications, and results were satisfactory in 5. In another study of

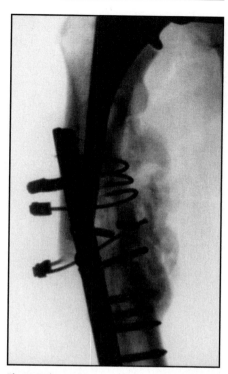

Fig. 8 Failure of fixation of a cable-plate system.

31 femoral fractures,[5] the worst results were noted in patients managed nonsurgically and the best results in patients receiving long-stem femoral prostheses.[24] In yet another study, 29 patients were evaluated; 21 fractures managed nonsurgically in traction. Results indicated that union could occur with the patient in traction. A high rate of malunion was reported, with six patients undergoing further surgery, along with high rate of nonunion, with three of eight fractures not uniting despite surgical fixation. Somers and associates[55] have recently reported on 34 fractures managed nonsurgically over a 20-year period. Despite obtaining union in 33 fractures, the prolonged periods of traction and/or cast immobilization caused high rates of complications, including malunion (Fig. 6). The authors no longer recommend this method of treatment.

Principles of Surgical Treatment Surgical treatment for the majority of

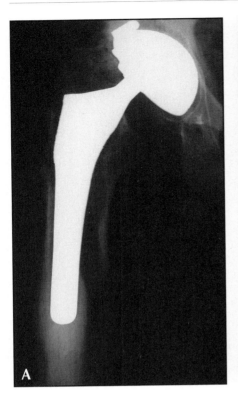
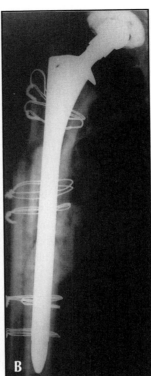
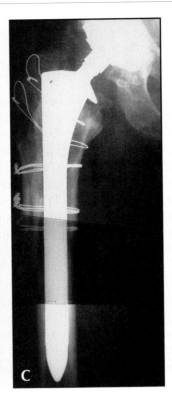

Fig. 9 A, Fracture around a loose cementless stem (Vancouver B$_2$). **B,** Segmental Vancouver B$_2$ fracture treated with long-stem fixation, allograft strut, and cerclage wires. **C,** Vancouver B$_2$ fracture treated with long-stem fixation, allograft strut, and cerclage.

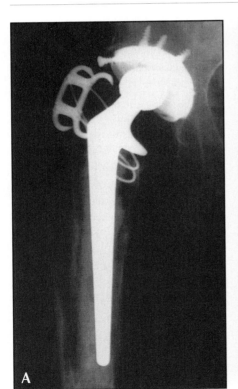
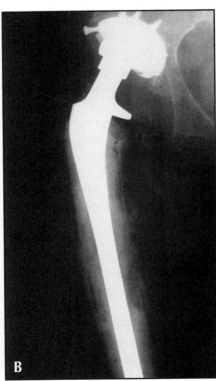

Fig. 10 A, Fracture around loose cemented stem (Vancouver B$_2$). **B,** Vancouver B$_2$ fracture treated with long-stem cemented fixation.

postoperative periprosthetic fractures is often preferable to accepting the inherent risks of nonsurgical treatment. Historical data suggest that a prolonged period of recumbency, possible traction, and hospitalization are required for successful nonsurgical treatment; even so, the rates of nonunion and malunion remain high. Furthermore, the majority of these fractures occur in elderly patients for whom the risks of prolonged bed rest are worse than the risks of surgery.

The surgeon should be familiar with the extensile approaches to the hip and femur. The lateral approach to the femur is often used in conjunction with the posterior approach to the hip or modified lateral approach to the hip. Fracture fragments can occasionally be separated to enhance canal débridement and to facilitate reaming and implant fit in patients treated with long-stem bypass fixation. Intraoperative tissue samples should be obtained for culturing and intraoperative prophylactic antibiotics administered.

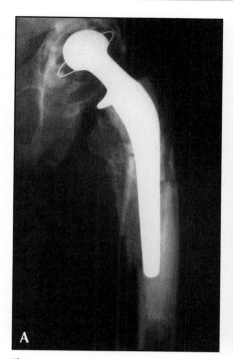
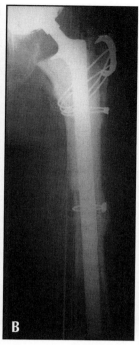
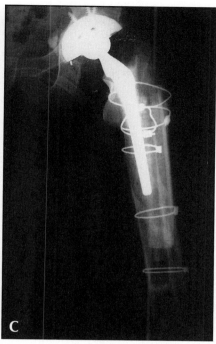

Fig. 11 A, Comminuted fracture with inadequate proximal femoral bone stock (Vancouver B₃). **B,** Vancouver B₃ fracture treated with proximal femoral allograft replacement and long-stem fixation. **C,** Vancouver B₃ fracture treated with impaction allografting and cemented fixation.

Intraoperative radiographs can assist in delineating of fracture repair and the integrity of the construct prior to wound closure. Postoperatively, management and mobilization are individualized as necessary for both fracture and implant stability. Thromboprophylaxis and antibiotic prophylaxis are administered per protocol for revision hip arthroplasty. For most procedures, protected weight bearing is recommended for 12 weeks or until there is convincing clinical and radiographic evidence of union.

Several methods are used to accomplish surgical treatment. Open reduction and internal fixation is appropriate for fractures in which the stem remains stable. Although standard plates and screws may be used, they tend to violate the cement mantle if the existing stem was inserted with cement. Furthermore, if a canal-filling cementless stem is present, it may be difficult to insert screws around the implant. As an alternative, specially designed plates that can accommodate

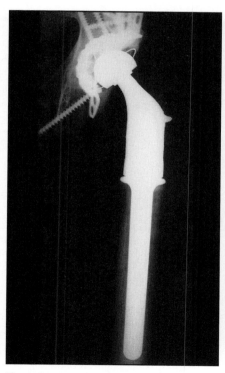

Fig. 12 Vancouver B₃ fracture treated with cemented proximal femoral replacement prosthesis.

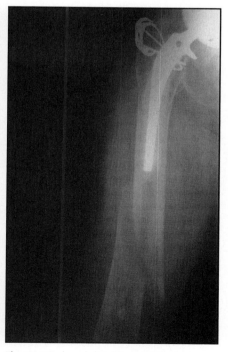

Fig. 13 Displaced distal femoral fracture without interference with proximal femur and hip arthroplasty (Vancouver C) amenable to open reduction and internal fixation.

Table 2
Postoperative Periprosthetic Fracture Management and Results Summary*

Author	Year	Number	Classification System	Treatment Methods	Excellent-Good	Fair-Poor
Macdonald et al[66]	2001	14	Johansson	Long-stem cementless revision	14	0
Venu et al[56]	2001	13	Vancouver (variety)	Plate and cable systems	10	3
Tadross et al[59]	2000	8	Vancouver (B1)	Plate and cable systems	2	6
Kamineni et al[57]	1999	15	Beals and Tower (IIIB)	Plate and cable systems	13	2
Kamineni and Ware[58]	1999	5	Beals and Tower (IIIA & IIIB)	Mennen plate	0	5
Wong and Gross[69]	1999	15	Vancouver (B3)	Proximal femoral allograft	13	2
Sandhu et al[67]	1999	5	Not mentioned	Long-stem cemented revision	5	0
Tower and Beals[65]	1999	86 (77 with follow-up)	Beals and Tower			
		22	Loose stem	Nonsurgical	0	5
				Long-stem revision	13	4
		55	Stable stem			
		2	Type I	Nonsurgical	2	0
		7	Type II	Nonsurgical	3	0
				ORIF	2	0
				Long-stem revision	2	0
		15	Type IIIA	Nonsurgical	4	2
				ORIF	1	2
				Long-stem revision	6	0
		18	Type IIIB	Nonsurgical	1	1
				ORIF	2	4
				Long-stem revision	5	5
		13	Type IIIC / IV	Nonsurgical	7	0
				ORIF	2	4
Somers et al[55]	1998	35	Whittaker	Nonsurgical		34
Lewallen and Berry[35]	1997	97	Vancouver	Various	65	32
Mont and Maar[72]	1994	487	Mont & Maar	Meta-analysis		
		10	Type 1	Nonsurgical	10	0
		125	Type 2	Nonsurgical	26	20
				ORIF	28	11
				Long-stem revision	29	7
				Girdlestone	1	3
		142	Type 3	Nonsurgical	25	33
				ORIF	31	18
				Long-stem revision	26	6
				Girdlestone	0	3
		200	Type 4	Nonsurgical	59	18
				ORIF	37	36
				Long-stem revision	37	13
		19	Type 5	Nonsurgical	1	2
				ORIF	1	1
				Long-stem revision	11	3

cables and screws are available from most implant manufacturers. These plates can be used in isolation or augmented with an allograft strut[48] (Fig. 7). Alternatively, the fracture may be fixed with two onlay cortical struts placed on the anterior and lateral aspects of the femur and held with cerclage cables. Regardless of the method of fixation, the fracture site should be bone grafted with morcellized bone. Allograft bone may be used to avoid the morbidity associated with harvesting autogenous bone grafts.

Cable-plate systems are commonly used for the fixation of periprosthetic fractures. The Ogden plate (Zimmer, Warsaw, IN) was one of the first systems in which either cables or screws were used with the plate to optimize fixation around and adjacent to the femoral prosthesis.[48] Several modifications on the same treatment modality have been developed since the inception of this technique.

Venu and associates[56] used the Dall-Miles cable-plate system (Howmedica, Rutherford, NJ) for the fixation of 12 periprosthetic hip fractures. Morcellized morselised autograft, allograft, or cortical strut allograft was used for all fractures. Nine of these 12 fractures achieved successful union, with three requiring further intervention for nonunion. Two of

Table 2 (Continued)
Postoperative Periprosthetic Fracture Management and Results Summary*

Author	Year	Number	Classification System	Treatment Methods	Excellent-Good	Fair-Poor
Missakian and Rand[44]	1993	7	Johansson	Nonsurgical	1	2
				Long-stem revision	2	1
Chandler et al[61]	1993	19	Vancouver (B1)	Cortical strut allograft	17	2
Roffman and Mendes[37]	1989	7	Roffman and Mendes			
		5	Type 1	Nonsurgical	4	0
				ORIF	1	0
		2	Type 2	Long-stem revision	1	1
Zenni et al[48]	1988	19	Zenni	ORIF	17	2
Cooke and Newman[34]	1988	75	Modified Bethea			
		8	Type 1	Long-stem revision/ORIF	5	3
		13	Type 2	Nonsurgical	1	5
				Long-stem revision/ORIF	4	3
		30	Type 3	Nonsurgical	5	7
				ORIF	7	0
				Long-stem revision	5	6
		24	Type 4	Nonsurgical	20	0
				Surgical	4	0
Wang et al[49]	1985	6	None	ORIF	5	1
Bethea et al[24]	1982	31	Bethea			
		14	Type A	Nonsurgical	4	3
				ORIF	1	1
				Long-stem revision	4	1
		7	Type B	Nonsurgical	1	5
				ORIF	1	0
				Long-stem revision	4	0
		10	Type C	Long-stem revision	6	0
Johansson et al[5]	1981	14	Johansson			
		5	Type I	Nonsurgical	1	1
				Long-stem revision	2	1
		7	Type II	Nonsurgical		7
		2	Type III	Nonsurgical	1	
				ORIF	1	

*ORIF = open reduction and internal fixation

the fractures that failed to unite were at the distal tip of the femoral stem. Kamineni and associates[57] described their experience with 15 femoral fractures in association with loose cemented stems that were treated with cable and plate fixation. Thirteen fractures were treated with a Dall-Miles cable-plate system, and two were treated with the Zimmer Cable-Ready system (Zimmer, Warsaw, IN). All 15 patients were allowed partial weight bearing until radiographic evidence of union was noted. There were four subsequent femoral prosthetic revisions: three fracture unions and one at the time of treatment for nonunion and plate failure. The one nonunion occurred

when internal fixation was used to treat a fracture caused by a loose stem (type B_2) which should have been an indication for immediate revision THA. One additional patient developed a fracture at the distal tip of the plate, which was treated successfully with a longer plate. The same authors reported on a separate cohort of five patients treated with the Mennen plate.[58] Because fracture fixation failed and reoperation was required in all five patients, the use of this plate to treat any periprosthetic fractures was discouraged.

Tadross and associates[59] reported on seven hip periprosthetic fractures managed with the Dall-Miles cable-plate system. Three of the fractures achieved

union with satisfactory results; however, the other four cases were considered failures because of nonunion in two cases and malunion in two cases. The authors associated the high failure rate in part to a varus position of the femoral prosthesis, which may have altered the biomechanics at the fracture site. Bone graft was not used in all cases, and its use did not appear to correlate with success. The high rate of failure in this series may suggest that additional fixation, such as onlay cortical struts, may be required (Fig. 8).

The use of cortical strut allograft in femoral reconstruction was first reported by Chandler and Penenberg in 1989.[60] In another study of 19 periprosthetic femoral fractures treated with massive cortical onlay grafts, 16 of 19 fractures united at a mean of 4.5 months. One malunion and two nonunions required further surgery.[61] Additionally, Chandler and associates have described the use of a metal plate on one cortex and an allograft strut on the other, with union and clinical success achieved in 21 of 22 patients. All of Chandler's reports confirm union of the allograft with host bone.[62] The basic science and clinical results of strut allografting have been described in the literature.[63,64] The advantages of a strut allograft are that it can be customized to fit any femur because the allograft shares the same modulus of elasticity as the host bone, and through union with host bone the allograft can augment host bone stock and strength.

Revision THA

Several authors have reviewed the literature on periprosthetic fractures and provided a statistical analysis of the outcome data. Mont and Maar[12] reported on 487 patients from 26 reports published over a 28-year period. The authors could not stratify the data on several important factors, including cemented versus cementless long-stem revisions, the use of bone grafting and type of bone graft used, and the status of fixation of the indwelling femoral implant, because of the inconsistency of statistical documentation in the original published reports. The authors were, however, able to successfully stratify data regarding location of the fracture and type of treatment and concluded that proximal trochanteric fractures did well with nonsurgical treatment. For mid-stem and distal-stem fractures, cerclage wire cables and bone graft or revision to a longer stem were more effective than screw-plate fixation or traction. Fractures below the stem tip generally responded well to long-stem revision or traction, whereas results were worse with screw/plate fixation. In addition, a trend toward poor results with cerclage wire

fixation was noted. Comminuted fractures appeared to do better with long-stem revision; however, statistical significance was not attained in comparison with the other methods of treatment.

In 1996, Beals and Tower[33,65] reported on a total of 102 interventions in 93 periprosthetic fractures of the femur by 30 different surgeons. Classifying surgical outcome as excellent (healed and stable implant), good (healed with mild-to-moderate deformity), or poor (loose stem, nonunion of fracture, deep infection, new fracture, or severe deformity), they found that outcome was excellent in 32% of interventions, good in 16% outcomes, and poor in 52% (numerator and denominator not reported). A stratified analysis of the location of the fracture and the type of fixation revealed that cementless revision implants had a better success rate than cemented implants. Furthermore, a high complication rate was reported across all treatment methods. Implant loosening occurred in 19% of cases for which nonsurgical treatment was used, in 33% of cases for which interfragmentary fixation was used, and in 13% of cases for which plate fixation was used; plate-fixation interventions were further complicated by a 7% rate of infection. Cemented revisions had a 62% complication rate (plate loosening occurred in 38% and other complications such as infection, dislocation, or trochanteric nonunion occurred in 24%.) Cementless revisions resulted in an 18% rate of subsidence (some of which stabilized), a 7% rate of implant loosening, and a 9% rate of dislocation, trochanteric nonunion, or infection.

According to a review of the Mayo Clinic Joint Registry, 97 postoperative fractures occurred in 94 patients from 1971 to 1993 and were treated with various methods.[35] Approximately 85% of these fractures united and 15% did not. Fifty percent of patients did not have stable, long-term fixation. Thirty-three percent of patients at latest follow-up had

implant loosening and severe pain. Because up to 50% of these fractures occurred without any inciting trauma or event, the authors highlighted the importance of regular preventive radiographic follow-up for all patients who have received primary and revision hip arthroplasties. This catastrophic rate of femoral failure is attributed to the progressive compromise of host bone caused by implant loosening or osteolysis.

Extensively porous-coated femoral implants have been popularized by Paprosky, Moreland, and Engh in revision hip arthroplasty as a method of bypassing proximal bone deficiency. Recently, there has been increased interest in using intramedullary fixation for complex periprosthetic fractures.[18,21,65,66] Macdonald and associates[66] recently reported on 14 cases of postoperative fracture that were treated with extensively coated cementless stems. All 14 fractures united and the deformity was corrected. (One stem, however, was not osseointegrated and was not revised.) Tower and Beals[65] also achieved their best results using cementless long-stem fixation. This technique can be used in conjunction with cortical onlay allograft or plate and cerclage cables/wires to provide maximal stability and fracture control (Fig. 9).

Long-stem cemented femoral revision for periprosthetic fracture has not become popular because of its high failure rate and the potential for the cement to interfere with fracture union. Sandhu and associates[67] described a case series of five patients who were treated with a new cement technique. They applied a split, 60-mL syringe, fashioned it as a sleeve around the fractured femur to contain the liquid cement, and then cemented the canal and inserted a long stem. The patients in this case series were elderly, with ages ranging from 82 to 94 years. Despite the short follow-up, this case series illustrates the usefulness of long-stem cemented femoral fixation in elderly patients with type B_2 fractures in whom bone stock is adequate for cemented fixation (Fig. 10). The authors also describe the benefits of early weight bearing and discharge from the acute-care hospital.

Major Allograft and Proximal Femoral Replacements Segmental allograft can also be used to treat bone deficiency at the time of revision hip arthroplasty for type B₃ fractures[68] (Fig. 11). Impaction allografting can also be used to reconstruct fractured femur. Wong and Gross[69] described the use of proximal structural allograft in patients with periprosthetic fracture and severe bone loss. Nineteen patients were treated using this technique, 15 of whom were available for review, with a mean follow-up of 5 years. Thirteen patients had a good result and two required further surgery (one required plating for nonunion and the other required a revision to a similar construct). For older patients, the authors prefer the use of proximal femoral replacement prostheses because of the shortened rehabilitation period and the immediate weight bearing that these implants allow (Fig. 12). Proximal femoral replacements have been demonstrated to be effective, with survivorship at 12 years reported to be 64%[70-72] (Fig. 13). A summary of results of postoperative periprosthetic fracture management is found in Table 2.

Summary

Periprosthetic femoral fractures present a difficult treatment challenge and their management has been associated with many complications.[73] Although many fracture configurations exist, the many treatment options as well as published results are available to guide surgical decision making. The use of a systematic approach to the diagnosis, classification, and treatment of these fractures can assist the surgeon in managing both intraoperative and postoperative periprosthetic fractures and help ensure optimal patient function and outcome.

References

1. Berry DJ: Epidemiology: Hip and Knee. *Orthop Clin North Am* 1999;30:183-190.

2. Fitzgerald RH Jr, Brindley GW, Kavanagh BF: The uncemented total hip arthroplasty: Intraoperative femoral fractures. *Clin Orthop* 1988; 235:61-66.

3. Morrey BF, Kavanagh BF: Complications with revision of the femoral component of total hip arthroplasty: Comparison between cemented and uncemented techniques. *J Arthroplasty* 1992;7:71-79.

4. Khan MA, O'Driscoll M: Fractures of the femur during total hip replacement and their management. *J Bone Joint Surg Br* 1977;59:36-41.

5. Johansson JE, McBroom R, Barrington TW, Hunter GA: Fracture of the ipsilateral femur in patients with total hip replacement. *J Bone Joint Surg Am* 1981;63:1435-1442.

6. Taylor MM, Meyers MH, Harvey JP Jr: Intraoperative femur fractures during total hip replacement. *Clin Orthop* 1978;137:96-103.

7. Schwartz JT Jr, Mayer JG, Engh CA: Femoral fracture during non-cemented total hip arthroplasty. *J Bone Joint Surg Am* 1989;71:1135-1142.

8. Mallory TH, Kraus TJ, Vaughn BK: Intraoperative femoral fractures associated with cementless total hip arthroplasty. *Orthopedics* 1989;12:231-239.

9. Stuchin SA: Femoral shaft fracture in porous and press-fit total hip arthroplasty. *Orthop Rev* 1990;19:153-159.

10. Kavanagh BF: Femoral fractures associated with total hip arthroplasty. *Orthop Clin North Am* 1992;23:249-257.

11. Duncan CP, Masri BA: Fractures of the femur after hip replacement. *Instr Course Lect* 1995;44:293-304.

12. Mont MA, Maar DC: Fractures of the ipsilateral femur after hip arthroplasty: A statistical analysis of outcome based on 487 patients. *J Arthroplasty* 1994;9:511-519.

13. Younger TI, Bradford MS, Magnus RE, Paprosky WG: Extended proximal femoral osteotomy: A new technique for femoral revision arthroplasty. *J Arthroplasty* 1995;10:329-338.

14. Larson JE, Chao EY, Fitzgerald RH: Bypassing femoral cortical defects with cemented intramedullary stems. *J Orthop Res* 1991;9: 414-421.

15. Chandler HP, Tigges RG: The role of allografts in the treatment of periprosthetic femoral fractures. *Instr Course Lect* 1998;47:257-264.

16. Christensen CM, Seger BM, Schultz RB: Management of intraoperative femur fractures associated with revision hip arthroplasty. *Clin Orthop* 1989;248:177-180.

17. Lawrence JM, Engh CA, Macalino GE, Lauro GR: Outcome of revision hip arthroplasty done without cement. *J Bone Joint Surg Am* 1994;76:965-973.

18. Moreland JR, Bernstein ML: Femoral revision hip arthroplasty with uncemented, porous-coated stems. *Clin Orthop* 1995;319:141-150.

19. Malkani AL, Lewallen DG, Cabanela ME, Wallrichs SL: Femoral component revision using an uncemented, proximally coated, long-stem prosthesis. *J Arthroplasty* 1996;11:411-418.

20. Paprosky WG, Greidanus NV, Antoniou J: Minimum 10-year-results of extensively porous-coated stems in revision hip arthroplasty. *Clin Orthop* 1999;369:230-242.

21. Paprosky WB, Aribindi R: Hip replacement: Treatment of femoral bone loss using distal bypass fixation. *Instr Course Lect* 2000;49: 119-130.

22. Chen WM, McAuley JP, Engh CA Jr, Hopper RH Jr, Engh CA: Extended slide trochanteric osteotomy for revision total hip arthroplasty. *J Bone Joint Surg Am* 2000;82:1215-1219.

23. Adolphson P, Jonsson U, Kalen R: Fractures of the ipsilateral femur after total hip arthroplasty. *Arch Orthop Trauma Surg* 1987;106:353-357.

24. Bethea JS III, DeAndrade JR, Fleming LL, Lindenbaum SD, Welch RB: Proximal femoral fractures following total hip arthroplasty. *Clin Orthop* 1982;170:95-106.

25. Fredin H: Late fracture of the femur following perforation during total hip arthroplasty: A report of 2 cases. *Acta Orthop Scand* 1988;59: 331-332.

26. Garcia-Cimbrelo E, Munuera L, Gil-Garay E: Femoral shaft fractures after cemented total hip arthroplasty. *Int Orthop* 1992;16:97-100.

27. Lowenhielm G, Hansson LI, Karrholm J: Fracture of the lower extremity after total hip replacement. *Arch Orthop Trauma Surg* 1989;108:141-143.

28. Scott RD, Turner RH, Leitzes SM, Aufranc OE: Femoral fractures in conjunction with total hip replacement. *J Bone Joint Surg Am* 1975;57: 494-501.

29. Garbuz DS, Masri BA, Duncan CP: Periprosthetic fractures of the femur: Principles of prevention and management. *Instr Course Lect* 1998;47:237-242.

30. Pazzaglia U, Byers PD: Fractured femoral shaft through an osteolytic lesion resulting from the reaction to a prosthesis: A case report. *J Bone Joint Surg Br* 1984;66:337-339.

31. Elting JJ, Mikhail WE, Zicat BA, Hubbell JC, Lane LE, House B: Preliminary report of impaction grafting for exchange femoral arthroplasty. *Clin Orthop* 1995;319:159-167.

32. Gie GA, Linder L, Ling RS, Simon JP, Slooff TJ, Timperley AJ: Impacted cancellous allografts and cement for revision total hip arthroplasty. *J Bone Joint Surg Br* 1993;75:14-21.

33. Beals RK, Tower SS: Periprosthetic fractures of the femur: An analysis of 93 fractures. *Clin Orthop* 1996;327:238-246.

34. Cooke PH, Newman JH: Fractures of the femur in relation to cemented hip prostheses. *J Bone Joint Surg Br* 1988;70:386-389.

35. Lewallen DG, Berry DJ: Periprosthetic fracture of the femur after total hip arthroplasty: Treatment and results to date. *Instr Course Lect* 1998;47:243-249.

36. Brady OH, Garbuz DS, Masri BA, Duncan CP: Classification of the hip. *Orthop Clin North Am* 1999;30:215-220.

37. Roffman M, Mendes DG: Fracture of the femur after total hip arthroplasty. *Orthopedics* 1989;12:1067-1070.

38. Brady OH, Garbuz DS, Masri BA, Duncan CP: Classification of the hip. *Orthop Clin North Am* 1999;30:215-220.

39. Brady OH, Garbuz DS, Masri BA, Duncan CP: The reliability and validity of the Vancouver classification of femoral fractures after hip replacement. *J Arthroplasty* 2000;15:59-62.

40. Spangehl MJ, Masri BA, O'Connell JX, Duncan CP: Prospective analysis of preoperative and intraoperative investigations for the diagnosis of infection at the sites of two hundred and two revision total hip arthroplasties. *J Bone Joint Surg Am* 1999;81:672-683.

41. Younger AS, Duncan CP, Masri BA, McGraw RW: The outcome of two-stage arthroplasty using a custom-made interval spacer to treat the infected hip. *J Arthroplasty* 1997;12:615-623.

42. Younger AS, Duncan CP, Masri BA: Treatment of infection associated with segmental bone loss in the proximal part of the femur in two stages with the use of an antibiotic-loaded interval prosthesis. *J Bone Joint Surg Am* 1998;80:60-69.

43. Dysart SH, Savory CG, Callaghan JJ: Nonoperative treatment of a postoperative fracture around an uncemented porous-coated femoral component. *J Arthroplasty* 1989;4:187-190.

44. Missakian ML, Rand JA: Fractures of the femoral shaft adjacent to long stem femoral components of total hip arthroplasty: Report of seven cases. *Orthopedics* 1993;16:149-152.

45. Dave DJ, Koka SR, James SE: Mennen plate fixation for fracture of the femoral shaft with ipsilateral total hip and knee arthroplasties. *J Arthroplasty* 1995;10:113-115.

46. Ogden WS, Rendall J: Fractures beneath hip prostheses: A special indication for Parham bands and plating. *Orthop Trans* 1978;2:70.

47. Partridge AJ, Evans PE: The treatment of fractures of the shaft of the femur using nylon cerclage. *J Bone Joint Surg Br* 1982;64:210-214.

48. Zenni EJ Jr, Pomeroy DL, Caudle RJ: Odgen plate and other fixations for fractures complicating femoral endoprostheses. *Clin Orthop* 1988;231:83-90.

49. Wang GT, Miller TO, Stamp WG: Femoral fracture following total hip arthroplasty: Brief note on treatment. *J Bone Joint Surg Am* 1985;67:956-958.

50. Radcliffe SN, Smith DN: The Mennen plate in periprosthetic hip fractures. *Injury* 1996;27:27-30.

51. Kelley SS: Periprosthetic femoral fractures. *J Am Acad Orthop Surg* 1994;2:164-172.

52. Kolstad K: Revision THR after periprosthetic femoral fracture: An analysis of 23 cases. *Acta Orthop Scand* 1994;65:505-508.

53. Ries MD: Intraoperative modular stem lengthening to treat periprosthetic femur fracture. *J Arthroplasty* 1996;11:204-205.

54. Mihalko WM, Beaudoin AJ, Cardea JA, Krause WR: Finite-element modelling of femoral shaft fracture fixation post total hip arthroplasty. *J Biomech* 1992;25:469-476.

55. Somers JF, Suy R, Stuyck J, Mulier M, Fabry G: Conservative treatment of femoral shaft fractures in patients with total hip arthroplasty. *J Arthroplasty* 1998;13:162-171.

56. Venu KM, Koka R, Garikipati R, Shenava Y, Madhu TS: Dall-Miles cable and plate fixation for the treatment of peri-prosthetic femoral fractures: Analysis of results in 13 cases. *Injury* 2001;32:395-400.

57. Kamineni S, Vindlacheruvu R, Ware HE: Periprosthetic femoral shaft fractures treated with plate and cable fixation. *Injury* 1999;30:261-268.

58. Kamineni S, Ware HE: The Mennen plate: Unsuitable for elderly femoral periprosthetic fractures. *Injury* 1999;30:257-260.

59. Tadross TS, Nanu AM, Buchanan MJ, Checketts RG: Dall-Miles plating for periprosthetic B1 fractures of the femur. *J Arthroplasty* 2000;15:47-51.

60. Chandler HP, Penenberg BL (eds): *Bone Stock Deficiency in Total Hip Replacement: Classification and Management*. Thorofare, NJ, Slack Inc, 1989, pp 103-164.

61. Chandler HP, King D, Limbird R, et al: The use of cortical allograft struts for fixation of fractures associated with well-fixed total joint prostheses. *Semin Arthroplasty* 1993;4:99-107.

62. Chandler HP, Tigges RG: The role of allografts in the treatment of periprosthetic femoral fractures. *Instr Course Lect* 1998;47:257-264.

63. Emerson RH Jr, Malinin TI, Cuellar AD, Head WC, Peters PC: Cortical strut allografts in the reconstruction of the femur in revision total hip arthroplasty: A basic science and clinical study. *Clin Orthop* 1992;285:35-44.

64. Head WC, Wagner RA, Emerson RH Jr, Malinin TI: Restoration of femoral bone stock in revision total hip arthroplasty. *Orthop Clin North Am* 1993;24:697-703.

65. Tower SS, Beals RK: Fractures of the femur after hip replacement: The Oregon experience. *Orthop Clin North Am* 1999;30:235-247.

66. Macdonald SJ, Paprosky WG, Jablonsky WS, Magnus RG: Periprosthetic femoral fractures treated with a long-stem cementless component. *J Arthroplasty* 2001;16:379-383.

67. Sandhu SS, Fern ED, Parsons SW: An improved cementing technique for revision hip surgery after peri-prosthetic fractures. *Injury* 1999;30:195-198.

68. Gross AE: Revision arthroplasty of the hip using allograft bone, in Czitrom AA, Gross AE (eds): *Allografts in Orthopaedic Practice*. Baltimore, MD, Williams & Wilkins, 1992, pp 147-173.

69. Wong P, Gross AE: The use of structural allografts for treating periprosthetic fractures about the hip and knee. *Orthop Clin North Am* 1999;30:259-264.

70. Sim FH, Chao EY: Hip salvage by proximal femoral replacement. *J Bone Joint Surg Am* 1981;63:1228-1239.

71. Malkani AL, Settecerri JJ, Sim FH, Chao EY, Wallrichs SL: Long-term results of proximal femoral replacement for non-neoplastic disorders. *J Bone Joint Surg Br* 1995;77:351-356.

72. Malkani AL, Paiso JM, Sim FH: Proximal femoral replacement with a megaprosthesis. *Instr Course Lect* 2000;49:141-146.

73. Crockarell JR Jr, Berry DJ, Lewallen DG: Nonunion after periprosthetic femoral fracture associated with total hip arthroplasty. *J Bone Joint Surg Am* 1999;81:1073-1079.

SECTION
4

Returning Function Through Revision Surgery

Returning Function Through Revision Surgery

The four articles in this section of *Instructional Course Lectures Hip* are of great relevance to surgeons who perform revision arthroplasty. Together, these articles, written by world authorities on the subject, offer a succinct technique manual and highlight key concepts for any surgeon who performs what often can be a challenging operation. The tips offered and techniques described in these articles are invaluable to anyone attempting revision hip arthroplasty. The information is current and allows the surgeon to tackle a revision arthroplasty in a rational, stepwise manner.

Any successful revision operation requires adequate work-up and planning. This point is well emphasized in the articles by Duffy and associates and Barrack and Burnett. Both emphasize the importance of thorough examination and history to sort out the reasons for pain and laboratory studies to rule out infection. Once these steps have been completed, a surgical plan can be developed. Factors associated with implant removal, especially well-fixed implants, also are key considerations, particularly in patients with infection or instability. These may make revision surgery challenging. For this reason, the article by Andrew Glassman on the removal of well-fixed cementless components is particularly important. Once implants

are removed, the surgeon may be faced with significant bone loss, which is the worst-case scenario in a revision total hip arthroplasty.

The article by Sporer and associates is a well-written discussion regarding options and techniques of reconstructing the acetabulum and managing bone loss on the acetabular side. The final article in the section by Gross and associates addresses the role of allografts in revision hip arthroplasty.

Duffy and associates point out in their article on patient evaluation that despite the fact that hip arthroplasty is one of the most successful operations in medicine, some patients experience persistent pain postoperatively. This result is particularly puzzling, especially when the implants appear to be well fixed and there appears to be no radiographic evidence of mechanical complications. In many of these patients, infection will be the most likely diagnosis; however, this is not always the case. The authors provide an excellent framework for thinking about these patients. They emphasize the importance of examining areas that might cause referred pain and will act as a confounding variable. They also discuss problems related to the hip, both extrinsic and intrinsic. A nice summary of the differential diagnosis and a detailed review of various laboratory and imaging studies needed to

diagnose infection also are provided. A very simple algorithm is presented that organizes information obtained from the various tests to diagnose infection, when necessary.

Barrack and Burnett's article on preoperative planning is certainly one of the best written articles on the topic. Although this is not addressed much in the literature, it is extremely important in the context of revision hip arthroplasty. The authors offer numerous helpful tips, discuss perioperative medical management, and describe how to identify and manage postoperative pain. They also discuss ways in which to rule out infection, what to look for on physical examination, and key findings on radiographs before undertaking revision hip arthroplasty. The article also is well illustrated with educational examples.

The importance of obtaining the implant labels from the hospital where the initial operation was performed is emphasized, and the authors illustrate how this information can be helpful in obtaining the necessary tools to perform a safe reconstruction. Some of the special techniques required to remove implants are described, particularly well-fixed cementless acetabular implants, which are not covered elsewhere in this volume. Preoperative templating also is described in a step-by-step manner.

Andrew Glassman provides an excellent, practical review of how to remove well-fixed cementless femoral components. The article is extremely well illustrated and very easy to follow. I believe that it should be recommended reading to anyone who is about to remove an implant, particularly surgeons who do not perform the procedure regularly. If the steps outlined by Dr. Glassman are followed in detail, implants will be removed with very little damage to the existing bone stock. The article also describes how to diagnose a loose stem and details the instrumentation required to remove well-fixed stems. Various surgical approaches, including the trochanteric slide and the extended trochanteric osteotomy, are described as are techniques and the different instruments required to remove implants, including proximally and distally fixed stems.

The article by Sporer and associates describes ways in which to determine whether an implant is loose or stable. The authors also describe the concept of inherent stability as it relates to revising the acetabular component, a topic of great importance to the practicing surgeon. Briefly, if a trial component is fully stable when gentle force is applied to the superior rim, then reconstruction with a standard cementless acetabular implant is appropriate. However, if the trial implant is not in the inheritably stable as described above,

then additional techniques to achieve inherent stability are required. These techniques are described in the article.

The authors comment on both the AAOS and Paprosky classification systems of bone loss in an effort to help the reader better understand the various principles. All necessary techniques for reconstruction of these defects are described, including newer techniques such as trabecular metal cups, with or without augmentation. The appropriate use of reconstruction cages in patients with severe bone loss also is described, as is the management of patients with pelvic discontinuity. The use of allografts for reconstruction is significantly emphasized, specifically distal femoral structural allografts. The techniques are well described and easy to follow, and the authors summarize outcomes of these operations.

The article by Gross and associates focuses principally on the use of allografts for reconstruction of femoral and acetabular defects. In this article, the authors classify bone stock defects on both femoral and acetabular sides and then discuss the classification system in the context of the use of allografts. The indications, risks, techniques, and results of reconstruction with allografts are clearly described. The risks of nonunion and resorption, as well as other risks of the operation, are discussed as

well. These are high-risk operations, and the results are not as good as those of other revision procedures. Nevertheless, they remain important techniques for the salvage of failed hip replacements with severe bone loss. When using proximal femoral allograft-prosthetic composites, the authors stress that the femur should be retained as a vascularized sleeve around the allograft femur. In addition to allografts on the femoral side, the authors discuss the use of massive allografts in the reconstruction of acetabular bone loss. They stress the importance of using a reconstruction cage to neutralize the allograft and reduce the stress transferred directly to the allograft.

The articles in this section address the entire gamut of revision total hip arthroplasty, beginning with indications, diagnosing ongoing pain and ruling out infection, preoperative planning, implant removal, and managing bone deficiency. The authors have done a fantastic job describing the topics in a very understandable manner. Put together, these articles should be required reading for any surgeon attempting revision total hip arthroplasty.

Bassam A. Masri, MD, FRCSC
Professor and Chairman
Department of Orthopaedics
University of British Columbia
Vancouver, British Columbia,
   Canada

Evaluation of Patients With Pain Following Total Hip Replacement

Patrick Duffy, MBBCh, FRCS(Orth)
Bassam A. Masri, MD, FRCSC
Donald Garbuz, MD, FRCSC
Clive P. Duncan, MD, FRCSC

Abstract

Ongoing pain after total hip replacement is a source of frustration to both the patient and the surgeon. A structured approach to the evaluation of patients with postoperative pain is essential. The key to such an approach is a meticulous patient history and physical examination. The results of relevant investigations allow an effective treatment plan to be quickly implemented.

The number of total hip replacements performed worldwide continues to rise annually, and total hip replacement is undoubtedly one of the most successful orthopaedic procedures of the last 40 years. Annually, more than 168,000 primary and 30,000 revision total hip replacements are performed in the United States.[1]

Patient satisfaction is generally high following this procedure, which provides excellent pain relief and an increased level of function.[2,3] Unfortunately, some patients have persistent or new pain and some have disability after surgery; these complications remain a challenge.[4] This chapter is a guide to the evaluation of these patients.

The evaluation should be structured in such a way that relevant and timely investigations are undertaken to allow an effective treatment plan to be implemented. Because the patient's expectations play a major part in the perceived success of the hip replacement,[5] it is important for the surgeon to address those expectations before surgery to ensure that they are realistic and to reinforce awareness of the more common complications. Comorbidities, particularly those affecting other joints, have a marked effect on the results of total hip replacement. Also, problems with the cardiovascular and respiratory systems may impair function and confound the results of total hip replacement.

Britton and associates[4] recommended using the presence or absence of pain as an indicator of the success of total hip replacement.

However, pain following total hip replacement is difficult to assess because it is subjective and is often underweighted on commonly used hip scoring systems.[3,6] The Pain and Function of the Hip Scale,[3] developed on the basis of the recommendation of the Société Internationale de Chirurgie Orthopédique et de Traumatologie, represents an attempt to overcome these limitations by more careful weighting and measurement of pain.

History

The cornerstone of diagnosis is an in-depth history combined with a thorough physical examination. The history should enable the clinician to narrow the differential diagnosis, allowing subsequent cost-effective and focused investigations. The most important feature is determining the nature of the patient's pain—that is, the temporal onset, severity, site, character, and duration. If the patient was never pain free after the operation, the initial diagnosis might have been incorrect and other local disorders or referred pain might have been the cause of the symptoms. Alternately, this may indicate that initial implant stability was never achieved or that infection is the cause of the ongoing pain. A pain-free interval after the operation is more suggestive of an implant-related cause of the pain, such as loosening, late-onset infection, or osteolysis.

The site of the pain may be indicative of the underlying diagnosis. Pain localized to the trochanteric region suggests bursitis, irritation secondary to underlying sutures or wires, osteolysis, or a fracture.[7,8] Pain felt in the buttock or groin suggests vascular[9] or neurogenic claudication, acetabular loosening, or osteolysis. Less frequently, it may indicate iliopsoas impingement or tendinitis secondary to acetabular retroversion; hematoma; an inguinal, femoral, or obturator hernia; or one of a variety of gynecologic or genitourinary causes.[10-13] Pain from nerve root involvement is also commonly felt in the buttock but tends to radiate distal to the knee. A patient who has iliopsoas tendinitis often will describe discomfort when getting in and out of an automobile or a chair, a maneuver that requires active flexion and rotation of the hip.

Thigh pain may be secondary to a loose femoral implant[14] or a mismatch in the modulus of elasticity between the host femur and the stiff femoral stem, although the literature is inconclusive regarding the prevalence of the latter condition.[14-16] It is, however, well recognized that some patients with a well-fixed cemented or cementless stem still experience some thigh pain.

Pain felt at rest or during the night should raise the suspicion of underlying infection or a malignant tumor. In particular, persistent low-level pain following a hip replacement is consistent with an occult infection.[12] Activity-related pain that is relieved by rest suggests loosening, subtle fracture, or vascular or neurogenic claudication. So-called start-up pain, which subsides after the first few steps, has been associated with early loosening and micromotion of either component but may be secondary to modulus mismatch, spondyloarthrosis, or iliopsoas tendinitis.[17]

Any precipitating causes should also be sought. If the pain started after a recent fall, traumatic loosening and fracture need to be excluded as causes. A history of persistent wound drainage, hematoma, or a prolonged course of antibiotics following surgery should increase the index of suspicion for infection as a cause of the pain. Other factors that increase the index of suspicion for infection include systemic illness; a recent dental, gastrointestinal, or genitourinary procedure; immunosuppression; obesity; and inflammatory arthritis.[18]

Finally, symptoms such as weight loss, general malaise, and loss of appetite should prompt a detailed systemic inquiry to ensure that an underlying generalized infectious or malignant condition is not overlooked.

Physical Examination

A comprehensive musculoskeletal examination should be undertaken. This examination should include determination of potential sources of referred pain as well as local examination of the hip joint. The spine, contralateral hip, and both knees should be examined. Gait should be carefully observed to look for antalgic gait, limb-length discrepancy, or abductor deficiency. The onset of limb-length inequality should be related to the time of the operation, as progressive shortening and muscle weakness may indicate subsidence of one of the components.[19]

Inspection of the skin and the surgical scar will reveal inflammation, drainage, or healed sinus tracks. Tenderness on palpation may indicate a neuroma, an actual or impending fracture, an area of osteolysis, or a metastatic deposit. Palpation may also reveal any hernias or defects in the deep fascia.

Pain at the extremes of the range of motion is suggestive of loosening of one or both components or, if it is reproducible in one particular position, of instability or impingement.[17] Pain with any motion is more suggestive of infection.[20] Radicular pain from sciatic nerve entrapment is usually exacerbated by passive straight-leg raising, whereas iliopsoas irritation tends to be painful with resisted flexion.[10]

A neurovascular examination of both lower limbs is mandatory, and abdominal, pelvic, and rectal examinations should be done when indicated to rule out causes of referred pain.

Differential Diagnosis

The differential diagnosis of hip pain can be divided into extrinsic and intrinsic causes, as listed in Table 1.

Extrinsic Causes

The most common confounding factor in an assessment of hip pain is low back disease. Spinal stenosis and nerve root irritation can cause discomfort in the buttock, thigh, and sometimes the groin. It is not unusual for there to be interplay of spondylogenic and coxogenic causes of pain in the same patient. Spondylogenic symptoms can sometimes be "unmasked" by a hip operation because of the resolution of the hip-related causes and an increase in the patient's activity level, which worsens the back-related symptoms.[21] In such cases, an intra-articular injection of a local anesthetic into the hip can be helpful. The local anesthetic usually eliminates pain that is related to the hip joint and allows distinction between hip-related and other symptoms.

Neurologic complications occur following less than 1% of primary total hip replacements.[22] They can be caused by a direct injury from a surgical instrument, a hematoma, cement, or scar entrapment, or they can be caused indirectly, usually by limb lengthening. They generally occur in the immediate or early postoperative period. Causalgic pain may be related to such injuries. In particular, with the increasing popularity of anterior approaches to the hip, there will be an increasing prevalence of injuries to the lateral cutaneous nerve of the thigh, which may be associated with lateral thigh pain.

Vascular insufficiency commonly causes buttock or thigh pain. Herald and associates[9] described a case of stenosis of both the superior and the inferior gluteal artery in a patient who presented with groin pain, which then resolved after angioplasty. Vascular complications following primary total hip replacement are infrequent, but injury to the femoral artery can result in a painful false aneurysm.

A malignant primary bone tumor and, much more commonly, metastasis around the pelvis and proximal part of the femur can cause symptoms suggestive of pain associated with a total hip replacement. A high index of suspicion is necessary to avoid missing these malignant conditions as they may not be obvious on plain radiographs; lucent le-

Table 1
Differential Diagnosis of Pain Following Hip Replacement

Intrinsic Causes	Extrinsic Causes
Infection: acute, delayed, late hematogenous	Lumbar spine disease: stenosis, disk herniation, spondylolysis/spondylolisthesis
Aseptic loosening	Malignant tumor: primary, secondary
Pain at stem tip (modulus mismatch)	Peripheral vascular disease
Greater trochanter nonunion	Metabolic disease
Wear debris synovitis	Stress and insufficiency fracture
Periprosthetic fracture Trochanteric fixation bursitis Osteolysis Occult instability	Nerve injury: sciatic, femoral, lateral cutaneous
	Iliopsoas tendinitis
	Hernia: femoral, inguinal, obturator
	Complex regional pain syndrome
	Other gastrointestinal, genitourinary, or gynecologic disease

sions may be obscured by orthopaedic implants. Supplementary tests, such as measurement of the prostate-specific antigen level and serum protein electrophoresis, and imaging, such as chest radiography or mammography, should be readily used when indicated.

Metabolic bone disorders such as Paget disease are generally apparent on preoperative radiographs. This condition often results in secondary osteoarthritis and, during its active phase, it also causes symptoms on its own, which may persist after a total hip arthroplasty. If a hip replacement is to be performed during the active phase of Paget disease, medical management should be instituted preoperatively both to decrease the symptoms caused by metabolic disease and to reduce the risk of intraoperative bleeding.

Intrinsic Causes
The reported rate of deep infection after total hip arthroplasty is less than 1%.[23] When infection does develop, it is a major complication. Be-

fore the patient has a revision hip replacement, the infection must be eradicated to prevent reinfection at the site of the new implant.

Aseptic loosening of both cemented and cementless implants remains a major cause of pain following total hip replacement. Radiographs may show characteristic features such as progressive lucent lines, migration, and cement fracture, but often changes are subtle or even absent.

The etiology of thigh pain can be multifactorial. It can be caused by a mismatch in the modulus of elasticity between a stiff, large-diameter cementless femoral implant and the surrounding, less stiff host bone.[15] Use of this type of implant is usually necessary only for a revision surgery. Thigh pain can also occur because stability of the implant was not achieved initially, with resultant motion at the stem tip.[24] Micromotion of radiographically stable implants is thought to be a potential source of pain, particularly when the implant has only fibrous ingrowth.[25] Occasionally, thigh pain can arise secondary to a vastus muscle hernia through a defect in the fascia lata; such a hernia can generally be palpated as a tender soft-tissue mass when the muscle is tensed.[26]

Periprosthetic fractures may occur intraoperatively or postoperatively. An intraoperative fracture is usually obvious but occasionally may go unrecognized initially and cause pain in the immediate postoperative period. A postoperative fracture may result from a traumatic incident or occur through an area of osteolysis with little or no warning. Osteolysis alone is rarely painful until there is an impending or actual fracture.

Stress fractures can develop at sites of cortical perforation (usually in revision arthroplasty) and also in the pubic ramus secondary to a combination of disuse osteopenia and increased patient activity after the total hip arthroplasty.[27,28] The fractures at the latter site may not be seen on radiographs until fracture callus has formed.

Instability can result in pain from capsular stretch and from soft-tissue impingement. The symptoms can usually be reproduced by placing the limb in a certain position and usually recur each time that position is recreated.

Soft tissues can occasionally become irritated by the prosthesis. This situation can occur where wires have been used to reattach the greater trochanter or an extended trochanteric osteotomy fragment. The psoas tendon may also become irritated by the prominent anterior flange of an insufficiently anteverted acetabular component[10,29] or by extruded cement in a patient with a cemented component.

There is controversy regarding whether trochanteric nonunion causes pain. Pritchett[7] reported on a series of 30 patients who had a fracture of the greater trochanter following a total hip arthroplasty. He found that, even when the fracture was markedly displaced, the symptoms usually eventually decreased and that surgical intervention did not reliably alleviate symptoms.

Imaging Studies
Plain Radiographs
A plain AP radiograph of the pelvis, AP and lateral radiographs of the hip, and AP and lateral radiographs of the femur should be made for all patients with symptoms following a hip replacement. They should be compared with serial radiographs made since the time of the surgery, because radiographic signs are often subtle and progress slowly.

There are radiographic criteria for predicting loosening of both cemented and cementless implants. O'Neill and Harris[30] defined the criteria for definite loosening of a cemented implant as migration or fracture of the stem or cement mantle or as a continuous radiolucent line that is, in part, 2 mm. It should be noted that these criteria have been found to be more accurate for the femoral component than the acetabular component. Other authors have questioned the usefulness of identifying radiolucent lines at the bone-cement interface. A study of specimens retrieved at autopsy indicated that these lines represent internal bone remodeling rather than a deterioration of the bone-cement interface.[31] It is generally agreed, however, that a radiolucent line at the prosthesis-cement interface represents debonding of the implant, which may indicate loosening if the implant is designed to bond to the cement mantle.

The stability of cementless implants is assessed according to different criteria. Engh and associates[14] defined major and minor criteria for predicting osseointegration of cementless stems: major signs are an absence of reactive lines and endosteal "spot welds" around the porous-coated part of the prosthesis. Minor signs of osseointegration are calcar atrophy, the absence of bead-shedding, and the absence of a pedestal, indicating a stable distal part of the stem. The presence of a pedestal does not necessarily indicate instability, provided that it is not associated with radiolucent lines. Reactive lines adjacent to the porous surface, bead-shedding, and an unstable distal part of the stem with a pedestal separated by a lucent line are minor signs of instability of the femoral stem. The only major (and only reliable) sign indicating acetabular instability is migration of the component.

Differentiation between septic and aseptic loosening on plain radiographs is difficult. However, certain features such as endosteal scalloping, generalized osteolysis, osteopenia, and periosteal new bone formation are more indicative of infection, especially if they are rapidly progressive.

Plain radiographs should also be scrutinized for marked wear of the polyethylene liner, which can highlight the need to look for associated osteolytic lesions. These lesions are often clinically silent but can become symptomatic in severe cases in which there is a risk of an impending pathologic fracture.

Fluoroscopy
An image intensifier can occasionally be useful when impingement and subluxation are suspected. The hip can be moved through a range of motion until the symptoms are re-

produced and the likely cause of the instability is identified.

Arthrography

This technique is rarely used currently, except in the context of joint aspiration. This lack of use is partly due to a lack of conformity in the performance of the technique and in the interpretation of the results. O'Neill and Harris indicated that arthrography was better than plain radiography for the detection of loose acetabular components;[30] however, Murray and Rodrigo[32] found that 7 of 12 components that had been identified as loose with arthrography were later shown to be firmly fixed at the time of surgery. It appears that arthrography generally leads to an overestimation of acetabular loosening and an underestimation of femoral loosening.[33]

Nuclear Imaging

A range of radioisotopes and a variety of techniques are now available to image the painful hip. Nonspecific tracers include technetium-99 methylene diphosphonate, gallium-67 citrate, technetium-99 nanocolloid, and nonspecific immunoglobulin-G (IgG). Technetium-99 methylene diphosphonate is bound to the hydroxyapatite crystal and is therefore taken up preferentially in areas of increased bone turnover (Figure 1). It is highly sensitive but not specific, as increased uptake is seen in various conditions, including infection, loosening, heterotopic bone formation, stress fracture, modulus mismatch, reflex sympathetic dystrophy, tumor, and metabolic bone disease. In addition, increased uptake of technetium-99 methylene diphosphonate can be seen up to 24 months after implantation in a patient with an asymptomatic hip replacement,[34] which

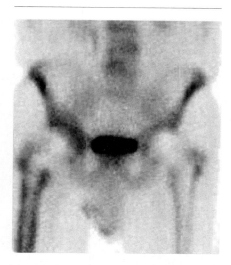

Figure 1 Technetium-99 methylene diphosphonate-labeled scan showing increased uptake around a cemented femoral implant.

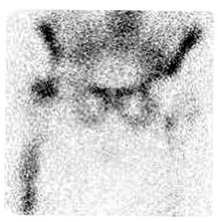

Figure 2 Indium-labeled white blood cell scan showing increased uptake around the same implant as shown in Figure 1.

limits the usefulness of the technique in the early postoperative period. The technetium-99 methylene diphosphonate scan is most useful when it reveals normal findings, which allows elimination of many of the potential component-related causes of pain at the site of a hip replacement. When the technetium-99 methylene diphosphonate scan is positive, a gallium-67 citrate scan can help in the evaluation.

Gallium-67 citrate is preferentially taken up in areas of infection and inflammation, and it has been reported to increase specificity when it is used in conjunction with a technetium-99 methylene diphosphonate scan; however, the sensitivity of the combined technique is poor,[35] which limits its usefulness. Piriou and associates[36] found that this combined scanning method was helpful in determining the appropriate interval between staged reconstructions in a patient with an infection at the site of an arthroplasty. When the second stage was delayed until the findings on the gallium

scan reverted to baseline, the infection did not recur.

The introduction of labeled leukocyte scans such as indium-111 and technetium-99m hexamethylpropylene amine oxime scans (Figure 2) has attracted a large amount of interest in the hope that they can overcome the limitation of gallium and technetium-99 methylene diphosphonate scans. In theory, labeled leukocyte tracers should not accumulate at sites of increased bone turnover in the absence of infection. When a dual-tracer technique is used—such as when a labeled leukocyte scan is performed simultaneously with a technetium-99 methylene diphosphonate scan—sensitivity (88% compared with 57%) and specificity (95% compared with 89%) are generally better than those associated with a combination of technetium-99 methylene diphosphonate and gallium scans,[37] although the reported results have varied.[38] It should also be noted that cementless implants tend to cause false-positive results.

Combined indium and bone marrow scintigraphy was developed

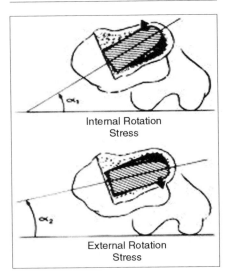

Figure 3 CT evaluation of the rotational stability of a femoral prosthesis. The test is positive for loosening if there is any difference between α_1 and α_2 beyond 2° of rotation. (Reproduced with permission from Berger R, Fletcher F, Donaldson T, Wasielewski R, Peterson M, Rubash H: Dynamic test to diagnose loose cementless femoral total hip components. *Clin Orthop Relat Res* 1996;330:118.)

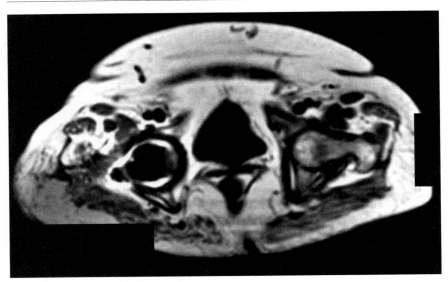

Figure 4 Magnetic resonance arthrogram showing the acetabular component and the femoral head of a right total hip replacement.

on the basis of the fact that both sulfur colloid and white blood cell tracers accumulate in normal bone marrow but sulfur colloid does not accumulate in the presence of infection, leaving only the white blood cell tracers. The diagnosis of infection is based, therefore, on the relative difference in the uptake of the two tracers. The reported accuracy of this technique ranges from 89% to 98%.[38]

More recent developments include the use of indium-labeled polyclonal IgG, which behaves in much the same way as the combination of indium and white blood cell tracers and has many of the same inherent drawbacks.[39] Other agents, including labeled monoclonal antibodies and chemotactic peptides, are under development but are not yet licensed for use in North America.

Ultrasound

Ultrasound has several uses in investigations of the painful hip. It can be used to image soft tissues around the joint, such as the psoas tendon, when impingement is suspected[40] as well as to guide aspiration of the joint.[41] Tunney and associates[42] used ultrasound to disrupt the bacterial biofilm before culture. They found that when an explanted prosthesis had been subjected to ultrasonification in a bath of lactated Ringer's solution, bacterial aggregates were observed in cultures of material dislodged from the prosthesis. In contrast, if the prosthesis had been just soaked in the lactated Ringer's solution, no bacteria were seen. This enhanced yield after ultrasonification was confirmed by Nguyen and associates;[43] however, the clinical relevance of these findings remains unclear.

Computed Tomography

This technique has been used to identify the inflammatory lesion in patients with iliopsoas impinge-

ment.[40] It has also been used to assess potential loosening of femoral implants before changes are visible on plain radiographs. Axial cuts are made through the implant and the surrounding femur in full internal and then full external rotation, and any difference in the relative position of the implant and the osseous femur beyond 2° of rotation is said to indicate loosening[44] (Figure 3).

Magnetic Resonance Imaging

Multiplanar MRI of a painful hip following total hip replacement has several theoretical benefits (Figure 4). It allows evaluation of the soft-tissue envelope, including the neurovascular structures, particularly where there is concern about entrapment by heterotopic bone or extravasated cement. The abductor muscle attachment can be visualized and osteolytic defects around the femoral implant can be quantified to some degree. Artifact generated by ferrous components is a problem with the technique, necessitating altered pulse sequences, and visualization of periacetabular structures is generally suboptimal.[45,46]

Laboratory Tests

Baseline blood work including a complete blood cell count, measurement of the erythrocyte sedimentation rate, and measurement of the C-reactive protein level should be performed for all patients being evaluated for pain after total hip arthroplasty. Although these tests do not yield a definite diagnosis of infection, they allow patients with a high likelihood of infection to be selected to undergo aspiration of the hip in an attempt to isolate an infecting organism.

The leukocyte count is of little use for diagnosing infection at the site of a total hip replacement. Canner and associates[18] found that only 15% of 52 patients with a confirmed infection following a total hip replacement had an elevated leukocyte count. This finding was confirmed by Spangehl and associates,[47] who reported that an elevated leukocyte count had a sensitivity of only 20% for predicting infection. At best, the complete blood cell count is useful only as a baseline hemoglobin count in patients who potentially may require surgical intervention in the future.

The erythrocyte sedimentation rate and C-reactive protein level are nonspecific but highly sensitive markers of inflammation. Forster and Crawford[48] found that, in the absence of other inflammatory processes, the erythrocyte sedimentation rate falls to less than 20 mm/h within 6 months following an uncomplicated total hip arthroplasty. They also documented a similar value for most patients with aseptic loosening of the prosthesis. Moreover, patients with known infection had a substantially higher erythro-

cyte sedimentation rate (mean, 60 mm/h) than those with either a well-fixed or a loose prosthesis and no infection.

The C-reactive protein level may be a more reliable indicator of infection in that it returns to normal more rapidly after total hip arthroplasty. Aalto and associates[49] noted that levels consistently returned to normal within 3 weeks after a successful hip replacement. Sanzen and Carlsson[50] found that measurement of both the erythrocyte sedimentation rate and the C-reactive protein level had only one false-negative result in a series of 23 patients with an infection. The combined efficacy of these two measurements was also confirmed by Spangehl and associates,[47] who found that a normal C-reactive protein level and a normal erythrocyte sedimentation rate were 100% specific for excluding infection.

Aspiration

Aspiration should not be performed routinely for all patients with pain at the site of a hip arthroplasty because the false-positive rate has proved to be unacceptably high. In a series in which aspiration was performed before 270 revision hip replacements, Barrack and Harris[51] reported that only 2 of 34 positive aspirations correctly identified an infection. This finding indicates that the procedure has poor specificity when performed routinely. In addition, all of the patients who had a true infection had clinical and radiographic evidence of it.

Aspiration has proved to be more sensitive and specific when there is radiographic or clinical evidence of infection or elevation of either the C-reactive protein level or the erythrocyte sedimentation rate. Spangehl and associates[47] found that

when the erythrocyte sedimentation rate and C-reactive protein level were both elevated, the probability that a positive aspirate would confirm an infection was 89%. Furthermore, they recommended that in the event of a "dry tap" during an attempted aspiration, nonbacteriostatic saline solution should be injected and the joint should be aspirated. In addition, they recommended that three biopsy specimens be taken from the capsule. All of these aspirates and biopsy specimens should be cultured in broth and solid media, with infection defined as growth in any sample including those in subculture. A potential drawback of this approach is that the broth culture is susceptible to contaminants. One advantage of aspiration is that it can be combined with injection of a local anesthetic to determine whether the hip pain is related to the hip replacement or to another source. This is particularly helpful when hip and lumbar spine disease coexist. Braunstein and associates[52] reported that 10 of 11 patients who had relief of hip pain following intra-articular injection were later confirmed to have an intrinsic cause of the pain.

Molecular Biology

Bacterial identification by polymerase chain reaction analysis has been reported to have better specificity and sensitivity than standard culture methods.[42,53] The technique involves the identification and amplification of the bacterial ribosomal RNA 16S fragment. Issues such as potential contamination can be addressed by direct immunologic detection of bacteria with use of antibodies and antiserum prepared against the bacteria implicated in the clinical infection; this allows comparison with potential contaminants.

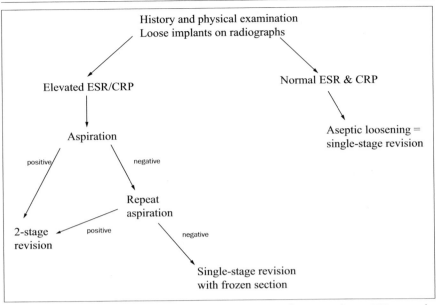

Figure 5 Algorithm for evaluation of radiographically loose implants. ESR = erythrocyte sedimentation rate, and CRP = C-reactive protein level.

In a series of 120 patients treated with revision total hip arthroplasty, Tunney and associates[42] reported that 26 periprosthetic infections were identified with standard culture methods, whereas polymerase chain reaction identified an additional 59 possible infections for which cultures were negative. It is unclear whether those were true infections or whether the positive results were related to contaminants. A drawback of this technique is that it does not allow identification of the bacteria or allow differentiation between live and dead bacteria. It is safe to say that, at present, polymerase chain reaction has no role in the routine investigation of pain associated with a hip replacement.

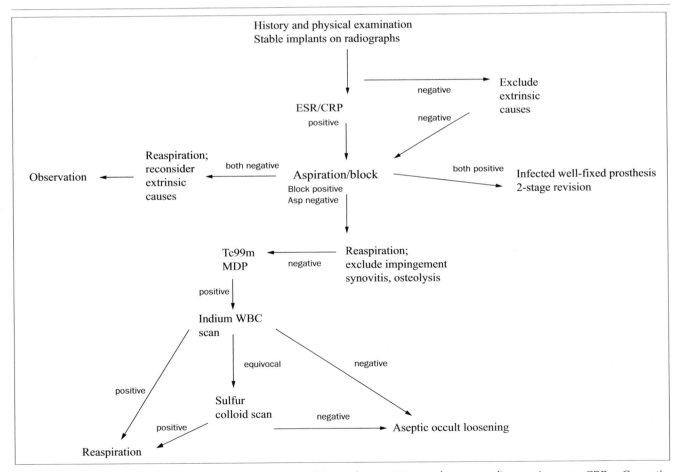

Figure 6 Algorithm for evaluation of radiographically stable implants. ESR = erythrocyte sedimentation rate, CRP = C-reactive protein level, WBC = white blood cell count, and Tc99m MDP = technetium-99 methylene diphosphonate scan.

Summary

The importance of a thorough history and physical examination cannot be overemphasized in the setting of pain following a total hip replacement. They allow focused and cost-effective investigations, minimizing the time needed for workup and increasing the diagnostic yield. It is critical that the surgeon have a high index of suspicion for both referred sources of pain and occult infection when examining these patients. If, despite a systematic workup (Figures 5 and 6), no obvious cause for the pain is found, then a period of observation is probably indicated. Exploratory operations have little if any role for these patients.

References

1. Hall MJ, Owings MF: *2000 National Hospital Discharge Survey.* Hyattsville, MD, US Department of Health and Human Services, Centers for Disease Control and Prevention, National Center for Health Statistics, 2002.

2. Visuri T, Koskenvuo M, Honkanen R: The influence of total hip replacement on hip pain and the use of analgesics. *Pain* 1985;23:19-26.

3. Alonso J, Lamarca R, Marti-Valls J: The pain and function of the hip (PFH) scale: A patient-based instrument for measuring outcome after total hip replacement. *Orthopedics* 2000;23:1273-1278.

4. Britton AR, Murray DW, Bulstrode CJ, McPherson K, Denham RA: Pain levels after total hip replacement: Their use as endpoints for survival analysis. *J Bone Joint Surg Br* 1997;79:93-98.

5. Mancuso CA, Salvati EA, Johanson NA, Peterson MG, Charlson ME: Patients' expectations and satisfaction with total hip arthroplasty. *J Arthroplasty* 1997;12:387-396.

6. Ritter MA, Fechtman RW, Keating EM, Faris PM: The use of a hip score for evaluation of the results of total hip arthroplasty. *J Arthroplasty* 1990;5:187-189.

7. Pritchett JW: Fracture of the greater trochanter after hip replacement. *Clin Orthop Relat Res* 2001;390:221-226.

8. Heekin RD, Engh CA, Herzwurm PJ: Fractures through cystic lesions of the greater trochanter: A cause of late pain after cementless total hip arthroplasty. *J Arthroplasty* 1996;11:757-760.

9. Herald J, Macdessi S, Kirsh G: An unusual cause of groin pain following hip replacement: A case report. *J Bone Joint Surg Am* 2001;83:1392-1395.

10. Jasani V, Richards P, Wynn-Jones C: Pain related to the psoas muscle after total hip replacement. *J Bone Joint Surg Br* 2002;84:991-993.

11. Ankarath S, Campbell P: Psoas hematoma presenting as hip pain. *Orthopedics* 2001;24:689-690.

12. Smith PN, Rorabeck CH: Clinical evaluation of the symptomatic total hip arthroplasty, in Steinberg ME, Garino JP (eds): *Revision Total Hip Arthroplasty.* Philadelphia, PA, Lippincott Williams & Wilkins, 1999, pp 109-120.

13. Gaunt ME, Tan SG, Dias J: Strangulated obturator hernia masquerading as pain from a total hip replacement. *J Bone Joint Surg Br* 1992;74:782-783.

14. Engh CA, Massin P, Suthers KE: Roentgenographic assessment of the biologic fixation of porous-surfaced femoral components. *Clin Orthop Relat Res* 1990;257:107-128.

15. Brown TE, Larson B, Shen F, Moskal JT: Thigh pain after cementless total hip arthroplasty: Evaluation and management. *J Am Acad Orthop Surg* 2002;10:385-392.

16. McAuley JP, Culpepper WJ, Engh CA: Total hip arthroplasty: Concerns with extensively porous coated femoral components. *Clin Orthop Relat Res* 1998;355:182-188.

17. White RE Jr: Evaluation of the painful total hip arthroplasty, in Callaghan JJ, Rosenberg AG, Rubash HE (eds): *The Adult Hip.* Philadelphia, PA, Lippincott-Raven, 1998, pp 1377-1385.

18. Canner GC, Steinberg ME, Heppenstall RB, Balderston R: The infected hip after total hip arthroplasty. *J Bone Joint Surg Am* 1984;66:1393-1399.

19. Cuckler JM, Star AM, Alavi A, Noto RB: Diagnosis and management of the infected total joint arthroplasty. *Orthop Clin North Am* 1991;22:523-530.

20. Bozic KJ, Rubash HE: The painful total hip replacement. *Clin Orthop Relat Res* 2004;420:18-25.

21. Bohl WR, Steffee AD: Lumbar spinal stenosis: A cause of continued pain and disability in patients after total hip arthroplasty. *Spine* 1979;4:168-173.

22. Johanson NA, Pellicci PM, Tsairis P, Salvati EA: Nerve injury in total hip arthroplasty. *Clin Orthop Relat Res* 1983;179:214-222.

23. Phillips CB, Barrett JA, Losina E, et al: Incidence rates of dislocation, pulmonary embolism, and deep infection during the first six months after elective total hip replacement. *J Bone Joint Surg Am* 2003;85-A:20-26.

24. Whiteside LA: The effect of stem fit on bone hypertrophy and pain relief in cementless total hip arthroplasty. *Clin Orthop Relat Res* 1989;247:138-147.

25. Engh CA Sr, Culpepper WJ II: Femoral fixation in primary total hip arthroplasty. *Orthopedics* 1997;20:771-773.

26. Higgs JE, Chong A, Haertsch P, Sekel R, Leicester A: An unusual cause of thigh pain after total hip arthroplasty. *J Arthroplasty* 1995;10:203-204.

27. Christiansen CG, Kassim RA, Callaghan JJ, Marsh JL, Schmidt AH: Pubic ramus insufficiency fractures following total hip arthroplasty: A report of six cases. *J Bone Joint Surg Am* 2003;85-A:1819-1822.

28. Courpied JP, Watin-Augouard L, Postel M: Femoral fractures in subjects with total prostheses of the hip or knee. *Int Orthop* 1987;11:109-115.

29. Ala Eddine T, Remy F, Chantelot C, Giraud F, Migaud H, Duquennoy A: Anterior iliopsoas impingement after total hip arthroplasty: Diagnosis and conservative treatment in 9 cases. *Rev Chir Orthop Reparatrice Appar Mot* 2001;87:815-819.

30. O'Neill DA, Harris WH: Failed total hip replacement: Assessment by plain radiographs, arthrograms, and aspiration of the hip joint. *J Bone Joint Surg Am* 1984;66:540-546.

31. Jasty M, Maloney WJ, Bragdon CR, Haire T, Harris WH: Histomorphological studies of the long-term skeletal responses to well fixed cemented femoral components. *J Bone Joint Surg Am* 1990;72:1220-1229.

32. Murray WR, Rodrigo JJ: Arthrography for the assessment of pain after total hip replacement: A comparison of arthrographic findings in patients with and without pain. *J Bone Joint Surg Am* 1975;57:1060-1065.

33. Robbins GM, Masri BA, Garbuz DS, Duncan CP: Evaluation of pain in patients with apparently solidly fixed total hip arthroplasty components. *J Am Acad Orthop Surg* 2002;10:86-94.

34. Oswald SG, Van Nostrand D, Savory CG, Callaghan JJ: Three-phase bone scan

and indium white blood cell scintigraphy following porous coated hip arthroplasty: A prospective study of the prosthetic tip. *J Nucl Med* 1989;30:1321-1331.

35. Kraemer WJ, Saplys R, Waddell JP, Morton J: Bone scan, gallium scan, and hip aspiration in the diagnosis of infected total hip arthroplasty. *J Arthroplasty* 1993;8:611-616.

36. Piriou P, de Loynes B, Garreau de Loubresse C, Judet T: Use of combined gallium-technetium scintigraphy to determine the interval before second-stage prosthetic reimplantation in hip arthroplasty infection: A consecutive series of 30 cases. *Rev Chir Orthop Reparatrice Appar Mot* 2003;89:287-296.

37. Tehranzadeh J, Gubernick I, Blaha D: Prospective study of sequential technetium-99m phosphate and gallium imaging in painful hip prostheses: Comparison of diagnostic modalities. *Clin Nucl Med* 1988;13:229-236.

38. Palestro CJ, Torres MA: Radionuclide imaging in orthopedic infections. *Semin Nucl Med* 1997;27:334-345.

39. de Lima Ramos PA, Martin-Comin J, Bajen MT, et al: Simultaneous administration of 99Tcm-HMPAO-labelled autologous leukocytes and 111In-labelled non-specific polyclonal human immunoglobulin G in bone and joint infections. *Nucl Med Commun* 1996;17:749-757.

40. Rezig R, Copercini M, Montet X, Martinoli C, Bianchi S: Ultrasound diagnosis of anterior iliopsoas impingement in total hip replacement. *Skeletal Radiol* 2004;33:112-116.

41. Eisler T, Svensson O, Engstrom CF, et al: Ultrasound for diagnosis of infection in revision total hip arthroplasty. *J Arthroplasty* 2001;16:1010-1017.

42. Tunney MM, Patrick S, Curran MD: Ramage: Detection of prosthetic hip infection at revision arthroplasty by immunofluorescence microscopy and PCR amplification of the bacterial 16S rRNA gene. *J Clin Microbiol* 1999;37:3281-3290.

43. Nguyen LL, Nelson CL, Saccente M, Smeltzer MS, Wassell DL, McLaren SG: Detecting bacterial colonization of implanted orthopaedic devices by ultrasonication. *Clin Orthop Relat Res* 2002;403:29-37.

44. Berger R, Fletcher F, Donaldson T, Wasielewski R, Peterson M, Rubash H: Dynamic test to diagnose loose uncemented femoral total hip components. *Clin Orthop Relat Res* 1996;330:115-123.

45. Sofka CM, Potter HG: MR imaging of joint arthroplasty. *Semin Musculoskelet Radiol* 2002;6:79-85.

46. White LM, Kim JK, Mehta M, et al: Complications of total hip arthroplasty: MR imaging- initial experience. *Radiology* 2000;215:254-262.

47. Spangehl MJ, Masri BA, O'Connell JX, Duncan CP: Prospective analysis of preoperative and intraoperative investigations for the diagnosis of infection at the sites of two hundred and two revision total hip arthroplasties. *J Bone Joint Surg Am* 1999;81:672-683.

48. Forster IW, Crawford R: Sedimentation rate in infected and uninfected total hip arthroplasty. *Clin Orthop Relat Res* 1982;168:48-52.

49. Aalto K, Osterman K, Peltola H, Rasanen J: Changes in erythrocyte sedimentation rate and C-reactive protein after total hip arthroplasty. *Clin Orthop Relat Res* 1984;184:118-120.

50. Sanzen L, Carlsson AS: The diagnostic value of C-reactive protein in infected total hip arthroplasties. *J Bone Joint Surg Br* 1989;71:638-641.

51. Barrack RL, Harris WH: The value of aspiration of the hip joint before revision total hip arthroplasty. *J Bone Joint Surg Am* 1993;75:66-76.

52. Braunstein EM, Cardinal E, Buckwalter KA, Capello W: Bupivicaine arthrography of the post-arthroplasty hip. *Skeletal Radiol* 1995;24:519-521.

53. Mariani BD, Martin DS, Levine MJ, Booth RE Jr, Tuan RS: Polymerase chain reaction detection of bacterial infection in total knee arthroplasty. *Clin Orthop Relat Res* 1996;331:11-22.

Preoperative Planning for Revision Total Hip Arthroplasty

Robert L. Barrack, MD
R. Stephen J. Burnett, MD, FRCSC

Abstract

Revision total hip arthroplasty is associated with more perioperative complications and unexpected findings than are encountered during primary total hip arthroplasty. Special instruments, implants, bone grafts, and other accessories may be required to treat complex problems that arise during revision surgery. Preoperative planning is important to anticipate potential complications and to ensure that all possible needed materials are readily available during surgery. Patients and their families also should be counseled on the specific additional risk factors involved in this complex surgery. An organized approach to revision total hip arthroplasty helps to reduce surgical time, minimize risks, decrease the stress level of the entire surgical team, and to increase the rate of successful outcomes for patients.

Perioperative complications and unexpected surgical findings are much more common in revision total hip arthroplasty than they are in primary total hip arthroplasty. There are often complications during surgery that require special instruments, implants, bone grafts, or other accessories that may not be available unless the potential need for these items was anticipated. Anticipation of possible complications also is crucial so that the patient can provide informed consent. Preoperatively, patients and their families should be counseled regarding the specific additional risks associated with revision total hip arthroplasty. Preoperative planning is the first and most

important step in performing a revision total hip arthroplasty. An organized approach reduces surgical time, minimizes risks, decreases stress, and increases the success rate.

It is important to consider the entire patient rather than just the hip so that the risk of major perioperative complications can be minimized. Preoperative planning entails numerous crucial steps before the surgeon decides which instruments, implants, bone grafts, and accessories will be required. The preoperative planning includes obtaining a thorough history, a physical examination, appropriate preoperative imaging and laboratory studies, and establishing an accurate diagnosis.

Preoperative templating is recognized as an important step. It helps to ensure that any required implants will be immediately available. Templating for more than one surgical option and anticipating intraoperative technical considerations must be a part of the preoperative planning process as well.

Preoperative Diagnosis

Although total hip arthroplasty is successful in more than 90% of patients,[1] revision surgery is becoming more common. Establishing an accurate diagnosis is the first step in successful planning for revision surgery. Details of the patient's history, a review of symptoms, and physical examination help to ensure that an accurate diagnosis is formulated. A detailed history of all prior surgeries and perioperative treatments should be obtained. A history of hip surgery (following trauma, with internal fixation, or for infection) should alert the surgeon to consider the case as a revision, which often requires additional information for planning. Hospital records from previous surgeries may provide important information. Records that list implanted components are especially helpful.

Patients should be questioned regarding "red flags" in their history, including persistent postoperative drainage, multiple surgical procedures, prior thromboembolism, or the evacuation of a hematoma.

The review of systems is important. Patients treated with revision total hip arthroplasty frequently are elderly and have associated medical comorbidities that require evaluation and, occasionally, treatment and medical optimization before surgery is performed. Any potential source of future or concurrent infection must be identified during the review of systems so that it may be evaluated and treated in advance. Urologic disorders are frequently encountered in this population. Men with prostate disease and women with recurrent urinary tract infections or incontinence should be evaluated by a urologist preoperatively. Patients should have a dental examination so that any potential or ongoing dental infection can be treated. Not only is a dental infection a potential source of infection at the site of a hip arthroplasty, but there is also the potential for the perioperative complication of fractured teeth and aspiration during intubation. Patients with chronic venous stasis ulcers, absent pulses, or previous lower extremity vascular bypass surgery should be evaluated by a vascular surgeon. A history of cardiac bypass surgery, angioplasty, or stenting often requires a preoperative stress test or cardiac catheterization. When advanced cardiovascular or respiratory monitoring is indicated, coordination with an anesthesiologist (and the intensive care unit) is suggested.

The patient's preoperative ambulatory status should be evaluated. Patients who have been immobilized are particularly prone to thromboembolic events (pulmonary embolism and deep vein thrombosis), and preoperative screening for deep vein thrombosis may be prudent for such patients. If a deep vein thrombosis is present, preoperative treatment is advised. If a semiurgent procedure is necessary, such as in a patient with a periprosthetic fracture or a chronic dislocation, it is acceptable to insert an inferior vena cava filter, perform the surgery, and use anticoagulation only in the postoperative period.

Ruling out infection is an important step in the planning for every revision procedure. Most deep infections associated with a total hip arthroplasty can be diagnosed by obtaining a thorough history and performing a physical examination. Certain historic factors suggest infection, including a history of delayed wound healing, persistent drainage, a prolonged course of postoperative antibiotics, or night pain, particularly if it was relieved by antibiotics. Routine hip aspiration is not recommended; it should be used only when an infection is suspected.[2-5] If a hip aspiration is to be performed, antibiotic therapy should be discontinued for at least 4 weeks[6] before the procedure to improve the sensitivity of the test. A lack of growth on culture of preoperative aspirate and normal laboratory values do not rule out an infection. Intraoperative tissue sampling is recommended to help determine the likelihood that an infection is present. It is prudent to plan for an analysis of intraoperative frozen sections by alerting the pathology department in advance and ensuring that they are familiar with the specific requirements for frozen-tissue analysis for diagnosis of infection at the site of a total joint arthroplasty.[7]

The patient's medical history can influence the decision regarding implant selection. Patients who have had high-dose pelvic irradiation are not good candidates for porous-coated implants.[8] A cemented all-polyethylene acetabular component with or without a protrusio ring is probably a better choice in this situation.

Patients with a history of subluxation or dislocation require special preparation and preoperative planning. A sensation of popping or clicking or a report that the hip is coming in and out of the joint suggests that the hip is subluxating. When the history of subluxation and dislocation is questionable, a preoperative fluoroscopic evaluation should be planned before the revision procedure is performed. A fluoroscopic evaluation also is valuable for patients who have documented dislocations and seemingly well-positioned components. Before a revision is done in this setting, it is advisable to have available special implants such as large femoral heads, constrained liners, and bipolar components.

The location and nature of pain may influence the preoperative plan. Groin pain is more typical of loosening of the acetabular component and, if it is present, particular attention should be given to exposing the entire rim of the acetabulum to detect micromotion at the interface between the component and the host bone. Similarly, pain that is well localized to the thigh and is worst with start-up (getting out of a chair) or going up and down stairs is more typical of femoral loosening. Suggested methods of detecting occult loosening on the femoral side have included the use of dynamic CT scanning with the hip in internal and external rotation[9] or the intraoperative use of a torque wrench.[10]

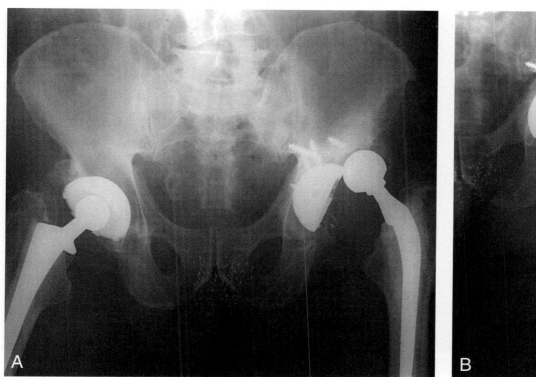
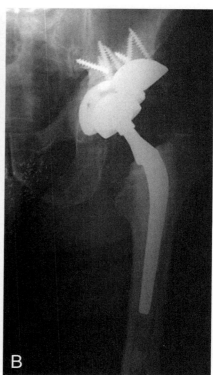

Figure 1   **A,** AP radiograph of a chronically unstable left total hip replacement, which had been inserted with acetabular bulk structural allograft. The cup placement is vertical, with limited anteversion. **B,** AP radiograph made following a revision in which a trabecular metal structural augment was used to allow placement of the revision cementless cup in a more horizontal position. A modular exchange to a larger head diameter was also performed to improve stability.

Physical Examination

The first useful step in the physical examination is to observe the patient's gait. A marked Trendelenburg gait indicates that the abductors are nonfunctional, which may be caused by paralysis or loss of continuity. If the greater trochanter is intact radiographically, preoperative electromyography can be performed to determine whether denervation of the abductor muscles has occurred. If the revision is being done because of instability and the abductors are absent or nonfunctional, the hip is particularly prone to recurrent dislocations. Use of special components such as a constrained liner or a large femoral head should be considered (Figure 1). If the trochanter is detached or has migrated, instruments

and implants to reattach the trochanter should be available at surgery.

Observation of gait should be followed by inspection of the wound. It is important to plan the surgical incision relative to previous incisions. It is not advisable to make a second, parallel incision, especially if the previous incision was posterior.[11]

The active and passive ranges of motion should be determined. Patients who have a partially or completely ankylosed hip and those with medial migration or protrusio can require an extensile exposure. If a trochanteric osteotomy or a trochanteric slide is planned, trochanteric reattachment equipment and implants must be available.

Measurement of limb length is a standard part of the physical examination, and it also is relevant to preoperative planning. Limb-lengthening frequently occurs during a revision procedure. When several centimeters of lengthening are anticipated, it is particularly important to evaluate the neurologic status of the limb. Partial sciatic nerve palsy is the most common nerve injury in total hip arthroplasty.[12] At least partial recovery occurs in 70% to 80% of patients, but the remainder are frequently dissatisfied with the result of the surgery. Somatosensory evoked potentials can be monitored intraoperatively, and when such monitoring is planned, the potentials should be recorded preoperatively so that intraoperative changes

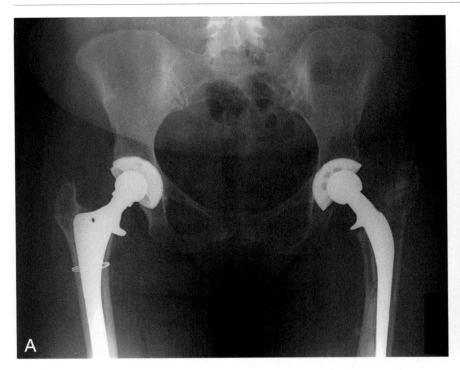
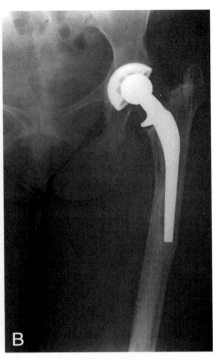

Figure 2 **A,** AP pelvic radiograph showing a symptomatic, subsided, loose cemented stem. **B,** The extent of the cement column and femoral remodeling is seen on a longer AP radiograph of the femur.

can be appreciated. The lumbar spine should also be examined before surgery. Patients with lumbar radiculopathy or spinal stenosis probably are at higher risk for nerve palsy (double-crush phenomenon), particularly if lengthening of, or traction on, the nerve is anticipated.

In patients with absent pulses or previous vascular bypass surgery, the surgical approach can be modified to minimize kinking of the femoral vessels or grafts.[13] Intraoperative heparin therapy and vascular assessment before and immediately after surgery also may be advisable for these patients. Vascular injury occurs most often with the use of screws for fixation of structural grafts, acetabular components, and protrusio rings and cages. An understanding of the acetabular quadrant system is crucial to minimize these potentially catastrophic complications.

Radiographic Examination

The radiographs should be of good quality. A low AP radiograph of the pelvis is useful for determining relative limb length by comparing the interischial line with a fixed point on the lesser trochanter. Radiographic measurements should be correlated with findings on physical examination. Judet radiographs are useful for assessing acetabular bone stock and the interface between the implant and bone. Lucent lines are frequently more apparent on a Judet radiograph than they are on an AP radiograph. A cross-table lateral radiograph of the acetabulum is useful for evaluating acetabular version, which is an important factor if instability is suspected. The shoot-through lateral radiograph also is useful for templating the acetabulum to ensure that the shell diameter estimated on the AP radiograph will fit without reaming away the anterior and posterior walls.

One should look specifically for intrapelvic cement or components. Components that are medial to Köhler's line may require additional evaluation. A CT scan usually reveals the proximity of major vascular structures to host bone, cement, screws, or acetabular components, but occasionally angiography is necessary.

AP and lateral radiographs of the femur are necessary to assess the femoral component and any cement that is present. The radiograph must extend beyond the tip of the component and cement (Figure 2). If there has been a femoral fracture, or if an osteotomy or another surgical procedure has been performed on the femur, AP and lateral radiographs of the entire femur are needed. Radiographs of the femur should be scrutinized to assess for areas of perforation, thinning, or osteolysis. It is important to evaluate the bow of the

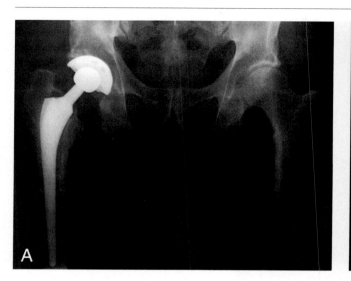
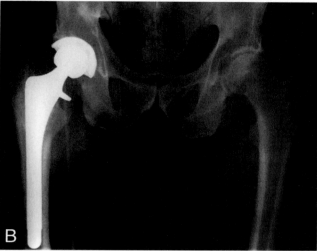

Figure 3 **A,** Preoperative AP radiograph of a right total hip replacement with aseptic loosening of the femoral component and a well-fixed cementless acetabular implant. **B,** AP radiograph made 6 months following revision of the femoral component to a fully porous-coated stem and modular exchange of the acetabular liner. A new locking mechanism was inserted at the time of the revision of the polyethylene liner.

femur on the lateral view, particularly if a stem that is more than 15 cm long might be used. In shorter patients, the bow of the femur may be encountered even with the use of primary cementless stem lengths. To assess the bow of the femur, a so-called table-down or Lowenstein lateral radiograph is more accurate than the traditional frog-leg lateral radiograph.[14]

Heterotopic ossification seen on plain radiographs should be graded.[15] The presence of grade 3 or grade 4 ossification should alert the surgeon to the possible need for prophylactic radiation or medication. To prevent recurrent heterotopic ossification most effectively, radiation must be administered either preoperatively[16] or within 48 hours postoperatively.[17] Cementless components and the sites of trochanteric osteotomies should be shielded to minimize the risk of nonunion or failure of bone ingrowth.[18]

It is important to specifically identify the components to be re-

moved. This is particularly true if any components are to be left in place. It is crucial that the characteristics and design of a retained component are compatible with those of the new components. A review of a large series of revision total hip arthroplasties revealed that at least one component was retained in 50% of the patients.[19] The most accurate information is the company implant record in the patient's medical record. This includes the sizes, manufacturer, and lot numbers of the components.

If the acetabular component is well fixed and aligned, it may be appropriate to exchange only the liner.[20] The appropriate modular liner should be available. Special tools may be required to remove the liner and to insert a second liner and/or a new locking mechanism (Figure 3). It may not be advisable to insert a second liner if the locking mechanism is damaged; in such a case, an all-polyethylene liner, which can be cemented into the well-fixed acetabular implant, should be available.[21]

Seating the liner, with avoidance of rim elevation, and scoring the back of the liner with a high-speed burr may improve cement interdigitation and fixation.

It is important to know whether the stem is a fixed head (monoblock) or modular design. If the stem is monoblock, the diameter of the head should be known so that, in the event that the stem is retained, the appropriate acetabular component liner can be available (Figure 4). If the stem is modular, the appropriate modular heads and trial implants should be available in case the head is damaged. In addition, longer head lengths (or offset liner options) are frequently necessary to restore tissue tension and stability after acetabular revision. Many implant manufacturers provide more than one modular head taper, so it is important to know which components are in place.

An acetabular component may have screws that require a special screwdriver for removal. Special osteotomes are available for removing,

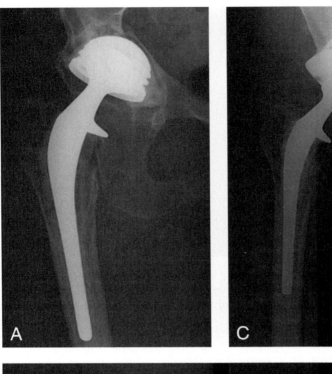

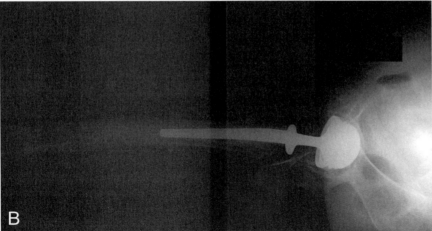

Figure 4 **A,** Preoperative AP radiograph showing a right hip with a loose acetabular component and an associated protrusio defect. The femoral component consists of a well-fixed monoblock Harris Design-2 stem (Howmedica, Rutherford, NJ) with a 26-mm head. **B,** Cross-table lateral radiograph showing a narrow anterior column and a contained acetabular defect. **C,** Radiograph made following acetabular revision to a large cementless cup with screw fixation and impaction of cancellous allograft medially. A 26-mm modular polyethylene liner for this shell was used, and the monoblock femoral component was retained.

components may require special equipment for removal such as high-speed burrs or trephines. A well-fixed cementless fully porous-coated stem may require an extended trochanteric osteotomy, sectioning of the stem, and trephining, which must be done with numerous high-speed carbide cutting tools and trephines. Similarly, removal of cementless acetabular components may be facilitated by the use of sharp curved osteotomes that match the diameter of the implant (Figure 5). Modular femoral components can require special tools to disassemble or retrieve their modular portions (Figure 6). Removal of well-fixed cemented stems can be facilitated by the use of special equipment such as ultrasonic tools, but this requires advance planning because most hospitals do not own such special equipment.

Radiographs should be reviewed not only to identify the components, but also to determine the adequacy of their position and fixation. This information then should be correlated with the findings at the time of the surgery. An analysis of sequential radiographs is the most accurate means of estimating the fixation status. Radiographs also should be reviewed for the location and extent of osteolysis. Large amounts of bone graft and/or bone graft substitute frequently are necessary to treat lytic lesions at the time of a revision total hip arthroplasty. After a general review of the radiographs, adjunctive laboratory studies, imaging, and aspiration may be considered.

Laboratory Tests

Once the surgeon has obtained an initial history, performed a physical examination, and carefully reviewed the radiographs, adjunctive testing often is required to establish or con-

with minimal bone damage, a well-fixed porous-coated ingrown shell that is malpositioned or complicated by infection. More commonly, the modular liner can be exchanged or a new liner can be cemented into a well-fixed cementless acetabular implant with a proven track record and appropriate orientation and version. Well-fixed cementless femoral

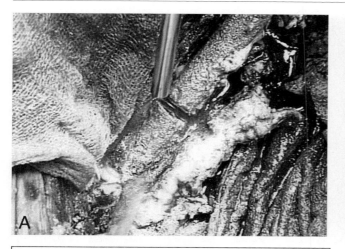

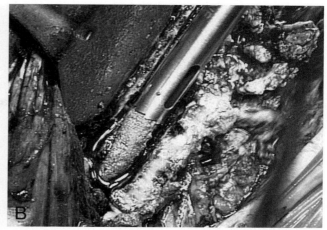

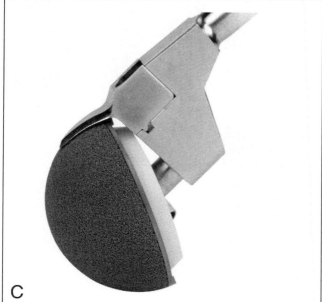

Figure 5   A, Intraoperative photograph showing use of a high-speed carbide disk-cutting wheel to cut across a well-fixed cobalt-chromium femoral stem. **B,** Trephining over the distal portion of a transected fully porous-coated stem to remove the stem. **C,** The Explant Acetabular Cup Removal System (Zimmer, Warsaw, IN) for removing a well-fixed cementless acetabular implant.

firm a definitive diagnosis. Blood testing is frequently performed preoperatively, most commonly to assess for possible infection related to the total hip arthroplasty. The hemoglobin level, hematocrit, and mean cell volume can reveal anemia, and this finding should guide preoperative treatment or additional investigations. Malnutrition is a risk factor for infection and should be corrected, if possible, before elective surgery. The preoperative nutritional status can be evaluated on the basis of serum protein levels and the total lymphocyte

count. Serum total protein, albumin and prealbumin, and transferrin levels are useful preoperative markers of nutritional status in patients undergoing total joint arthroplasty.[22-27] The white blood cell count is rarely elevated, even in the presence of obvious infection and thus is unreliable for the assessment of infection after total hip arthroplasty.[4,28,29] The erythrocyte sedimentation rate is a nonspecific inflammatory marker, which normalizes between 6 and 12 months following total hip arthroplasty.[30,31] Several authors have re-

ported that using an erythrocyte sedimentation rate of greater than 30 mm/hr as a cutoff provides increased sensitivity and specificity in the diagnosis of infection at the site of a total hip arthroplasty.[3,29,31] C-reactive protein is an acute-phase reactant that increases normally within hours after total hip arthroplasty and returns to normal within 3 months.[32] In a study of the sensitivity and specificity of investigations for diagnosing infection in patients being treated with revision total hip arthroplasty, a combination of a C-reactive protein

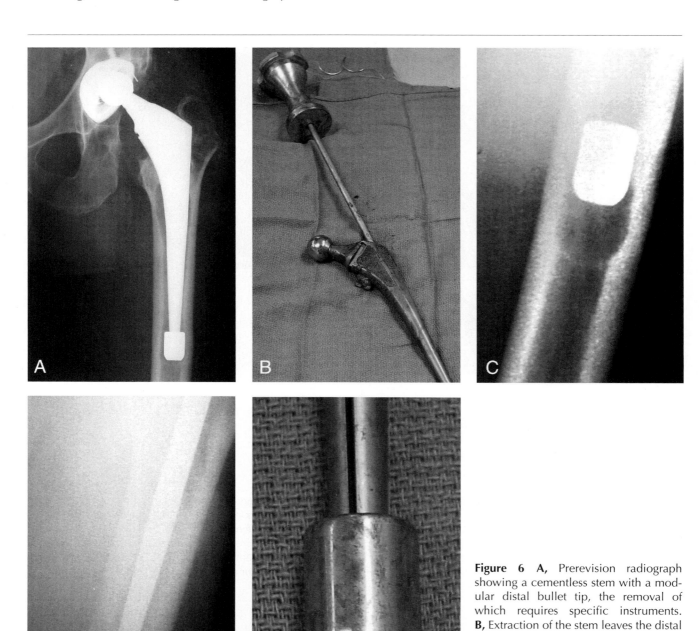

Figure 6 A, Prerevision radiograph showing a cementless stem with a modular distal bullet tip, the removal of which requires specific instruments. **B,** Extraction of the stem leaves the distal bullet tip remaining within the canal. **C,** Radiograph showing the distal bullet tip after the stem has been removed. **D** (radiograph) and **E** (photograph), Extraction of the bullet with the appropriate three-pronged device, which expands once the instrument is screwed into the bullet, allowing safe removal.

level of greater than 10 mg/L and an erythrocyte sedimentation rate of greater than 30 mm/hr was found to be most useful.[29] Values below normal or in the normal range were most valuable for excluding the diag-nosis of infection after total hip arthroplasty, whereas elevation of both values increased the probability of an infection.

Hip aspiration improves the accuracy of diagnosing infection and is recommended when the erythrocyte sedimentation rate and C-reactive protein level are elevated.[29,33] Although hip aspiration has been reported to have a sensitivity of 67% to 92% and a specificity of 94% to

97%,[29] its usefulness is primarily in combination with a review of the patient's history, a physical examination, and measurements of the erythrocyte sedimentation rate and C-reactive protein level. Aspiration and arthrography may be useful for defining a pseudocapsule, joint space extension, and sinus tracts in the setting of infection.

Nuclear medicine imaging may occasionally be useful for evaluating pain at the site of a total hip arthroplasty before a revision. To more accurately differentiate infection from loosening, indium-111-labeled leukocyte scans have been combined with technetium-99 sulfur colloid imaging. The uptake on a technetium-99 sulfur colloid image is similar to that on a 111-indium-labeled leukocyte scan when the bone is normal, but the uptake of technetium-99 sulfur colloid is inhibited by infection. These complementary scans improve the sensitivity and specificity for distinguishing between infection and aseptic loosening of implants after total hip arthroplasty.[34]

Templating

Careful preoperative templating of an adequate set of radiographs is crucial to preoperative planning for revision total hip arthroplasty. The sequence of steps, which is analogous to those used before a primary total hip arthroplasty, begins on the acetabular side. A porous-coated hemispheric component is most commonly used in revision total hip arthroplasty. The first step is to place an acetabular template against the host bone on the radiograph to maximize coverage and attempt to place the inferomedial edge adjacent to the teardrop. Often the template must extend superior to the prior implant because of bone loss or os-

teolysis. Fortunately, this is frequently offset by the use of a larger acetabular component, which often brings the center of rotation close to normal, as opposed to the use of a smaller cup at a higher hip center. It is helpful when a template of the size that was planned on the basis of the AP radiograph is placed on a cross-table lateral radiograph to ensure that the size of the selected implant will fit on both views.

Overreaming can remove most or all of the bone of the anterior and posterior parts of the acetabular rim, making it difficult to obtain a press-fit. When the component template has been placed in the desired position on the radiograph, the amount of the component that is not covered laterally should be determined. Minor amounts of as much as 20% generally can be ignored, but when 20% to 40% of the acetabular component is not covered, a structural graft or augment should be used. A distal femoral allograft is preferred. When contact between the porous-coated component and the host bone is anticipated to be less than 50% to 60%, an antiprotrusio cage and a structural bone graft or trabecular metal augments should be available.

If pelvic discontinuity is suspected, a CT scan should be performed. Signs of pelvic discontinuity on a true AP radiograph include a visible fracture line through the anterior and posterior columns, medial translation of the inferior aspect of the hemipelvis relative to the superior aspect (seen as a break in Köhler's line), and rotation of the inferior aspect of the hemipelvis relative to the superior aspect (seen as asymmetry of the obturator rings).[35] A protrusio cage can be used in this situation; however, alternatives such as posterior column plates also should be available.

After the acetabular side has been templated, the center of rotation is marked and the femoral templating is planned around this center of rotation. As is the case with a primary total hip arthroplasty, restoring hip biomechanics is the ultimate goal. This goal is achieved by restoring limb length, femoral offset, and the center of rotation. The center of rotation is the most difficult to replicate because it depends on the placement of the acetabular component, which often is nonanatomic. Specifically, with very large revision cup diameters, the center of rotation moves proximally. Eccentric, oblique, anteverted, or other special liner options can be used, especially in the case of a jumbo acetabular component, to restore the center of rotation to a more anatomic level. Special femoral components must also be available to restore length and offset when there is a nonanatomic center of rotation. This frequently requires calcar replacements and stems with increased offset. It is important to have appropriate radiographs to determine the offset. Typically, the hip should be internally rotated 15° to compensate for the typical amount of femoral anteversion and to accurately reflect the offset of the femur. This rotation places the femoral neck in a plane 90° to the radiograph and more accurately depicts the femoral offset and the area of the intertrochanteric region, thereby allowing more accurate femoral templating. If the affected hip cannot be rotated internally by 15°, templating should be done on the unaffected side. The center of rotation is raised vertically by the amount of lengthening that is planned. Generally, approximately two thirds of shortening is corrected at the time of surgery. This is a practical consideration as it is often diffi-

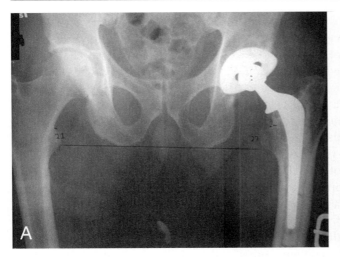

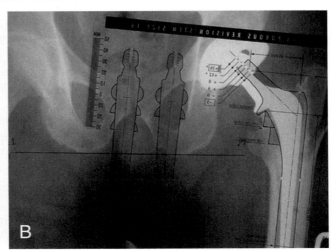

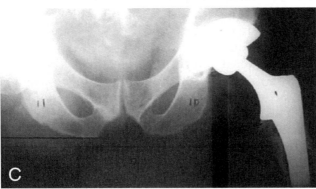

Figure 7 **A,** AP radiograph showing a loose cemented stem. The surgical side was 6 mm short as measured radiographically. **B,** The template indicates that a 15-mm calcar replacement set on the lesser trochanter will restore limb length. **C,** Postoperative radiograph showing restoration of limb length with a 15-mm calcar replacement.

cult to overcome excessive tissue tension associated with chronic shortening. When there is substantial distortion in offset and/or length, it also may be advisable to template the uninvolved side. In such a case, the center of rotation should be transposed from the surgically treated side to the uninvolved side, and then templating on the femoral side can proceed around that point, thereby reproducing more normal length and offset.

The femoral template then is placed over the center of rotation of the acetabular component at the level of the plus-zero head to allow for sizing above or below this point. Generally, a stem length is chosen to bypass any femoral defects by 2 to 3 canal diameters. When an extensive-

ly coated stem is used, approximately 6 cm of direct cortical contact with the porous coating is desirable. The stem diameter that most effectively achieves this contact is selected. Attention then is directed to the proximal fill and the point of contact with the collar relative to the available calcar bone. Invariably, there is some degree of bone loss in the area of the lesser trochanter, and it is frequently necessary to place a component on the lesser trochanter. As a general rule, this requires a 15-mm adjustment in vertical height. Most systems have calcar replacements that restore 15 to 30 mm of length. Bone loss to the bottom of the lesser trochanter generally requires a 30-mm calcar replacement (Figure 7). If more than 30 or

40 mm of length must be restored, options include proximal femoral replacement or an allograft-prosthesis composite. If there is a cortical shell of bone for several centimeters proximally followed by a short or narrow isthmus beyond this point, the situation is not ideal for either a cemented or a cementless conventional stem. In this setting, impaction grafting should be considered. This grafting requires an array of bone grafting instruments and implants, for which there must be additional planning, including surgeon education.

It is important to perform templating on lateral radiographs. Stems that are more than 175 mm long frequently impinge on the anterior cortex distally. Longer stems frequently

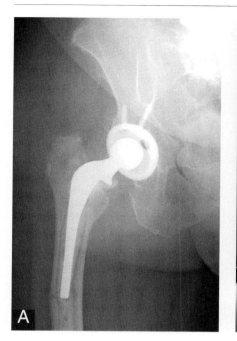 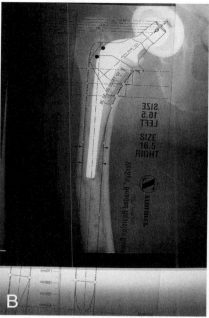 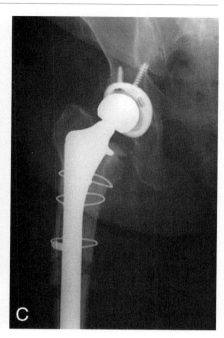

Figure 8 **A,** Preoperative radiograph showing a right total hip replacement with aseptic loosening of a cemented stem. **B,** There is varus remodeling of the femur, with an associated fracture, and templating shows that a long cementless stem inserted without an osteotomy will result in perforation. **C,** Radiograph made after revision of the femoral component, which required an extended trochanteric osteotomy. The varus remodeling necessitated completion of a transfemoral osteotomy to allow the stem to pass into the distal part of the canal. Strut allografting was used to reinforce the osteotomy sites.

require a bow to avoid eccentric reaming or perforation. The AP radiograph also must be reviewed for varus remodeling. Such remodeling frequently necessitates an extended trochanteric femoral osteotomy to safely insert a long cementless stem and occasionally may require a transfemoral osteotomy[36] (Figure 8). Templating for a cemented stem requires provision for room for a cement mantle, which should be approximately 2 mm circumferentially. In addition, it generally is desirable to have several centimeters of contact between the cement mantle and relatively healthy bone. It is difficult to introduce a cemented stem that is longer than 160 to 180 mm without an eccentric cement mantle and abutment of the tip of the cement on the femoral cortex. It generally is desirable to avoid cementing the stem beyond

the isthmus because of the difficulty with cement pressurization and with subsequent revision of such a stem.

Summary

Adequate preoperative planning is the first and most important step in the successful completion of a revision total hip arthroplasty. The many challenges that the surgeon faces exceed those posed by most primary total hip arthroplasties, although complex primary total hip arthroplasties may require a similar preoperative planning process. The planning process should be organized and include the recording of a history and a review of symptoms to ensure an accurate diagnosis as well as a physical examination to take into account the unique findings of each patient. Following the clinical encounter, a complete series of radiographs and the implant records should be carefully reviewed and ad-

junctive laboratory testing or imaging should be performed. Ruling out infection should be a part of every preoperative plan before a revision total hip arthroplasty. Templating to devise a clear plan for selection of implants, instruments, other equipment, and bone grafts is essential to a successful outcome. Removal of well-fixed implants often requires specialized instruments that may not be immediately available. A backup plan or a second line of reconstructive options should always be considered and be in place before surgery. Communication with the surgical team in advance of the procedure facilitates efficient surgery. Such an organized approach helps the patient and family to provide more specific informed consent and prepares the surgeon and the surgical team for the surgery. These steps help to reduce the surgical time, minimize the risk of complications, and improve the chances of success of a revision total hip arthroplasty.

References

1. Mancuso CA, Salvati EA, Johanson NA, Peterson MG, Charlson ME: Patients' expectations and satisfaction with total hip arthroplasty. *J Arthroplasty* 1997;12:387-396.

2. Barrack RL, Harris WH: The value of aspiration of the hip joint before revision total hip arthroplasty. *J Bone Joint Surg Am* 1993;75:66-76.

3. Levitsky KA, Hozack WJ, Balderston RA, et al: Evaluation of the painful prosthetic joint: Relative value of bone scan, sedimentation rate, and joint aspiration. *J Arthroplasty* 1991;6:237-244.

4. Lachiewicz PF, Rogers GD, Thomason HC: Aspiration of the hip joint before revision total hip arthroplasty: Clinical and laboratory factors influencing attainment of a positive culture. *J Bone Joint Surg Am* 1996;78:749-754.

5. Moeckel B, Huo MH, Salvati EA, Pellicci PM: Total hip arthroplasty in patients with diabetes mellitus. *J Arthroplasty* 1993;8:279-284.

6. Barrack RL, Jennings RW, Wolfe MW, Bertot AJ: The value of preoperative aspiration before total knee revision. *Clin Orthop Relat Res* 1997;345:8-16.

7. Della Valle CJ, Bogner E, Desai P, et al: Analysis of frozen sections of intraoperative specimens obtained at the time of reoperation after hip or knee resection arthroplasty for the treatment of infection. *J Bone Joint Surg Am* 1999;81:684-689.

8. Jacobs JJ, Kull LR, Frey GA, et al: Early failure of acetabular components inserted without cement after previous pelvic irradiation. *J Bone Joint Surg Am* 1995;77:1829-1835.

9. Berger R, Fletcher F, Donaldson T, Wasielewski R, Peterson M, Rubash H: Dynamic test to diagnose loose uncemented femoral total hip components. *Clin Orthop Relat Res* 1996;330:115-123.

10. Harris WH, Mulroy RD Jr, Maloney WJ, Burke DW, Chandler HP, Zalenski EB: Intraoperative measurement of rotational stability of femoral components of total hip arthroplasty. *Clin Orthop Relat Res* 1991;266:119-126.

11. Rothman RH, Hozack WJ: Early complications, in Rothman RH, Hozack WJ (eds): *Complications of Total Hip Arthroplasty*. Philadelphia, PA, WB Saunders, 1988, pp 14-30.

12. Barrack RL: Neurovascular injury: Avoiding catastrophe. *J Arthroplasty* 2004;19(4 suppl 1)104-107.

13. Cameron HU: Hip surgery in aortofemoral bypass patients. *Orthop Rev* 1988;17:195-197.

14. Barrack RL: Preoperative planning for revision total hip arthroplasty, in Steinberg ME, Garino JP (eds): *Revision Total Hip Arthroplasty*. Philadelphia, PA, Lippincott Williams and Wilkins, 1998, pp 151-165.

15. Brooker AF, Bowerman JW, Robinson RA, Riley LH Jr: Ectopic ossification following total hip replacement: Incidence and a method of classification. *J Bone Joint Surg Am* 1973;55:1629-1632.

16. Schneider DJ, Moulton MJ, Singapuri K, et al: Inhibition of heterotopic ossification with radiation therapy in an animal model. *Clin Orthop Relat Res* 1998;355:35-46.

17. Pellegrini VD Jr, Gregoritch SJ: Preoperative irradiation for prevention of heterotopic ossification following total hip arthroplasty. *J Bone Joint Surg Am* 1996;78:870-881.

18. Jasty M, Schutzer S, Tepper J, Willett C, Stracher MA, Harris WH: Radiation-blocking shields to localize periarticular radiation precisely for prevention of heterotopic bone formation around uncemented total hip arthroplasties. *Clin Orthop Relat Res* 1990;257:138-145.

19. Jones DL, Vigna F, Barrack RL: The use of modularity in revision total hip replacement. *Am J Orthop* 2001;30:297-302.

20. Maloney WJ, Herzwurm P, Paprosky W, Rubash HE, Engh CA: Treatment of pelvic osteolysis associated with a stable acetabular component inserted without cement as part of a total hip replacement. *J Bone Joint Surg Am* 1997;79:1628-1634.

21. Jiranek WA: Acetabular liner fixation by cement. *Clin Orthop Relat Res* 2003;417:217-223.

22. Patterson BM, Cornell CN, Carbone B, Levine B, Chapman D: Protein depletion and metabolic stress in elderly patients who have a fracture of the hip. *J Bone Joint Surg Am* 1992;74:251-260.

23. Marin LA, Salido JA, Lopez A, Silva A: Preoperative nutritional evaluation as a prognostic tool for wound healing. *Acta Orthop Scand* 2002;73:2-5.

24. Lavernia CJ, Sierra RJ, Baerga L: Nutritional parameters and short term outcome in arthroplasty. *J Am Coll Nutr* 1999;18:274-278.

25. Greene KA, Wilde AH, Stulberg BN: Preoperative nutritional status of total joint patients: Relationship to postoperative wound complications. *J Arthroplasty* 1991;6:321-325.

26. Gherini S, Vaughn BK, Lombardi AV Jr, Mallory TH: Delayed wound healing and nutritional deficiencies after total hip arthroplasty. *Clin Orthop Relat Res* 1993;293:188-195.

27. Del Savio GC, Zelicof SB, Wexler LM, et al: Preoperative nutritional status and outcome of elective total hip replacement. *Clin Orthop Relat Res* 1996;326:153-161.

28. Canner GC, Steinberg ME, Heppenstall RB, Balderston R: The infected hip after total hip arthroplasty. *J Bone Joint Surg Am* 1984;66:1393-1399.

29. Spangehl MJ, Masri BA, O'Connell JX, Duncan CP: Prospective analysis of pre-operative and intraoperative investigations for the diagnosis of infection at the sites of two hundred and two revision total hip arthroplasties. *J Bone Joint Surg Am* 1999;81:672-683.

30. Shih LY, Wu JJ, Yang DJ: Erythrocyte sedimentation rate and C-reactive protein values in patients with total hip arthroplasty. *Clin Orthop Relat Res* 1987;225:238-246.

31. Forster IW, Crawford R: Sedimentation rate in infected and uninfected total hip arthroplasty. *Clin Orthop Relat Res* 1982;168:48-52.

32. Aalto K, Osterman K, Peltola H, Rasanen J: Changes in erythrocyte sedimentation rate and C-reactive protein after total hip arthroplasty. *Clin Orthop Relat Res* 1984;184:118-120.

33. Della Valle CJ, Zuckerman JD, Di Cesare PE: Periprosthetic sepsis. *Clin Orthop Relat Res* 2004;420:26-31.

34. Palestro CJ, Kim CK, Swyer AJ, Capozzi JD, Solomon RW, Goldsmith SJ: Total-hip arthroplasty: periprosthetic indium-111-labeled leukocyte activity and complementary technetium-99m-sulfur colloid imaging in suspected infection. *J Nucl Med* 1990;31:1950-1955.

35. Berry DJ, Lewallen DG, Hanssen AD, Cabanela ME: Pelvic discontinuity in revision total hip arthroplasty. *J Bone Joint Surg Am* 1999;81:1692-1702.

36. Della Valle CJ, Paprosky WG: The femur in revision total hip arthroplasty evaluation and classification. *Clin Orthop Relat Res* 2004;420:55-62.

The Removal of Cementless Total Hip Femoral Components

Andrew H. Glassman, MD

Introduction

Cementless fixation of total hip femoral components remains popular in both primary and revision arthroplasty. Fixation failure was common with many early designs of cementless stems; implant removal was most often required for symptomatic instability and posed few technical difficulties. With technological advances and improved understanding of the requirements for successful biologic fixation, osseointegration can now be achieved in a very high percentage of patients using a variety of contemporary implant designs. The responsible orthopaedist should be capable of removing whatever prostheses he or she implants and thus should be familiar with the special techniques necessary for the safe and expeditious removal of well-fixed cementless femoral stems.

The term cementless encompasses a variety of surface treatments. These include true porous coatings (those with a three-dimensional network of interconnecting pores), various surface textures (plasma spray, corundum), and biologically active coatings (hydroxyapatite, tricalcium phosphate). The removal techniques described are equally applicable to all of these.

Like most orthopaedic procedures, the successful removal of cementless total hip components depends on careful preoperative planning, adequate exposure, proper instrumentation, and appro-

priate technique. The methods presented here have been developed during the past decade and have proved to be both safe and effective.

Preoperative Planning
Indications

That implant removal is indicated is determined from a thorough history and physical and radiographic examinations, and occasionally through ancillary studies such as aspiration and nuclear scanning. The indications for the removal of cementless femoral components are summarized in Table 1.

Two important differences distinguish the approach to removing cementless components from that used for cemented femoral components. The first is that thigh pain associated with a cementless femoral component does not necessarily indicate that the implant is

loose or easily removable. Mechanically stable cementless stems, particularly those fixed by stable fibrous tissue encapsulation, may be associated with persistent thigh pain. Rarely is the same true for optimally fixed (bone-ingrown or bone-ongrown) stems. The pain associated with optimally fixed stems frequently abates or disappears after 2 years. Hence, once infection has been ruled out, patients with thigh pain and well-fixed stems should be reassured and treated symptomatically for 2 years before stem removal is considered. The second important difference is that, unlike cemented stems, well-fixed cementless stems do not loosen in the presence of infection.

Stem removal followed by revision with a longer stem may be indicated for some periprosthetic femoral fractures. However, if the prosthesis remains well

Table 1
Indications for Cementless Stem Removal

Symptomatic instability
Persistent thigh pain (stable stem)
Infection
Osteolysis
Component malposition
    Excessive leg lengthening
    Recurrent dislocation
Stem fracture
Femoral fracture
Accommodation of cup revision

(Adapted with permission from Glassman AH, Engh CA: The removal of porous-coated femoral hip stems. *Clin Orthop* 1992;285:164-180.)

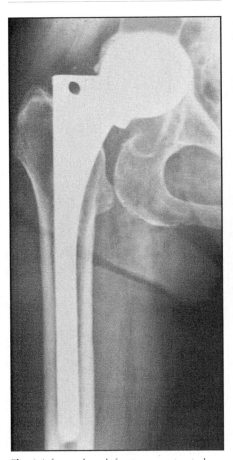

Fig. 1 A femoral neck fracture was treated with a monoblock, fully porous-coated endoprosthesis that became bone ingrowth. Painful acetabular cartilage erosion developed, necessitating femoral component removal to accommodate conventional total hip replacement.

Table 2 Radiographic Features of Implant Fixation	
Stable Fixation Modes	**Unstable Fixation Modes**
Bone-ingrown	Progressive implant motion
No implant motion (subsidence, tilting, rotation)	Divergent reactive lines surrounding the implant
No reactive lines adjacent to ingrowth surface	Pedestal formation at the stem tip
Endosteal hypertrophy at the distal limit of the ingrowth surface	Hypertrophy beneath the implant collar
Proximal atrophy	Bead shedding/delamination of porous surface
Stable bone-fibrous tissue encapsulation	
No implant motion, or minimal motion that ceases within 1 year	
Reactive lines parallel to the ingrowth surface	
Minimal proximal atrophy	

(Adapted with permission from Glassman AH, Engh CA: The removal of porous-coated femoral hip stems. *Clin Orthop* 1992;285:164-180.)

fixed and if the fracture is situated distally, then retention of the prosthesis with open reduction and internal fixation is preferable.

Component removal to accommodate acetabular revision refers to early monoblock designs, in which the diameter of the prosthetic head is incompatible with the new acetabular component (Fig. 1) or the fixed neck length does not allow for leg length correction or sufficient muscle tension to provide stability against dislocation.

Radiographic Evaluation
The most important determinant of the technical requirements for implant removal is the mode of implant fixation. Numerous retrieval studies correlating plain film and specimen radiographs with histologic studies of the bone-implant interface have confirmed that the mode of implant fixation can be determined radiographically by a trained observer.[1] Each mode of implant fixation has distinguishable radiographic features that should be recognized preoperatively (Table 2). The key features of each mode of implant fixation are illustrated in Figure 2.

The second major radiographic consideration is the degree of femoral canal filling by the implant (Fig. 3). Accessing and dividing the bone-implant interface is considerably easier for undersized than for canal-filling stems. The removal of bone-ingrown, canal-filling stems, particularly if extensively coated, requires special exposure, instrumentation, and techniques.

Implant Identification
The manufacturer and model of the implant must be identified. Although this can sometimes be accomplished by radiographic examination, a review of previous medical records is the most reliable means of positive identification. Precise identification is important for a variety of reasons. Many manufacturers provide implant-specific extraction handles that are invaluable for removing the implant. Also, because implant removal requires division of the bone-implant interface, the surgeon must be thoroughly familiar with the stem geometry as well as the extent and location of the ingrowth surfaces of components to be removed. If necessary, a sample of the implant should be obtained and inspected preoperatively.

Exposure
Proximal access to the bone-implant interface is sufficient for femoral implants with fixation surfaces limited to the metaphyseal region. Extensively coated stems, defined as those with the ingrowth surface extending into the diaphysis, require distal access as well. The sliding trochanteric osteotomy is particularly well suited to provide the exposure necessary to access these interfaces.[2] The key features of this approach include the creation of a longer, more vertically oriented osteotomy than that of a standard trochanteric osteotomy and the elevation of the vastus lateralis muscle in continuity with the distal aspect

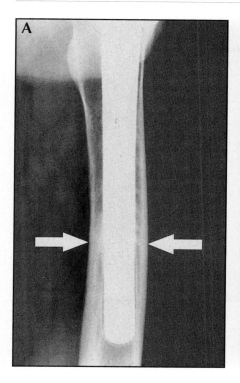
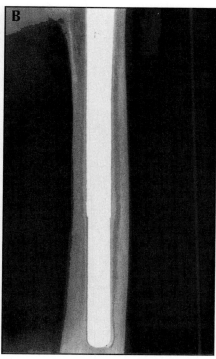
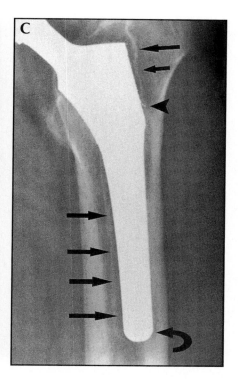

Fig. 2 Modes of cementless implant fixation. **A,** Bone ingrowth is typified by endosteal hypertrophy at the junction of the smooth and porous-coated regions of the stem (arrows). Note the reactive line surrounding the distal, uncoated portion of the stem. **B,** Stable fibrous encapsulation is characterized by reactive lines parallel to both the smooth and porous-coated regions of the stem. **C,** Unstable fixation. The implant has subsided and is surrounded by divergent reactive lines (straight arrows). There is a pedestal at the stem tip (curved arrow) and bead shedding proximal-laterally (arrowhead).

of the osteotomized fragment, thereby exposing the femoral shaft (Fig. 4). The longer osteotomy provides broad access to the bone-implant interfaces anteriorly, posteriorly, and laterally.

Exposure of the femoral shaft is essential for removing extensively porous-coated stems. Alternative exposures are suitable, including the extended trochanteric osteotomy.[3] For this approach, the lateral one third of the femoral diaphysis is osteotomized in continuity with the greater trochanteric fragment as far distally as desired (Fig. 5).

Instrumentation

It is strongly recommended that the full complement of instruments described here, designed specifically for the removal of cementless implants, be avail-able when revision arthroplasty is performed. Many of these special tools bear similarities to standard instruments, and there is a natural tendency among orthopaedists to improvise with standard instruments in their attempts at implant removal. Doing so, however, significantly increases the likelihood of failure in terms of unnecessary bone stock damage, fracture, or inability to remove the implant.

Many instruments are useful for division of the femoral bone-implant interface. Specially designed thin, flexible osteotomes are effective in the metaphyseal region (Fig. 6). These osteotomes are available in both flat and crescentic cross-sectional designs. A thin, mini-oscillating saw can be used as an alternative to the flat osteotomes. Finally, a very thin "pencil-tip" attachment can be used on a high-speed motor. Division of the interfaces with standard osteotomes should never be attempted because the greater thickness and wedge shape of standard osteotomes pose significant risk of fracture.

An overhanging collar will obscure access to the proximal medial bone-implant interface. One option is to notch or remove the collar with a tungsten carbide burr. Alternatively, a Gigli saw can be passed around the implant medially beneath the collar to divide the medial interface. This technique is recommended in conjunction with the extended trochanteric osteotomy.

The recommended technique for the removal of extensively coated femoral components requires stem transection using tungsten carbide burrs. Subsequent

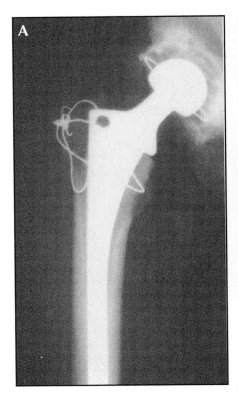

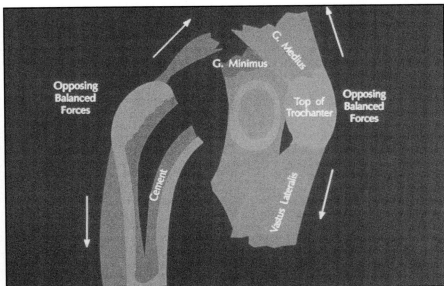

Fig. 4 The sliding trochanteric osteotomy features a longer, more vertically oriented osteotomy than does the standard osteotomy, and retention of the vastus lateralis muscle attachment, which resists trochanteric migration.

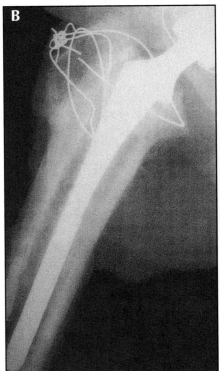

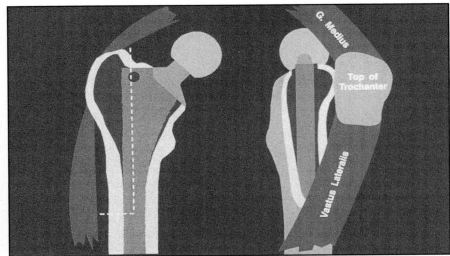

Fig. 5 The extended trochanteric osteotomy includes removal of the lateral one third of the femur as far distally as necessary.

Fig. 3 Differing degrees of femoral canal filling by two bone-ingrown stems. A, Canal-filling stem. B, Undersized stem.

removal of the distal stem segment is accomplished with specially designed hollow trephines (Fig. 7). These trephines must be available in a variety of diameters to accommodate different stem sizes while sacrificing a minimum amount of the surrounding endosteum. Tools used for cutting metal, or for cutting bone closely applied to metal, are subject to breakage and rapid dulling. Hence, several tungsten carbide bits, Gigli saws, and trephines must be available for each case.

After division of the bone-implant interface is completed, an extraction device must be used to remove the stem. Although

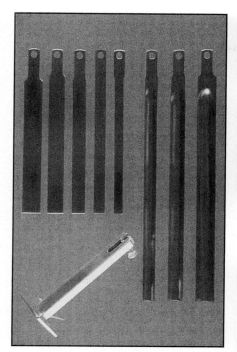

Fig. 6 Thin, flexible osteotomes for dividing the bone-implant interface are available in flat and crescentic (gutter-shaped) designs.

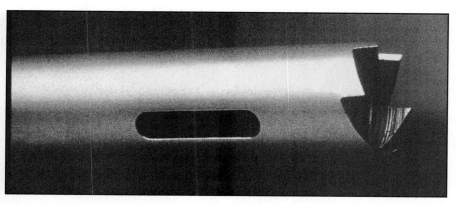

Fig. 7 A specially designed trephine for coring out the distal aspect of an extensively coated stem.

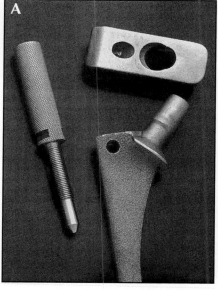
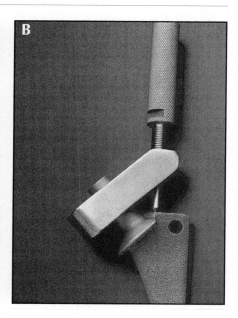

Fig. 8 Universal extraction device. **A,** Unassembled. **B,** Assembled. (Reproduced with permission from Glassman AH, Engh CA: The removal of porous-coated femoral hip stems. *Clin Orthop* 1992;285:164-180.)

some stems have points of attachment for implant-specific extraction devices, others do not. Therefore, a universal extraction device capable of firm attachment to any cementless stem is helpful (Fig. 8).

Certain modular femoral components are most easily removed if disassembled in situ. In such cases, implant-specific instruments for disengaging the modular junctions should be available.

Despite the use of appropriate instrumentation and careful technique, fractures can and do occur during implant removal. Hence, strut allografts, plates, cerclage wires or cables, and long-stem revision components should be available.

Techniques for the Removal of Cementless Femoral Components

The removal of an unstable stem generally can be accomplished with simple manual extraction without the necessity of trochanteric osteotomy. However, to

avoid fracture, care must be taken so that trochanteric overhang does not obstruct the pathway of stem exit during extraction.

Regardless of the preoperative radiographic prediction of implant fixation, mechanically stable implants are defined intraoperatively by their failure to move after several firm (but not violent) blows are applied to an extraction device secured to the implant. When this is the case, further attempts at forceful manual extraction must be abandoned and efforts

directed toward access to and division of the bone-implant interface. The approach to this task varies according to the extent of the ingrowth surface and the degree of femoral canal filling.

Proximally Coated Stems

For proximally porous-coated, mechanically stable stems, a sliding trochanteric osteotomy generally provides sufficient exposure. In the presence of an overhanging collar, a short extended trochanteric osteotomy may be preferable. The

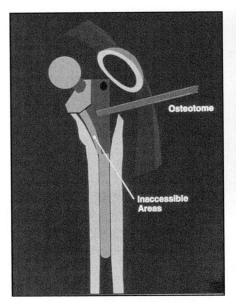

Fig. 9 The proximal bone-implant interface can be divided anteriorly, posteriorly, and laterally through a sliding or extended trochanteric osteotomy. Access to the proximal medial interface is obscured by an overhanging collar. (Reproduced with permission from Glassman AH, Engh CA: The removal of porous-coated femoral hip stems. *Clin Orthop* 1992;285:164-180.)

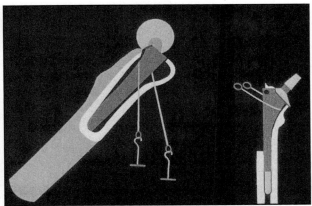

Fig. 10 In the presence of a collar, the proximal medial interface can be divided with a Gigli saw.

interface requiring division is situated in the metaphysis and therefore largely in cancellous bone. Although this bone may be densified, a thin, flexible osteotome usually can be passed through the interval between the cortex and the implant. This requires constant attention to the direction taken by the osteotomes because they are quite sharp and may veer off the implant surface to exit the surrounding bone. The flat osteotomes are passed anteriorly and posteriorly, both from proximal to distal and from lateral to medial, through the trochanteric osteotomy. Crescentic or "gutter" osteotomes are passed from proximal to distal along the lateral aspect of the implant to divide the interface in this area. Alternatively, a mini-oscillating saw can be passed from lateral to medial through the trochanteric osteotomy to divide the anterior and posterior inter-

faces in a fashion analogous to that described for the flat osteotomes. Finally, extra-thin cutting tools on a high-speed motor have been specially designed for division of the bone-implant interface. These tools are preferable to osteotomes in areas where the stem is in direct contact with cortical bone.

Although the anterior, posterior, and lateral bone-implant interfaces are accessible through the trochanteric osteotomy, the proximal medial interface is not (Fig. 9). For collarless implants, the interface is accessed from proximal to distal about the femoral neck. Direct contact between the implant and cortical bone is common in this area, and the thin, high-speed cutting tools generally are used. The presence of a collar will obscure access to this area. The most direct solution is to notch or remove the collar with a tungsten carbide bit and then proceed with interface division as described for collarless implants. This is particularly easy for implants fabricated of titanium alloy, which is easily cut. Cobalt-chromium stems are much more difficult to machine, and removal of their collars, although quite feasible, is time consuming, may require several cutting bits, and is therefore expensive. For these reasons, an alternative method using a Gigli saw in conjunction with an extended trochanteric osteotomy was developed.[4] The saw is passed around the

medial aspect of the femoral neck below the collar and its two limbs are brought out laterally, parallel to the anterior and posterior implant surfaces, to exit through the trochanteric osteotomy (Fig. 10). The handles are alternated back and forth and simultaneously drawn distally. Although this method is effective, the saw has a tendency to bind and/or break. This is especially true if the implant has very narrow anterior-posterior dimensions; the saw must therefore make two rather acute bends medially. In such cases, collar removal may be necessary.

Once all areas of the bone-implant interface have been divided, implant removal is usually easily achieved with an appropriate extraction device. Nonetheless, several precautions should be taken. As is true during the initial assessment of mechanical implant stability, if several firm blows to the extraction device fail to produce any implant movement, attempts at removal are stopped. The implant is, by definition, still stable, most likely because the interface has not been adequately divided. All interfaces should then be reassessed and divided with the techniques described above.

Sometimes, proximally coated implants will remain stable even after complete division of the interface between the primary fixation surface and the bone. In my experience, this has occurred with titanium stems in which the distal stem is not highly polished. These stems were eventually removed using the techniques described below for extensively porous-coated stems. Subsequent histologic examination confirmed prior reports of titanium's ability to become osseointegrated, even in the absence of a true porous surface.[5] This information must be taken into consideration when the removal of a proximally coated titanium stem is contemplated, especially if the stem is known to be grit blasted or otherwise roughened distally, is canal filling, and shows radiographic signs of osseointegration, such as endosteal hypertrophy and lack of reactive lines adjacent to the distal portion of the stem.

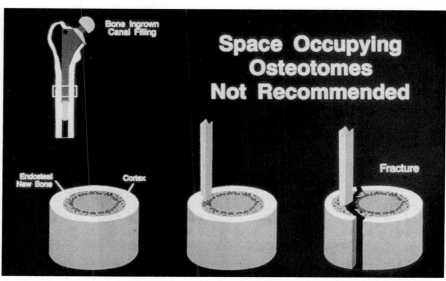

Fig. 11 Osteotomes, however thin, are not recommended for distal interface division when removing a canal-filling, extensively coated stem. (Reproduced with permission from Glassman AH, Engh CA: The removal of porous-coated femoral hip stems. *Clin Orthop* 1992;285:164-180.)

Extensively Coated Stems

Mechanically stable, extensively porous-coated femoral components are sometimes erroneously regarded as being distally fixed. Although adaptive remodeling about such implants may result in the most abundant ingrowth at the distal limit of the coating, such stems are in reality extensively fixed. Proximal interface access and division is therefore equally as critical to the removal of these stems as it is for proximally coated stems and is accomplished in exactly the same fashion. In addition, distal interface access and division are required.

The techniques for accomplishing distal interface access and division depend on the nature of the ingrowth (bone ingrowth versus stable bone-fibrous encapsulation) and on the degree of diaphyseal canal filling by the stem. Stable bone-fibrous tissue–encapsulated interfaces are characterized by a neocortex separated from the ingrowth surface, generally by 1 mm or less. Radiographically, this appears as a reactive line that parallels the implant surface (Fig. 2, *A*). For undersized, extensively coated stems

fixed by stable bone-fibrous tissue encapsulation, this neocortex is joined to the endosteum by less dense trabecular bone. In such cases, thin osteotomes can be passed along the length of the implant from proximal to distal to divide these trabeculae outside of the neocortex without incurring a fracture. For canal-filling stems, the neocortex is closely applied to the true endosteum, and passage of osteotomes is not only difficult but risks fracture. It is safer to remove such stems with the methods described for bone-ingrown, canal-filling stems.

Occasionally, significantly undersized, extensively porous-coated stems become fixed by bone ingrowth (Fig. 3, *B*). The trabeculae joining the endosteum to the surface of such stems can also be divided with osteotomes in areas where the implant is widely separated from the cortex. If the stem is well centered within the femoral canal, the entire interface can be divided in this fashion. If, however, the stem is in significant varus or valgus and there is direct contact

between the stem and the endosteum, osteotomes are not recommended, and these stems are treated as bone-ingrown, canal-filling stems.

Extensively porous-coated, canal-filling, bone-ingrown stems present the greatest difficulties for removal. The use of osteotomes distally, however thin, poses a high risk of fracture and is to be avoided (Fig. 11). Because no space is present between the stem and cortical bone, access and division of the bone-implant interface requires the use of an instrument capable of removing interface material as it is advanced distally. My preference in such cases is the so-called trephine technique.[6] This technique can be done using the sliding trochanteric osteotomy (Fig. 12). After proximal interface division, the anterior femoral cortex is exposed. The junction between the proximal triangular and distal cylindrical segments of the implant is estimated using an appropriately sized trial component placed over the anterior femur. This location is marked, and a transversely oriented window is created in the

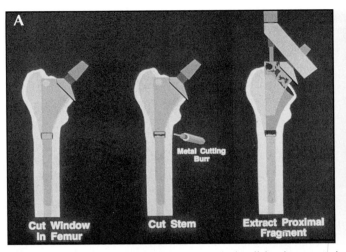
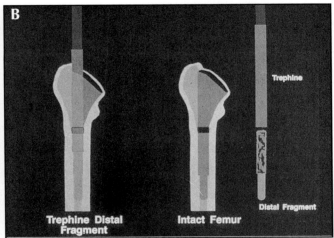

Fig. 12 The trephine technique for the removal of well-fixed, extensively coated stems. **A,** After proximal interface division, the stem is transected through a cortical window and the upper portion is removed. **B,** The remaining distal portion is cored out using a hollow trephine. (Reproduced with permission from Glassman AH, Engh CA: The removal of porous-coated femoral hip stems. *Clin Orthop* 1992;285:164-180.)

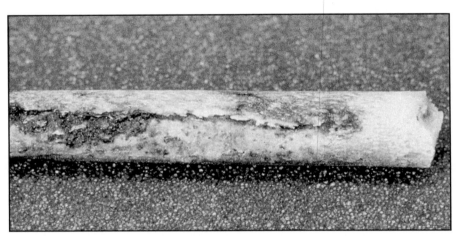

Fig. 13 The removed distal segment of an extensively coated stem demonstrating abundant ingrowth.

anterior femoral cortex with a burr. The window should be approximately 1.0 to 1.5 cm in width from medial to lateral, depending on the diameter of the stem. Next, the stem is transected using tungsten carbide cutting tools on a high-speed motor passed through the window. The surrounding soft tissue should be carefully protected using plastic surgical drapes or moistened towels to avoid metal contamination. Copious irrigation is required to speed cutting and to prevent rapid dulling of

the cutting tool and thermal damage to the surrounding bone. Several cutting bits may be required. The volume of metal removed increases with the square of the stem diameter. Hence, the transection of a 15-mm stem takes more than twice as long as does a 10.5-mm stem (and twice the number of tungsten carbide bits).

After the stem is transected, assuming that proximal interface division has been complete, the proximal segment of the implant can be removed using an appropri-

ate extraction device. The remaining distal segment is then "cored out" using the smallest available trephine that will fit over it. Copious irrigation is required. In addition, the trephine should periodically be removed from the femoral canal and the canal thoroughly flushed of debris before the trephine is advanced further. More than one trephine may be required, depending on the length of the stem. When interface division is complete, the distal segment of the stem will "seize" within the trephine, which is then withdrawn. The distal portion of the stem is then tapped out of the trephine (Fig. 12). When this technique is properly used, bone-ingrown, extensively porous-coated stems can be removed with minimal bone stock damage and without compromising the structural integrity of the cortical tube (Fig. 13).

The trephine technique also can be used in conjunction with an extended trochanteric osteotomy.[3] In general, the osteotomy is carried distally approximately 3 cm beyond the junction between the proximal metaphyseal and distal cylindrical portions of the stem (Fig. 14). When this approach is used, it is helpful to use a thin oscillating saw passed from lateral to medial through the osteotomy to divide the interfaces anteriorly and posteriorly (Fig. 15). The channels thus created facilitate subsequent passage of a Gigli saw medially to divide the bone-implant interface in that region. The stem is then transected through the distal portion of the osteotomy, eliminating the need to create a separate cortical window. The distal stem is then removed with the trephine. An alternative technique is to continue the extended trochanteric osteotomy all the way to the stem tip and use the Gigli saw to divide the entire medial interface, without the need to transect the stem. Although it is effective, this method disrupts the integrity of the cortical tube and compromises reconstruction. Its use is therefore reserved for septic patients with infected prostheses in whom the primary goal is to remove the prosthesis as quickly as possible.

Curved, extensively coated prostheses are best approached in a fashion similar to that just described. The extended trochanteric osteotomy should be used and carried distally, at least to the apex of the anterior bow of the stem. The stem is first transected at the same junctional level as described above. The trephine is advanced over the distal stem as far as possible, at which point it will bind on the curved portion of the stem. When this depth is attained, the stem is transected a second time at the apex of the curve. The remaining stem beyond the curve can then be removed with a trephine. It may be necessary to use a trephine one size larger to accommodate the bowed segments.

References

1. Engh CA, Bobyn JD, Glassman AH: Porous-coated hip replacement: The factors governing bone ingrowth, stress shielding, and clinical results. *J Bone Joint Surg Br* 1987;69:45-55.

2. Glassman AH, Engh CA, Bobyn JD: A technique of extensile exposure for total hip arthroplasty. *J Arthroplasty* 1987;2:11-21.

3. Younger TI, Bradford MS, Magnus RE, Paprosky WG: Extended proximal femoral osteotomy: A new technique for femoral revision arthroplasty. *J Arthroplasty* 1995;10:329-338.

4. Younger TI, Bradford MS, Paprosky WG: Removal of a well-fixed cementless femoral component with an extended proximal femoral osteotomy. *Contemp Orthop* 1995;30:375-380.

5. Branemark PI, Zarb GI, Albrektason T: *Tissue Integrated Prostheses: Osseointegration in Clinical Dentistry.* Chicago, IL, Quintessence Press, 1985.

6. Glassman AH, Engh CA: The removal of porous-coated femoral hip stems. *Clin Orthop* 1992;285:164-180.

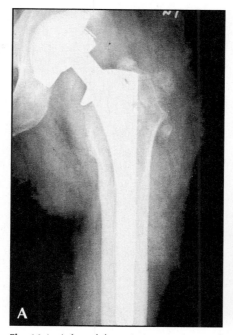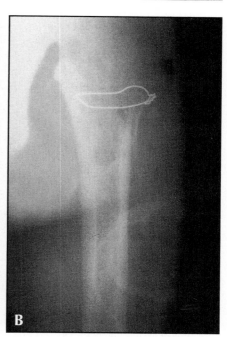

Fig. 14 An infected, bone-ingrown, extensively porous-coated stem. **A,** Preoperatively. **B,** Following removal with the trephine technique. The proximal femur remains intact. The anterior cortical window used for stem transection is visible in the metaphyseal-diaphyseal transition.

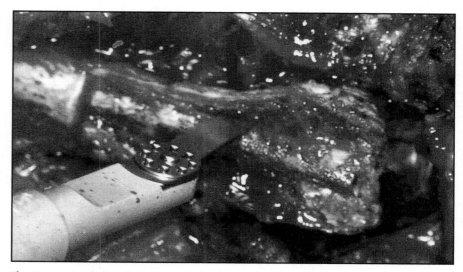

Fig. 15 An extended trochanteric osteotomy has been performed. The anterior and posterior bone-implant interfaces are divided with a thin oscillating saw in preparation for the passage of a Gigli saw medially.

21

The Role of Allografts in Revision Arthroplasty of the Hip

Allan E. Gross, MD, FRCSC
Hugh Blackley, MD, FRACS
Paul Wong, MD, MSc, BEng, FRCSC
Khal Saleh, MD, MSc(Epid), FRCSC
Ian Woodgate, MBBS(Hons), FRACS(Orth)

Although somewhat controversial in the past, the use of allograft tissue is now clearly indicated in lower extremity reconstructive surgery. Improved and safer availability of banked tissue has made the use of musculoskeletal allografts nearly universal. In lower extremity reconstructive surgery, allograft tissue is used in revision arthroplasty of the hip and knee and for the reconstruction of osteochondral joint defects. This chapter discusses the role of allografts in revision hip arthroplasty and reports the results of the authors' portion of a comprehensive transplant program.

Revision Arthroplasty of the Hip

Restoration of bone stock is an important goal in revision arthroplasty of the hip, particularly in patients likely to undergo further surgery.[1,2] In some patients with severe bone loss, stabilizing a new implant without restoring bone stock is not possible, even with implants designed to be used after tumor excision. Tumor implants can be used in some revision situations; generally, however, these mega-

One or more of the authors or the departments with which they are affiliated have received something of value from a commercial or other party related directly or indirectly to the subject of this chapter.

prostheses are more suitable after en bloc excision of bone tumors because the questionable prognosis necessitates faster rehabilitation, and chemotherapy and radiation have a deleterious effect on bone grafts.[2,3] In addition, these megaprostheses do not restore bone stock,[4] and they make further surgery more difficult because they violate residual host bone on the femoral side with cement or porous-coated implants. Also, these implants do not allow biologic reattachment of bone and muscle.[5] The use of these prostheses other than in en bloc excisions is therefore limited.

Classification of Bone Stock Deficiency

Classification of acetabular and femoral revisions is based on bone stock deficiency. The deficiency is defined radiographically by routine and Judet views.[6] Final verification of the bone deficiency is made intraoperatively, and the surgeon should anticipate that, after removal of the old components, the loss of bone may be worse than was apparent on radiograph. If the failed hip is infected, allograft bone still can be used, but the reconstruction must be done in two stages (excision arthroplasty, débridement, insertion of cement spacer, and antibiotic therapy, followed by revision arthroplasty).[7]

Acetabulum

Bone stock deficiency of the acetabulum is classified as being of four types.

Type 1 No significant loss of bone stock: Conventional cemented or uncemented acetabular components can be used.

Type 2 Contained (cavitary) loss of bone stock: The columns and acetabular rim are intact. Morcellized allograft bone is used with an uncemented cup if contact can be made with at least 50% of the host bone.[8,9] This may require the use of a jumbo cup.[10] If contact cannot be made with 50% of the host bone, then impaction grafting with mesh and a cemented cup,[11] or impaction grafting with a ring and a cemented cup, is necessary.[12,13]

Type 3 Uncontained loss of bone stock involving less than 50% of the acetabulum: This defect is segmental and may involve either the anterior or posterior column; posterior column defects are more significant. This defect can be managed by a high hip center,[14] an oblong cup,[15,16] or a structural allograft that supports less than 50% of the cup.[1]

Type 4 Uncontained defect involving more than 50% of the acetabulum: This is segmental loss of bone affecting both the anterior and posterior columns, and it may be associated with a pelvic discontinuity. This defect requires a structural allograft and a reconstructive ring that protects the graft.[17]

Femur

Bone stock deficiency of the femur is classified as being of five types.

Type 1 No significant loss of bone stock: This defect occurs only with loose cementless components and can be managed with cemented or cementless components.

Type 2 Contained (cavitary) loss of bone: This type of defect can be managed by proximal fixation with modular components,[18] proximal porous-coated components,[19] or impaction grafting using morcellized allograft bone.[20] It also can be managed by distal fixation with long-stem cemented[21] or uncemented components.[22] Long-stem uncemented components achieve biologic fixation by an extensive porous coating (ingrowth)[22] or roughened titanium (ingrowth).[23] A third method of managing this type of defect is extensive (proximal and distal) fixation using uncemented modular components.[18]

Type 3 Noncircumferential segmental loss of bone: This type of defect can be managed with cortical strut allografts.[24]

Type 4 Uncontained (segmental) loss of bone stock less than 5 cm in length: These defects involve the calcar and the lesser trochanter but do not extend into the diaphysis. These defects can be managed with calcar-replacing implants.[24]

Type 5 Uncontained (segmental) loss of bone stock more than 5 cm in length: This type of defect extends into the diaphysis and requires a structural allograft[25] or a tumor prosthesis.[2] Periprosthetic fractures may be associated with any type of bone loss on both the acetabular and femoral sides.

Authors' Techniques and Results: Acetabulum

At Mount Sinai Hospital, allograft bone is used to manage acetabular types 2, 3, and 4 bone stock deficiencies.

Approach and Graft Preparation

Reconstruction of the acetabulum with a contained defect (type 2) can be carried out through any conventional approach, often without the need for a trochanteric osteotomy. For structural defects (types 3 and 4), we prefer to have access to the anterior and posterior columns, and therefore we use a transtrochanteric approach. The trochanteric slide allows access to the posterior and anterior columns.[26] This osteotomy is more stable than the transverse trochanteric osteotomy because the trochanter remains in continuity with the abductor and vastus lateralis muscles and tendons, thus making trochanteric migration unlikely. (In our experience with the classic transverse osteotomy, the prevalence of nonunion and of trochanteric migration of 25% [32 of 130 hips] is unacceptably high.[25]) The trochanteric slide can be converted to a transverse osteotomy by releasing the vastus lateralis muscle if more exposure is required.

A pin is inserted into the iliac crest, and the distance between it and a fixed point on the resected trochanteric bed is measured as a reference for leg length. The sciatic nerve is identified in order to evaluate tension if leg lengthening of more than 3 cm is anticipated.

The acetabulum is prepared after the hip has been dislocated. After the acetabular component and the cement have been removed, the interface membrane is gently excised. The defect is then defined by visualization, palpation, and the use of a trial cup and is classified as contained or uncontained. The decision is then made regarding the type of reconstruction to be done and bone graft to be used. (Much of this decision-making can be done preoperatively based on radiographs, but the final decision is based on the intraoperative findings.)

The deep-frozen, irradiated (2.5 Mrad [25,000 Gray]) allograft bone comes from our hospital bone bank, which is accredited by the American Association of Tissue Banks.[27] The allograft bone is not opened until infection in the host joint has been ruled out by Gram stain, frozen section, and visual inspection and the bone defect defined. After the graft is unwrapped and cultured, it is thawed in a warm 50% povidone-iodine–and–saline solution. The thawed bone is prepared on a separate table while the revision is being done. When morcellized bone is needed, morcellization can be done manually with rongeurs or by a bone mill. (A bone mill that does not make the bone too mushy should be used.) Morcellized bone pieces should be 5 to 10 mm in diameter. Alternatively, prepared morcellized bone can be obtained from some bone banks in freeze-dried or deep-frozen forms. Structural grafts are prepared from acetabular allografts, male femoral heads, or distal femurs. All bone is rinsed with a mixture of one-third 3% hydrogen peroxide with two-thirds normal saline and finally with bacitracin (30,000 units in 1,000 mL normal saline) before the bone is placed into the acetabular bed.

Surgical Technique

Type 2 A central or superomedial protrusio may be associated with a loose acetabular prosthesis (Fig. 1, *A*). The bone stock is restored with impacted, morcellized, cancellous allograft bone. Female femoral heads should be used for morcellized bone. Some type 2 defects are so large that two or three femoral heads may be needed to obtain enough bone for morcellization. As mentioned, cemented or uncemented acetabular implants can be used.

Impacted morcellized bone with an uncemented large-diameter cup should be used in younger patients with higher demands. Contact with at least 50% of the host bone must be made. Some rim contact between the cup and the host bone is necessary (Fig. 1, *B* and *C*). Host bone contact can be evaluated using a trial cup placed in the correct anatomic

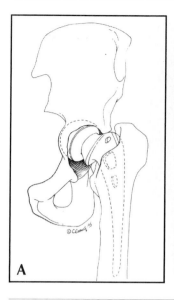

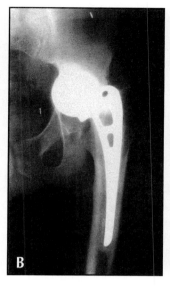

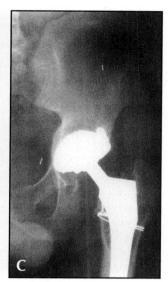

Fig. 1 A, An acetabular contained (cavitary) defect (type 2) (Copyright © 1995 Christine Chang, Medical Illustrator). **B,** AP radiograph of a 30-year-old man with a superomedial contained defect 10 years after a hemiarthroplasty for osteonecrosis of the femoral head. **C,** AP radiograph taken 11.5 years after revision surgery with morcellized allograft bone and an uncemented cup.

position and not in a high hip position. Some rim contact is important, particularly superiorly and posteriorly; rim contact is optimal if the 50% host-bone contact is superior and posterior.

When contact cannot be made with 50% of the host bone, a roof-reinforcement ring and a cemented cup are recommended. The ring must make rim contact with the host bone superiorly, posteriorly, and inferomedially and is fixed with at least three screws directed into the acetabular dome (Fig. 2). If a contained defect is global, involving all quadrants of the acetabulum, then a reconstruction ring that goes from ilium to ischium must be used.

Type 3 Obtaining good coverage of the new cup is difficult in some acetabular revisions because of superolateral bone loss, caused by loosening or by good coverage not having been obtained during the primary procedure (Fig. 3, *A*). In this situation, intact male femoral head segments or true acetabular allografts can provide good coverage of the acetabular implant. These shelf or minor column grafts are fixed with 4.5-mm cancellous screws placed in an oblique-to-vertical direction (Fig. 3, *B*). The junction of the shelf allograft and the pelvic wall is auto-

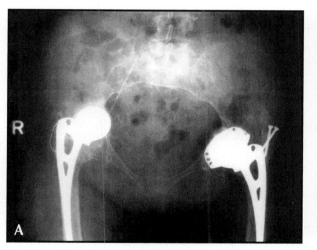

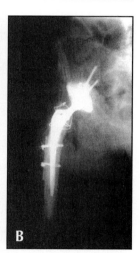

Fig. 2 A, AP radiograph of a 60-year-old woman with an acetabular contained defect (type 2) several years after a hemiarthroplasty for a fracture. **B,** AP radiograph 5 years after revision surgery with a roof-reinforcement ring and morcellized allograft bone. Note that the ring has made contact inferomedially with the host bone.

grafted with cancellous bone (a flying buttress graft). Cemented or uncemented acetabular implants can be used in combination with the shelf graft. There is contact with more than 50% of the host bone; therefore, an uncemented cup can be used, although technically it is easier to use a cemented cup (Fig. 3, *C* and *D*).

Type 4 Major column defects are best restored with true acetabular allografts. These major column grafts are fixed to

the host bone with cancellous screws and are protected by reconstruction rings that bridge the defect from host bone to host bone (Fig. 4, *A* and *B*). The cup must be cemented because there is no contact with the host bone. The reconstruction ring spans and protects the graft and also fixes a discontinuity when one exists. The ring reaches from ilium to ischium and is fixed by at least three cancellous screws inserted into the ilium and two

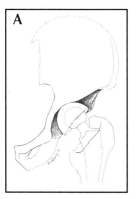
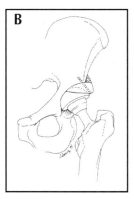
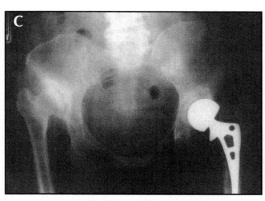
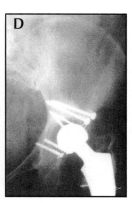

Fig. 3 A, An acetabular uncontained defect involving less than 50% of the acetabulum (type 3) (Copyright © 1995 Christine Chang, Medical Illustrator). **B,** A structural allograft (shelf or minor column) fixed by cancellous screws supports less than 50% of the cup. The stippled area above the shelf graft represents the flying buttress graft (morcellized autograft bone) (Copyright © 1995 Christine Chang, Medical Illustrator). **C,** AP radiograph of a 32-year-old woman who underwent bipolar arthroplasty for hip dysplasia and osteoarthritis. The poor coverage of the bipolar cup is visible. **D,** AP radiograph of the patient in panel C 14 years after revision surgery with a minor column (shelf) allograft and an uncemented cup.

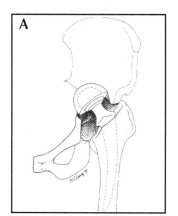
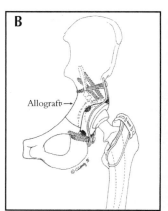
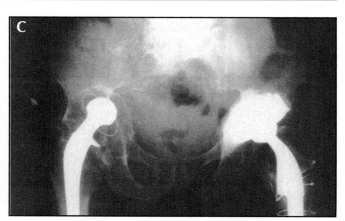

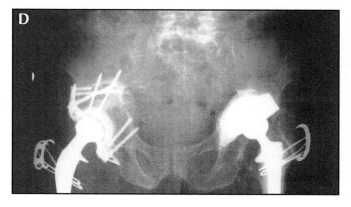

Fig. 4 A, An acetabular uncontained defect involving more than 50% of the acetabulum (type 4) with pelvic discontinuity (Copyright © 1995 Christine Chang, Medical Illustrator). **B,** Reconstruction with a structural allograft fixed by two cancellous screws and protected by a reconstruction ring fixed to the ilium and ischium (Copyright © 1995 Christine Chang, Medical Illustrator). **C,** AP radiograph of a 77-year-old man with a loose cemented cup and massive osteolysis of the right acetabulum involving more than 50% of the acetabulum and pelvic discontinuity. **D,** AP radiograph of the patient in panel C 5 years after reconstruction with a major column allograft protected by a reconstruction ring reaching from host ilium to host ischium.

cancellous screws inserted into the ischium. If good screw fixation cannot be achieved into the ischium, then the inferior flange can be slotted into or buttressed against the ischium (Fig. 4, C and D). If the inferior flange is slotted into the ischium, one or two inferior screws still may be used.

When stable fixation is achieved by screws in the ilium and the ischium, an associated pelvic discontinuity is stabilized. However, if stable fixation cannot be achieved, particularly in the ischium, then additional fixation must be provided by a plate, in addition to the ring if there is a pelvic discontinuity.

Results

Patients were evaluated prospectively using a modified Harris hip scoring system.[25] Success was defined as an increase in the hip score of 20 points, a stable cup (no migration of the cup or cement fractures), and no need for additional surgery on the acetabular side.[28]

Allograft bone was assessed radiographically for union, as evidenced by trabecular bridging of the donor-host interface; for allograft fracture and fragmentation (for the structural grafts); and for graft resorption. Resorption was measured on AP pelvic radiographs and graded as minor (less than one third of graft resorbed), moderate (one third to one half of graft resorbed), or severe (more than one half of graft resorbed). Migration was measured in superior and medial directions using the superolateral corner of the obturator foramen as a landmark. Loosening was defined as cup or ring migration of more than 4 mm or a fracture of screws or the cement mantle. Radiographs were reviewed by two unblinded orthopaedic surgeons (K.S. and I.W.); interobserver reliability was not assessed. As of October 1, 2000, 676 hips had been revised using allograft bone during a period of 18 years at Mount Sinai Hospital. Of these, 575 have required acetabular revision.

Type 2 Morcellized allograft bone was used in 297 hips in 281 patients. Of these, 20 hips in 17 patients required subsequent operations, for a rerevision rate of 6.7%. Seven hips were revised for recurrent dislocations and 13 for cup loosening. In a study by Garbuz and associates[28] of 51 hips in 51 patients with at least 5 years of follow-up (average, 6.8 years), the success rate was 90%. Four hips in four patients required an additional operation on the acetabular side.[28]

Twenty-five hips had uncemented cups (92% success rate); 16 hips had roof-reinforcement rings (100% success rate); 10 hips had bipolar acetabular components (70% success rate). Severe resorption was noted and revised in two of the 25 hips with uncemented cups and in three of the 10 bipolar cups, two of which were revised.[28] In the four hips rerevised because of severe graft resorption, additional morcellized grafting was necessary.

In a more recent study,[13] 43 hips were reconstructed with morcellized allograft bone, a roof-reinforcement ring, and a cemented cup because contact could not be made with 50% of the host bone. At an average follow-up of 5 years, one cup was revised for loosening; four hips that were radiographically loose, demonstrating migration of the ring, were asymptomatic.[13]

Type 3 As of October 1, 2000, 74 hips in 69 patients were revised with minor column allografts. Of these, eleven hips in 10 patients required additional operations, for a rerevision rate of 15%. Seven hips in six patients were revised for cup loosening. In addition, one hip was revised for infection, one for severe resorption, one for dislocation, and one for graft fracture. Of 29 hips in 28 patients with a minimum of 5 years of follow-up (average, 7.1 years), the success rate as defined above was 86%.[29] Sixteen cups were uncemented porous-coated, one was bipolar, eight were cemented all-polyethylene, and four were cemented into roof-reinforcement rings. Four patients required additional operations. Three grafts had severe resorption, with two (one cemented, one uncemented) requiring additional operations for cup loosening, and only one of the two requiring additional grafting. One patient had an excision arthroplasty for loosening of a cemented cup, and one patient had exploration of the joint for pain, although the graft was intact and the uncemented cup was solid. All but one graft united. There was no resorption in

9 patients, minor resorption in 17, and moderate resorption in 3.

In a more recent study[30] of 51 hips in 47 patients revised with minor column (shelf) allografts at an average follow-up of 10 years, 11 patients had required additional surgery. Three underwent excisional arthroplasty and eight were successfully revised, with only three of the eight requiring another structural graft. The cup aseptic survival rate was 80.4% and the graft survival rate, 94.1%.[30]

Type 4 As of October 1, 2000, 136 hips in 132 patients were revised with major column allografts. Of these, 38 hips in 37 patients required further surgery, for a rerevision rate of 28%. Excision arthroplasty was done in 11 hips in 10 patients because of nonunion in one hip, cup loosening in three (two patients), infection in three, fracture in one, and dislocation in three. Twenty-seven hips in 27 patients were revised successfully: 17 for cup loosening and 9 for dislocation, while 1 hip was explored for a sciatic nerve injury. In 33 hips in 31 patients with major column grafts and a minimum of 5 years of follow-up (average, 7.1 years), 18 hips in 17 patients had successful results, for a success rate of 55%.[28] Six hips in six patients required additional operations for cup loosening, but the grafts were intact and united. One hip required exploration for a sciatic nerve injury. These hips were considered a partial success because no additional grafting was necessary. The overall success rate, therefore, was 76% (25 of 33 hips). Eight of 33 hips required additional operations because of graft failure: seven underwent severe resorption and one had infection.[28]

The acetabular implants used were 14 cemented polyethylene cups, 7 cementless cups, 4 bipolar cups, and 8 reconstruction rings with cemented cups. Seven of eight reconstructions done with a ring and cemented cup were successful, with the only failure a result of infection. Two of seven cementless cups and three of four bipolar cups had moderate or severe resorption that required revision. Three of 14 cups in 13 patients that were cemented directly into the allograft were associated with severe resorption and required additional surgery. Cup loosening occurred only when cementless or cemented cups were inserted directly into the allograft.

Of the 15 hips in the 14 patients that required additional surgery, seven required no additional grafting, six required additional grafting because of severe graft resorption, and two underwent excision arthroplasty.

As mentioned, seven of eight reconstructions done with a protective ring were successful, with the only failure the result of infection. In a more recent study,[17] we examined results in 12 patients with 13 type 4 defects reconstructed with structural grafts protected by a ring. Three of these patients underwent resection arthroplasty, one for graft resorption and two for recurrent dislocation. Nine patients with 10 reconstructions were considered successes at an average follow-up of 10.5 years.[17]

Authors' Techniques and Results: Femur

Full circumferential structural femoral allografts are used for type 5 femoral defects. Noncircumferential allografts (cortical struts) are used for type 3 defects, which also are managed with biologic plates for periprosthetic fractures, reinforcement of windows, and adding to the fixation of proximal femoral allografts at the graft–host bone junction.

Structural Femoral Allografts

Full circumferential allografts are used for segmental defects more than 5 cm in length (type 5 defects). These grafts allow reattachment of the greater trochanter and soft tissue. The surgical technique described below does not violate the distal host canal by cement or a porous coating, thus facilitating future revision surgery, if necessary.

Surgical Technique The allograft is stored in the hospital bone bank at -70°C after being irradiated (2.5 Mrad). Preoperatively, the approximate allograft size is templated out, and a longer graft is ordered to allow for any intraoperative variations. As with the preoperative procedure described for acetabular reconstruction, the proximal femoral allograft is brought into the operating room only after possible infection has been ruled out. Any suspicion of infection requires a two-stage procedure. The graft is unwrapped and specimens obtained for culture; the graft is then placed in a warm solution of 50% povidone-iodine and saline. To reduce surgical time, preparation of the graft is carried out on a separate back table by part of the team while the revision is done.

In this study, the transtrochanteric approach was most commonly used because of the need for extensive exposure. However, either a longitudinal trochanteric splitting osteotomy or a sliding osteotomy are now preferred because both are more stable than a transverse osteotomy and have a lower risk of trochanteric migration.[26] The proximal femur is exposed by reflecting the vastus lateralis muscle off the intermuscular septum anteriorly, with care taken not to completely strip any residual bone of its soft tissue because this tissue is used later as a vascularized autogenous graft. Before dislocation, a Steinmann pin is inserted into the iliac crest, and the distance to the roof line (origin of the vastus lateralis) is measured as a reference point to determine limb length. In preparation for the femoral split, a transverse cut is made at the junction of deficient and healthy femur; it is to this level that the femoral split will extend distally. This transverse osteotomy, which extends just through the lateral half of the femur, must be done carefully with an oscillating saw, leaving the medial femur intact. Then a midline lateral femoral split is carried out, also with the oscillating saw. The split is gently spread open with multiple osteotomes, carefully levering against the femoral implant or cement in the canal. The deficient femur cracks anteriorly and posteriorly and falls open down to the transverse osteotomy. When this happens, a spike of femur, usually on the medial side, will remain attached to the healthy distal femur; this spike can be shaped into a step-cut or an oblique osteotomy to help stabilize the graft–host bone junction later. Care is taken to preserve the soft-tissue attachments to the split femur.

The acetabulum is reconstructed first so that the length of the femoral allograft can be determined. The host canal is nearly always larger than that of the allograft. A guide wire is inserted into the distal host femur and the canal is gently reamed. It is important to emphasize that press-fit of the implant into the host femur is not essential. A press-fit generally leads to a larger implant proximally, which reduces the cement mantle. It also results in excessive reaming of the allograft to fit the implant, which weakens the graft and reduces bone stock. Finally, a tight distal fit can result in distraction at the host bone–allograft junction, which increases the risk of nonunion.

The approximate length of the graft required is assessed by placing the femoral implant into the host femur and reducing it into the acetabulum. Stability and any preoperative limb-length discrepancy are taken into account in determining the allograft length. The allograft is cleaned of soft tissue, and the graft is reamed and broached until a good fit for the implant is achieved while allowing for at least a 2-mm cement mantle around the stem. The long-stem femoral prosthesis used is narrow proximally so that the graft does not have to be excessively reamed and so that there is at least a 2-mm cement mantle. The implant is long enough to reach the distal femoral

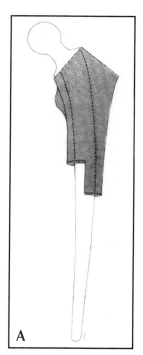
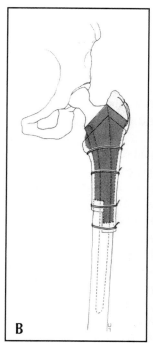
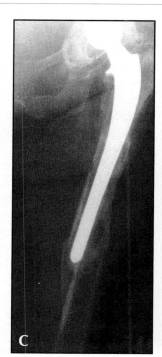
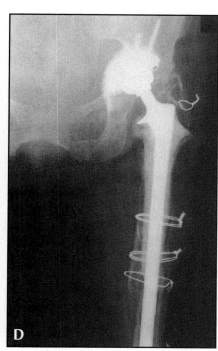

Fig. 5 A, Proximal femoral allograft with the implant cemented into allograft. **B,** The proximal femoral allograft implant composite has been inserted into the host canal without cement. The junction has been stabilized by a step-cut osteotomy and cerclage wires. Residual host femur has been cerclaged around the allograft, particularly at the graft–host bone junction, to enhance stability and union. (Figures 5, *A* and *B* are reproduced with permission from Gross AE, Hutchison CR: Proximal femoral allografts for reconstruction of bone stock in revision hip arthroplasty. *Orthopedics* 1998;21:999-1001.) **C,** AP radiograph of a 6-year-old girl with a periprosthetic fracture and loss of proximal femoral bone stock. **D,** AP radiograph of the patient in panel C. The femur has been reconstructed with a proximal femoral allograft. The implant has been cemented into the allograft but not the host bone. The patient's residual femoral bone has been wrapped around the host bone–allograft junction to enhance union and stability. At 4 years, the allograft was united and stable.

diaphyseal-metaphyseal junction. Trial reduction of the prosthesis-allograft composite is carried out, and a step-cut or oblique cut of approximately 2 × 2 cm is marked and cut, adjusting for correct anteversion and length.

On the back table, the graft canal is cleaned and dried; then cement is pressurized into the graft. The stem is inserted in the correct anteversion. Great care is taken to ensure that the cement is recessed around the step-cut to allow host bone contact (Fig. 5, *A*). The composite is then inserted into the host stem and the hip reduced. Wires are passed around or through the lesser trochanter of the allograft for later attachment of the host greater trochanter. The implant is always cemented to the allograft but not to the host bone. We have found that

cementing distally is unnecessary; doing so increases the risk of nonunion and makes further revision more difficult because of the added destruction of distal bone stock. Reamings and other available host bone are applied to the host bone–graft junction to encourage union.

The step-cut is stabilized with cerclage wires; increasingly, we are reinforcing this with cortical struts made from any remnants from the allograft or from the bone bank. When there is a large discrepancy between the diameters of the host femur and the allograft, stabilizing can be difficult; telescoping the graft inside the host bone is occasionally an option but may require trimming of host bone, which we try to avoid. Because we do not obtain a rigid press-fit distally, intraoperative rigid stabilization of the

graft–host bone junction is essential to prevent nonunion. The residual host proximal femur is wrapped around the allograft and held with cerclage wires (Fig. 5, *B* through *D*). An attempt is made to bring these vascularized pieces distally to wrap around the osteotomy junction to encourage union. Finally, the trochanter is reattached to the allograft with the previously placed wires and autografted, if bone is available. The average surgical time, including administration of anesthesia, positioning, and performing acetabular revision, is 4.2 hours (range, 3 to 6 hours).

Prophylactic intravenous antibiotics, usually a cephalosporin, are used postoperatively for 5 days, then orally for 10 days. If the patient is catheterized, gentamicin is added for 24 hours, then oral co-trimoxazole until the catheter is removed. The patient is mobilized with no weight bearing permitted on the treated side until evidence of allograft–host bone union, usually at 3 to 6 months.

Results Between April 1984 and December 1989, we performed 122 total hip arthroplasty revisions using allograft bone on the femoral side. This material included morcellized bone, cortical struts, calcar allografts (less than 5 cm long), and large proximal femoral allografts (more than 5 cm long).

In 60 patients (63 hips) with proximal femoral deficiencies longer than 5 cm, a proximal femoral allograft-prosthesis construct was used. The minimal length of the proximal femoral allograft was 10 cm. Of these 60 consecutive patients, 20 were men and 40, women. Average age at surgery was 62.5 years (range, 30.2 to 81.6 years). The primary diagnosis was osteoarthrosis (in 39 patients), posttraumatic arthritis (6), congenital hip dysplasia (5), rheumatoid arthritis (5), osteonecrosis (2), previous septic arthritis (1), poliomyelitis (1), and Legg-Calvé-Perthes disease (1). All patients had undergone at least one previous total hip arthroplasty of the studied side, with an average of 3.8 (range, one to nine total hip arthroplasties). Three patients had had a prior resection arthroplasty, two for infection and one for aseptic arthroplasty failure.

The mean length of the proximal femoral allograft was 15 cm (range, 10 to 22 cm). The proximal femoral defects were all circumferential cortical defects more than 5 cm long, ranging from 8 to 22 cm as measured from the tip of the greater trochanter.

Clinical and Radiographic Evaluation Each patient was evaluated before surgery with a modified Harris hip score protocol.[25] Living patients either returned for clinical and radiographic evaluation or saw a local orthopaedic surgeon for hip score assessment, and their radiographs were sent for review. Deceased patients'

radiographs and clinical notes were reviewed and relatives contacted when necessary to assess patient function before death. Clinical success was defined as a postoperative increase in the Harris hip score of more than 20 points, a stable implant, and no need for further surgery related to the allograft at the time of review.

Immediate postoperative and successive follow-up AP and lateral radiographs were examined for trochanteric union, allograft–host bone union, endosteal and periosteal resorption, component loosening, and fractures. The allograft was divided into zones similar to those described by Gruen and associates;[31] however, zones 1 and 4 were excluded because of the absence of an allograft trochanter (zone 1) and allograft–host bone junction (zone 4), resulting in five zones. Implant stability was assessed by lucent lines and implant migration: definite loosening was defined as more than 3 mm migration of the implant or fracture of the cement. Mild resorption was classified as partial-thickness resorption of less than 1 cm in length; moderate, as partial-thickness resorption of more than 1 cm in length; and severe, as full-thickness resorption of any length.[32]

Statistical Evaluation The Kaplan-Meier method was used for survivorship analysis, and the 95% confidence intervals (CIs) were calculated with the Greenwood formula for variance.[33] Statistical failure was defined as planned or actual removal of the original allograft-prosthesis construct or as severe radiographic resorption of the allograft. Patients who were deceased or lost to follow-up were censored as of their latest date of review.

Clinical Results At the time of follow-up, a minimum of 9 years 4 months after surgery, 45 patients (75%) were alive, 14 (23%) were deceased, and 1 was lost to follow-up.

The 14 deceased patients represented 14 allografts (22%), with an average dura-

tion from surgery to death of 5 years 7 months (range, 2 years 4 months to 8 years). The patient lost to follow-up moved 4 years after surgery but had had no complications up to that time. All deceased or lost patients thus had a minimum follow-up of 2 years 4 months. The failures or complications of these patients up to the last review are included below.

The living patients represented 48 allografts (76%), with a mean follow-up of 11 years and a median of 10 years 11 months (range, 9 years 4 months to 15 years). There were 28 women and 17 men, with an average age at follow-up of 73 years 11 months (range, 53 to 92 years). The average preoperative modified Harris hip score was 30 (range, 6 to 65); at the latest follow-up of those with the original graft in situ, the average score was 71 (range, 47 to 95), with a mean score of 70.

Radiographic Results Radiographic analysis disclosed four nonunions (6%) at the host bone–allograft junction. Two were treated at 6 months and a third at 12 months with cortical struts and bone grafting (autograft). All three went on to union. At surgery, the fourth patient (a woman aged 70 years) was only mildly symptomatic and declined further surgery. At the most recent follow-up, 11 years 6 months after surgery, the nonunion persisted; as of this writing, the patient has mechanical thigh pain and a Harris hip score of 57 (Fig. 5), and she still does not desire further surgery. Trochanteric escape of more than 1 cm was seen in 14 cases (22%). No fractures occurred.

Peripheral allograft resorption in some form was seen in 13 of the 40 surviving hips (33%) with more than 9 years 4 months of follow-up. Mild resorption occurred in 10 (25%) and moderate resorption in two (5%). Resorption was most common in zones 7 (10 hips) and 2 (6 hips), with three hips having resorption in both zones. In 9 of the 13 hips, this resorption occurred around the cerclage wires. Interestingly, the resorption took several years to become evident but was noted to be nonprogressive in 12 hips, compared with an extensive radiographic review performed on these patients in 1994. One hip showed progressive, full-thickness resorption of more than 1 cm in length; this was at the host bone–allograft nonunion site of the 70-year-old patient (Fig. 5). This full-thickness resorption was associated with subsidence of the allograft-prosthesis construct into the host femur.

One other patient showed subsidence; this was of 14 mm after 11 years and occurred at the prosthesis-cement interface. As of this writing, the graft remains intact with no evidence of resorption; the patient has a Harris hip score of 47 and is awaiting femoral revision. There were no cases of cement fracture or endosteal resorption. No revisions were done for graft resorption.

Rerevisions The total number of complications related to the allograft and requiring further surgery in hips with more than 2 years of follow-up was 13 (21%), including the patient eligible for revision. This total includes five infections, three nonunions, two dislocations, and three cases of late aseptic loosening at an average of 10 years postoperatively. One patient with a nonunion declined surgery, and two dislocations were treated with closed reductions. Thus, the total number of allograft complications is 16 (25%) over the average of 11 years of follow-up. In addition, six complications were related to the acetabular side of the revision surgery.

Overall Results According to our criteria for clinical success, 14 hips were deemed failures: five infections, three nonunions, two dislocations, and two cases of late aseptic loosening that resulted in further surgery, plus two unstable implants: the patient with persistent nonunion who declined surgery and a patient with aseptic loosening at 11 years who as of this writing is awaiting revi-

sion. The success rate of all patients (including deceased and lost patients) was 78% (49 of 63 hips) at an average follow-up of 9 years (range, 2 years 4 months to 15 years). The success rate of those alive at follow-up was 77% (37 of 48 hips) at an average follow-up of 11 years. Of these clinical failures, the three nonunions and two dislocations were treated successfully and retained their allografts without further complication. Four of the five infections and the two aseptic failures were successfully treated with new proximal femoral allografts.

In the statistical analysis, the recurrent dislocation treated with a hemiarthroplasty and the nonunion with severe resorption were recorded as failures. In both of these cases, the allograft has remained in situ for more than 10 years; however, we consider the overall revision arthroplasty to be a failure because of these complications. These two patients function with walking aids and do not desire further surgery. The estimated 5-year survival, according to the Kaplan-Meier method, was 90% (95% CI, 80% to 90%) and, at 10 years, was 86% (95% CI, 74% to 93%).

Cortical Strut Allografts

As previously mentioned, these noncircumferential structural grafts are used to augment bone stock for noncircumferential type 3 femoral defects to reinforce cortical windows and as biologic plates to stabilize periprosthetic fractures, osteotomies, and proximal femoral allograft–host bone junctions.

Surgical Technique Strut grafts were fashioned to fit to the femur where augmentation was necessary. Whole fibular diaphyseal segments usually are used; for larger defects, we use segments of tibia or humerus. Stable fixation of the strut grafts to the host femur usually was obtained with multiple 16-gauge cerclage wires. When available, autogenous morcellized graft was placed along the allograft–host bone junction to enhance

union. Excessive circumferential stripping of soft tissue was avoided to preserve as much periosteal circulation as possible (Fig. 6).

Results Between March 31, 1987, and April 1, 1996, 52 patients were identified with revision total hip arthroplasty using cortical strut allografts. Thirty-three patients had cementless porous-coated femoral components, five had press-fit stems, and seven had cemented stems, while seven revisions had been done in conjunction with proximal femoral allografts. The average follow-up was 4.8 years (range, 1.6 to 10.0 years). Average patient age was 65 years (range, 33 to 87 years). Allograft was harvested and stored according to the guidelines of the American Association of Tissues Banks,[27] deep-frozen to –70C°, and irradiated (2.5 Mrad). All cortical struts were fashioned from fibulae.

Radiographic analysis was carried out to determine the union rate, the remodeling, and incorporation of the strut grafts. The following radiographic factors were studied: location and dimension of the allografts, resorption and incorporation of the allografts, and union between the cortical strut allograft and host bone. In measuring the length of the cortical struts, the circumferential wires were used as reference points. All measurements were done on serial radiographs by two of the authors (K.S. and I.W.). Radiographic failure was defined as either nonunion, fractures of the strut grafts, or significant progressive graft resorption. The graft was considered united when there was bony bridging between any part of the graft and host bone. Resorption was considered significant when it involved any part of the grafts except the ends and was obviously not part of a remodeling process.

The clinical results were evaluated with the modified Harris hip score. The underlying diagnoses were osteoarthritis in 27 patients, hip dysplasia in 8, and femoral neck fractures in 6. Four patients

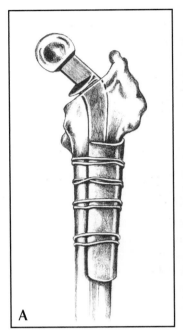
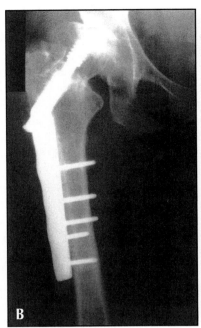
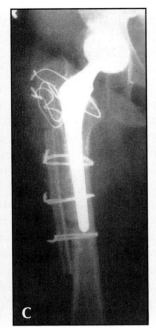
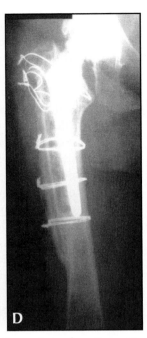

Fig. 6 A, A cortical strut allograft held by cerclage wires over a noncircumferential cortical defect. (Reproduced with permission from Gross AE: Revision arthroplasty of the hip using allograft bone, in Czitrom AA, Gross AE (eds): *Allografts in Orthopaedic Practice*. Baltimore, MD, Williams & Wilkins, 1992, pp 147-173.) **B,** AP radiograph of a 45-year-old woman with osteonecrosis after failed internal fixation of a subcapital fracture. **C,** The same patient as in panel *B*. A cortical strut allograft has been used to bypass stress risers in conjunction with an uncemented femoral component. **D,** The same patient as in panels *B* and *C*. Two years postoperatively, the cortical strut is united, with excellent remodeling.

had rheumatoid arthritis; the remaining diagnoses included osteonecrosis (three patients), infected total hip arthroplasties (two), and previous excisional arthroplasties (two). Many of the patients in this study had had multiple previous surgical procedures (average, two) in the hip.

Seven of the cortical struts were used to stabilize segmental femoral allograft–host bone junctions. Forty-five were used to graft noncircumferential femoral defects—for example, cortical windows, perforations, erosions, osteolysis. Most of the grafts (48) were placed laterally. Two grafts were placed medially; two were anterior strut grafts. There were no fractures of the strut grafts or infections.

Radiographically, the average length of the strut allografts immediately postoperatively was 154 mm (range, 66 to 280 mm). The length of the strut allografts at final follow-up was 143 mm (range, 54 to 258 mm). The percentage decrease in length of the struts was 8% (range, none to 48%) and in all but two cases appeared to be part of remodeling at the end of the grafts (ie, rounding off).

There were two nonunions (for a 96% union rate) but no graft fractures. The average time for union to occur was 10 months. In addition, two patients had significant progressive resorption of more than 50% of the grafts. Thus, the overall radiographic failure rate was 8% (4 of 52 patients). Resorption commonly occurred at the ends of the strut allograft and, except in the two previously mentioned cases, was not progressive and was part of the remodeling process. The process of incorporation in some patients took more than 2 years to complete.

Mean preoperative and postoperative Harris hip scores were 39.4 (range, 6 to 90) and 65.6 (range, 21 to 97), respectively. The average amount of femoral subsidence was 8.5 mm (range, none to 45 mm). Thirty-eight of the 52 patients had cementless femoral stems. The cemented stems did not subside; six cementless femoral stems had subsidence of more than 1 cm and had to be revised, for a rerevision rate of 12% for the entire series. All other cementless stems had subsidence of less than 5 mm. The cortical struts were not used to support the implant and were not considered a causative factor in the subsidence.

Summary

The role of allograft tissue, including bone, cartilage and soft tissue, has become more defined in lower extremity reconstructive surgery. Revision arthroplasty of the hip commonly requires restoration of bone stock using allograft bone. Morcellized bone is used for contained defects on both the acetabular and femoral sides. Structural allograft bone is used for uncontained or segmental defects, and the results are less predictable; therefore, its use is more controversial. Alternatives include the jumbo cup, oblong cup, and high hip center on the pelvic side and tumor prostheses or distal fixation on the femoral side. These alternatives do not, however, restore bone stock, thus making further surgery more difficult. Structural grafts allow attachment of bone and soft tissue and restoration of the correct anatomy and have been shown to restore bone stock for further surgery, particularly on the acetabular side. Improvements in the quality and safety of banked bone and the development of surgical techniques have enhanced the results of structural allograft bone grafting. Restoring bone stock in revision arthroplasty of the hip is an accepted standard for the patient likely to undergo further surgery. Continuing to develop technologies that will facilitate the use of allograft tissue is imperative.

References

1. Gross AE, Duncan CP, Garbuz D, Mohamed EM: Revision arthroplasty of the acetabulum in association with loss of bone stock. *J Bone Joint Surg Am* 1998;80:440-451.
2. Fabroni RH, Castagno A, Aguilera AL, Steverlynck AM, Zeballos J: Long-term results of limb salvage with the Fabroni custom made endoprosthesis. *Clin Orthop* 1999;358:41-52.
3. Sim FH, Chao EY: Hip salvage by proximal femoral replacement. *J Bone Joint Surg Am* 1981;63:1228-1239.
4. Shin DS, Weber KL, Chao EY, An KN, Sim FH: Reoperation for failed prosthetic replacement used for limb salvage. *Clin Orthop* 1999;358:53-63.
5. Clarke HD, Berry DJ, Sim FH: Salvage of failed femoral megaprostheses with allograft prosthesis composites. *Clin Orthop* 1998;356:222-229.
6. Judet R, Judet J, Letournel E: Fractures of the acetabulum: Classification and surgical approaches for open reduction: Preliminary report. *J Bone Joint Surg Am* 1964;46:1615-1646.
7. Alexeeff M, Mahomed N, Morsi E, Garbuz D, Gross A: Structural allograft in two-stage revisions for failed septic hip arthroplasty. *J Bone Joint Surg Br* 1996;78:213-216.
8. Heekin RD, Engh CA, Vinh T: Morselized allograft in acetabular reconstruction: A post-mortem retrieval analysis. *Clin Orthop* 1995;319:184-190.
9. Silverton CD, Rosenberg AG, Sheinkop MB, Kull LR, Galante JO: Revision of the acetabular component without cement after total hip arthroplasty: A follow-up note regarding results at seven to eleven years. *J Bone Joint Surg Am* 1996;78:1366-1370.
10. Tanzer M, Drucker D, Jasty M, McDonald M, Harris WH: Revision of the acetabular components with an uncemented Harris-Galante porous-coated prosthesis. *J Bone Joint Surg Am* 1992;74:987-994.
11. Slooff TJ, Buma P, Schreurs BW, Schimmel JW, Huiskes R, Gardeniers J: Acetabular and femoral reconstruction with impacted graft and cement. *Clin Orthop* 1996;324:108-115.
12. Zehntner MK, Ganz R: Midterm results (5.5-10 years) of acetabular allograft reconstruction with the acetabular reinforcement ring during total hip revision. *J Arthroplasty* 1994;9:469-479.
13. Wong P, Saleh KJ, King A, Gross AE: Acetabular revision with a roof reinforcement ring and impacted allograft bone. *Hip International* 2000;10:145-150.
14. Harris WH: Reconstruction at a high hip center in acetabular revision surgery using a cementless acetabular component. *Orthopedics* 1998;21:991-992.
15. DeBoer DK, Christie MJ: Reconstruction of the deficient acetabulum with an oblong prosthesis: Three-to-seven-year results. *J Arthroplasty* 1998;13:674-680.
16. Koster G, Willert HG, Kohler HP, Dopkens K: An oblong revision cup for large acetabular defects: Design rationale and two-to-seven-year follow-up. *J Arthroplasty* 1998;13:559-569.
17. Saleh KJ, Jaroszynski G, Woodgate I. Saleh L, Gross AE: Revision total hip arthroplasty with the use of structural acetabular allograft and reconstruction ring: A case series with a 10-year average follow-up. *J Arthroplasty* 2000;15:951-958.
18. Chandler HP, Ayres DK, Tan RC, Anderson LC, Varma AK: Revision total hip replacement using the S-ROM femoral component. *Clin Orthop* 1995;319:130-140.
19. Peters CL, Rivero DP, Kull LR, Jacobs JJ, Rosenberg AG, Galante JO: Revision total hip arthroplasty without cement: subsidence of proximally porous-coated femoral components. *J Bone Joint Surg Am* 1995;77:1217-1226.
20. Gie GA, Linder L, Ling RS, Simon JP, Slooff TJ, Timperley AJ: Impacted cancellous allografts and cement for revision total hip arthroplasty. *J Bone Joint Surg Br* 1993;75:14-21.
21. Estok DM II, Harris WH: Long-term results of cemented femoral revision surgery using second-generation techniques: An average 11.7-year follow-up evaluation. *Clin Orthop* 1994;299:190-202.
22. Paprosky WG: Distal fixation with fully coated stems in femoral revision: A 16-year follow-up. *Orthopedics* 1998;21:993-995.
23. Wagner H, Wagner M: Conical stem fixation for cementless hip prostheses for primary implantation and revisions, in Morscher E, Frey-Zund O (eds): *Endoprosthetics*. Berlin, Germany, Springer-Verlag, 1995, pp 258-267.
24. Head WC, Malinin TI, Mallory TH, Emerson RH Jr: Onlay cortical allografting for the femur. *Orthop Clin North Am* 1998;29:307-312.
25. Gross AE, Hutchison CR, Alexeeff M, Mahomed N, Leitch K, Morsi E: Proximal femoral allografts for reconstruction of bone stock in revision arthroplasty of the hip. *Clin Orthop* 1995;319:151-158.
26. Glassman AH, Engh CA, Bobyn JD: A technique of extensile exposure for total hip arthroplasty. *J Arthroplasty* 1987;2:11-21.
27. Jacobs NJ: Establishing a surgical bone bank, in Fawcett KJ, Barr AR (eds): *Tissue Banking*. Arlington, VA, American Association of Blood Banks, 1987, pp 67-96.
28. Garbuz D, Morsi E, Mohamed N, Gross AE: Classification and reconstruction in revision acetabular arthroplasty with bone stock deficiency. *Clin Orthop* 1996;324:98-107.
29. Morsi E, Garbuz D, Gross AE: Revision total hip arthroplasty with shelf bulk allografts: A long-term follow-up study. *J Arthroplasty* 1996;11:86-90.
30. Woodgate IG, Saleh KJ, Jaroszynski G, Agnidis Z, Woodgate MM, Gross AE: Minor column structural acetabular allografts in revision hip arthroplasty. *Clin Orthop* 2000;371:75-85.
31. Gruen TA, McNeice GM, Amstutz HC: "Modes of failure" of cemented stem-type femoral components: A radiographic analysis of loosening. *Clin Orthop* 1979;141:17-27.
32. Gross AE, Hutchison CR: Proximal femoral allografts for reconstruction of bone stock in revision hip arthroplasty. *Orthopedics* 1998;21:999-1001.
33. Kaplan EL, Meier P: Non-parametric estimation from incomplete observations. *J Am Stat Assoc* 1958;53:457-481.

Managing Bone Loss in Acetabular Revision

Scott M. Sporer, MD, MS
Wayne G. Paprosky, MD
Michael R. O'Rourke, MD

Abstract

The management of bone loss encountered during acetabular revision remains challenging. In order to obtain a successful surgical result, preoperative planning is required to estimate the severity and location of bone defects. Most acetabular revisions can be treated with the use of a cementless hemispherical component. However, a successful surgical reconstruction requires component stability. Depending on the degree of bone loss, the surgical reconstruction may require the use of cancellous or structural bone graft, acetabular augmentation, an acetabular cage, a custom implant, or an acetabular transplant.

Revision of cemented acetabular components is most commonly performed because of aseptic loosening with migration of the component. The most challenging aspect of acetabular revision is the management of bone loss compromising implant fixation and stability. The severity of bone loss can be pronounced, as a result of asymptomatic osteolysis and stress-shielding, before migration of cementless components. This bone loss is a common condition that is expected to become more common in the future.

The prevalence of revision hip arthroplasty is 18% in the United States and 8% in the Swedish registry. The indications for acetabular revision include symptomatic aseptic loosening, failure of fixation, infection, wear, osteolysis, and insta-

bility. Revision may be indicated for an asymptomatic patient who has progressive osteolysis, severe wear, or bone loss that could compromise a future reconstruction. Contraindications for revision of the acetabular component include severe bone loss precluding allograft fixation or implant fixation, uncontrolled infection, or medical comorbidities that preclude surgery.

Options for Acetabular Revision

Several options, including both nonbiologic and biologic fixation, are available for acetabular revision. Nonbiologic fixation refers to any method of reconstruction that achieves stability of the acetabular component through a mechanical construct without the need for os-

seointegration between the acetabular shell and the host bone. Biologic fixation refers to any surgical option that requires direct contact with host bone and osseointegration into the acetabular shell to provide long-term fixation. Nonbiologic fixation options include cementing of a polyethylene cup, use of a superior structural allograft and a cemented polyethylene cup with or without an antiprotrusio cage, impaction grafting with or without an antiprotrusio cage, and application of a total acetabular allograft. Biologic fixation options include use of a hemispherical cementless cup at the anatomic hip center or a high hip center (> 2 cm superior to the native hip center), a jumbo cup (66 to 80 mm), an oblong cup, a cementless hemispherical cup supported by structural allograft, and a modular cementless implant system.

Because the outcomes of acetabular revision have been better with cementless fixation than they have been with cement fixation, cementless fixation has become the preferred method for most acetabular revisions. Templeton and associates[1] and Gaffey and associates[2] reported no instances of aseptic loosening of cementless Harris-Galante I components used for revisions of cemented components, whereas cemented revision acetabular components had a 14% rate of revision for aseptic loosening and a 33% prevalence of radiographic evidence of aseptic loosening. Della Valle and associates,[3] in a study of the experience with cementless acetabular revision at the Rush University Medical Center, found aseptic loosening in 2 of 138 patients followed for a mean of 15 years, with revision (for any reason) reported in 19 of the 138 patients. In a study of the results of cementless revisions performed by Harris, Hallstrom and associates[4] reported a rate of aseptic loosening of 11% (13 of 122) and a rate of revision because of aseptic loosening of 4% (5 of 122).

Reliable and durable fixation of cementless acetabular components requires intimate contact between the implant and viable bone as well as mechanical stability (motion of less than 40 to 50 μm). Bone loss can compromise both of these prerequisites for successful use of cementless implants. The amount of host bone required to provide durable fixation is not known. Although it is difficult to measure the amount of bone supporting an implant, most surgeons believe that 50% to 60% is necessary. This value was derived from the literature and is a measure of the coverage of the acetabular component in the coronal plane as seen on an AP radiograph. However, the support of an implant is geometrically more complex than can be determined on a two-dimensional radiograph alone. The location of the remaining supportive bone probably has a more important role in providing durable fixation than does the quantity of bone. Finally, the percentage of bone necessary to support the implant probably decreases as the implant

size increases because of the increased surface area.

Inherent Stability

Although there are reports of the successful use of cementless cups in revision surgery without the achievement of an initial press-fit,[1,3] we believe that it is necessary to achieve inherent stability of the implant. Trial components are used to accomplish this goal and to assess the remaining bone stock properly. A trial implant can have full inherent stability, partial inherent stability, or no inherent stability. A trial component with full inherent stability will not be displaced by pushing on its rim or by trial reduction. A trial component with partial inherent stability will maintain its position while the inserter is removed, but it will be displaced by loading of its rim and by trial reduction. Finally, when a trial component has no inherent stability, support by host bone is inadequate to maintain placement of the component in the desired location once the inserter is removed.

Classification and Decision Making
AAOS Classification
The AAOS (American Academy of Orthopaedic Surgeons) classification of bone defects, described by D'Antonio and associates,[5,6] identifies the pattern and location of bone loss but does not quantify the defect. The bone loss is classified as contained, segmental, combined contained and segmental, pelvic discontinuity, and ankylosis. This is the most commonly used classification in the literature.

Paprosky Classification
This classification system is based on the severity of bone loss and the

ability to obtain cementless fixation for a given bone loss pattern.[7] The key to the classification is determining the ability of the remaining host bone to provide initial stability to a hemispherical cementless acetabular component until ingrowth occurs. Intraoperative decisions are based on the findings when trial components are used. The amount of rim that remains determines the stability of the trial implant and is one of the variables that identifies the type of acetabular defect. A type I defect has an undistorted rim; a type II defect, a distorted but intact rim with adequate remaining bone to support a hemispherical cementless implant; and a type III defect, a nonsupportive rim.

Radiographic Correlation Preoperative findings on the AP radiograph of the pelvis are used to predict the type of defect and allow the surgeon to plan for the acetabular reconstruction accordingly. The four criteria that are important to assess on the preoperative radiograph are: (1) superior migration of the hip center, (2) ischial osteolysis, (3) teardrop osteolysis, and (4) position of the implant relative to the Kohler line.

Superior migration of the hip center represents bone loss in the acetabular dome involving the anterior and posterior columns. Superior and medial migration indicates a greater involvement of the anterior column. Superior and lateral migration indicates a greater involvement of the posterior column. The amount of superior migration is measured as the distance in millimeters (adjusted for magnification) relative to the superior obturator line.

Ischial osteolysis indicates bone loss from the inferior aspect of the posterior column, including the posterior wall. The amount of ischial osteolysis is quantified by measuring the distance from the most inferior extent of the lytic area to the superior obturator line.

Teardrop osteolysis indicates bone loss from the inferior and medial aspect of the acetabulum, including the inferior aspect of the anterior column, the lateral aspect of the pubis, and the medial wall. Moderate osteolysis includes partial destruction of the structure with maintenance of the medial limb of the teardrop. Severe involvement means complete obliteration of the teardrop.

Medial migration of the component relative to the Kohler line represents a deficiency of the anterior column. The Kohler line is defined as a line connecting the most lateral aspect of the pelvic brim and the most lateral aspect of the obturator foramen on an AP radiograph of the pelvis. The medial aspect of the implant is lateral to the Kohler line with grade 1 migration and medial to the line with grade 3 migration. With grade 2, there is migration to the Kohler line or slight remodeling of the iliopubic and ilioischial lines without a break in continuity.

Type I Defect With a type I defect, the acetabular rim is intact and supportive without distortion (Figure 1). The acetabulum is hemispherical, and there may be small focal areas of contained bone loss (cement anchor sites). The anterior and posterior columns are intact. A hemispherical cementless implant is almost completely supported by native bone and has full inherent stability.

The preoperative radiograph shows no migration of the component and no evidence of osteolysis in the ischium or teardrop, and the Kohler line has not been violated (the medialmost aspect of the component is lateral to the Kohler line).

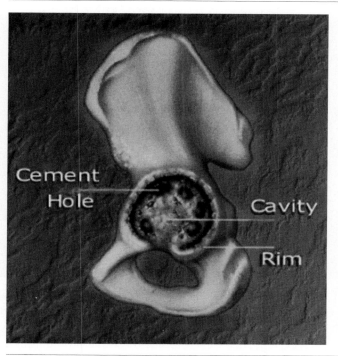

Figure 1 Type I acetabular defect. Note that the rim remains supportive and will provide full stability for a hemispherical component.

Type II Defect In a type II defect, the acetabulum is distorted but there is adequate host bone to support a cementless acetabular component (Figure 2, *A*). The trial component has full inherent stability. The distortion may be superior and lateral, superior and medial, or directly medial. At least 50% of the surface area of the component is in contact with host bone for potential ingrowth, and good mechanical support can be provided entirely by host bone. The anterior and posterior columns remain intact and supportive. The hip center can be elevated as much as 1.5 cm to achieve superior contact and support.

On the preoperative radiograph of a type II defect, the superior migration of the hip center is < 3 cm from the superior obturator line and there is no substantial osteolysis of the ischium or teardrop (ischial osteolysis extending < 7 mm distal to the obturator line).

In a type IIA defect, the pattern of bone loss is superior and medial, al-

lowing migration of the failed component into a cavitary defect medial to the thinned intact superior rim. In most patients, the defect is treated with particulate allograft because the defect is contained. The remaining superior rim provides a buttress for containment of the allograft.

In a type IIB defect, less than one third of the circumference of the superior rim is deficient, and the defect is not contained. The remaining anterior and posterior rims and columns can support an implant. Allograft is used to restore bone stock and not to support the implant. The defect is segmental, and a femoral head allograft may be chosen. The majority of reconstructions are done without grafting of the segmental defect.

In a type IIC defect, there is a medial wall defect and migration of the acetabular component medial to the Kohler line (Figure 2, *B*). The rim of the acetabulum is intact and will support a hemispherical component. Reconstruction of these de-

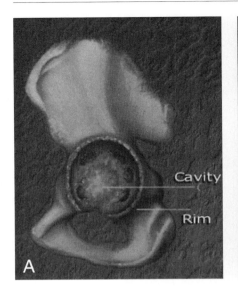
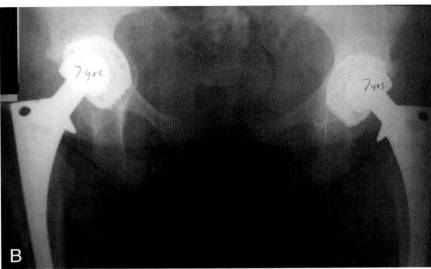

Figure 2 **A,** Type II acetabular defect. Note the rim defect. The remaining host bone is supportive and will provide full stability for a hemispherical component. **B,** Preoperative radiograph of a type IIC acetabular defect. Note the violation of the Kohler line.

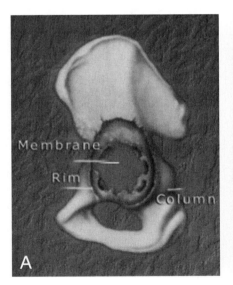
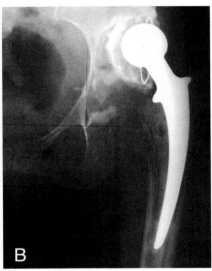
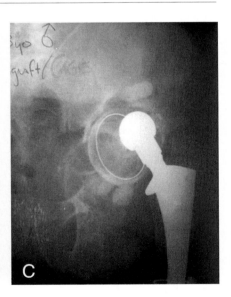

Figure 3 **A,** Type III acetabular defect. The remaining host bone is not supportive and will not provide full stability for a hemispherical component. **B,** Preoperative radiograph of a type IIIA acetabular defect. Note the superior-lateral migration and loss of the superior dome. **C,** Preoperative radiograph of a type IIIB acetabular defect. Note the superior-medial migration with disruption of the Kohler line.

fects is similar to the treatment of protrusio acetabuli in the setting of a primary arthroplasty. Sequentially larger reamers are used until the acetabular rim is engaged. Particulate bone graft can be placed medially to lateralize the hip center of rotation back to its anatomic position.

Type III Defect The remaining acetabular rim in a type III defect will not provide adequate initial component stability to achieve reliable biologic fixation (Figure 3, *A*). The trial implant lacks full intrinsic stability. The use of structural allograft is an option to restore the

center of rotation to the proper anatomic location and to provide mechanical stability for the implant.

In a type IIIA defect, there is adequate host bone in contact with the ingrowth surface of the implant to obtain durable biologic fixation (Figure 3, *B*)—that is, more than 40% to

60% of the surface area of the cementless cup is in contact with host bone. The trial component has partial inherent mechanical stability. Support of the implant with a structural augment or allograft is necessary in the short term to provide initial stability and thus allow ingrowth into the areas of the implant that are in contact with the host bone. The defect involves more than one third but not more than one half of the circumference and usually is located between the 10 o'clock and 2 o'clock positions. Preoperative radiographs show superior and lateral migration of the component < 3 cm above the obturator line (with adjustment for magnification). Ischial lysis is mild to moderate, extending <15 mm inferior to the obturator line. There is partial destruction of the teardrop, but the medial limb of the teardrop usually is present. The component is at or lateral to the Kohler line, and the ilioischial and iliopubic lines are intact.

In a type IIIB defect, host bone is in contact with < 40% of the ingrowth surface of the implant. Inherent stability is not achievable with a trial implant. The defect involves more than half of the circumference of the rim, and it usually extends from the 9 o'clock to the 5 o'clock position (Figure 3, C). Patients with a type IIIB defect are at high risk for occult pelvic discontinuity, and this possibility must be ruled out at the time of reconstruction. Preoperative radiographs show extensive ischial osteolysis (extending > 15 mm distal to the superior obturator line), complete destruction of the teardrop, migration medial to the Kohler line, and migration > 3 cm superior to the obturator line. With a type IIIB defect, the failed acetabular component migrates superiorly and medially, in contrast to the migration

with the type IIIA defect, which is superior and lateral.

Algorithmic Approach to Decision Making

An algorithmic approach to revision of the acetabulum is shown in Figure 4. We use a posterolateral approach to the hip for all acetabular revisions. The initial decision regarding how to proceed with the surgery depends on the superior migration of the hip center before the revision. If the hip center has not migrated > 3 cm above the superior obturator line, the surgeon determines whether full inherent stability can be achieved with a trial component. If it can, the defect is classified as type I or type II, and a hemispherical cementless implant is used. If there is migration medial to the Kohler line, the defect is classified as type IIC and the rim will support the hemispherical implant.

When the hip center has migrated > 3 cm superior to the superior obturator line or the surgeon is unable to achieve full inherent stability of the hemispherical trial component, the defect is classified as type III. If a trial component has partial inherent stability, there is generally enough contact with host bone to support ingrowth and therefore the defect is type IIIA. Type IIIA defects usually have an oblong shape, but occasionally they are spherical. If the defect is spherical, a jumbo cup may be appropriate. With oblong remodeling of the host acetabulum, the options include a structural distal femoral graft with a cementless hemispherical cup, a modular trabecular metal augment with a hemispherical cup, or a high hip center hemispherical cup. The former two options are appropriate when restoration of an anatomic hip center is desired. With both the structural distal femoral

graft and the modular augment, the goal is to provide support to a hemispherical implant that has partial inherent stability until there is adequate supportive ingrowth into the cup. The advantages of a distal femoral allograft are the good results that have been seen with longer follow-up and the restoration of bone for future reconstruction if necessary. The potential advantages of a modular cup-and-augment system include less stripping of the ilium and less mobilization of the abductors, a technically easier and faster procedure, and the fact that the augment does not have the potential for resorption. The disadvantages of this method include its unknown long-term durability, the potential for debris generation at the interface, the potential for fatigue failure, and the inability to restore bone stock for future revisions.

When the hemispherical trial component has no inherent stability, the defect is classified as type IIIB. When pelvic discontinuity has been ruled out, the options for treatment of such defects include (1) nonbiologic fixation with an impaction allograft supported with a cage or with a structural allograft (an acetabular allograft or a distal femoral allograft) supported with a cage and (2) biologic fixation with a modular trabecular metal system or a custom triflanged implant.

In the presence of pelvic discontinuity, we determine intraoperatively whether the discontinuity appears to be acute, with the potential for healing, or chronic, without the potential for healing. If healing is possible, we use a compression plate across the dissociation as well as one of the reconstructive approaches described for a type IIIB defect above. When there is no potential for healing, we distract the discontinuity and insert

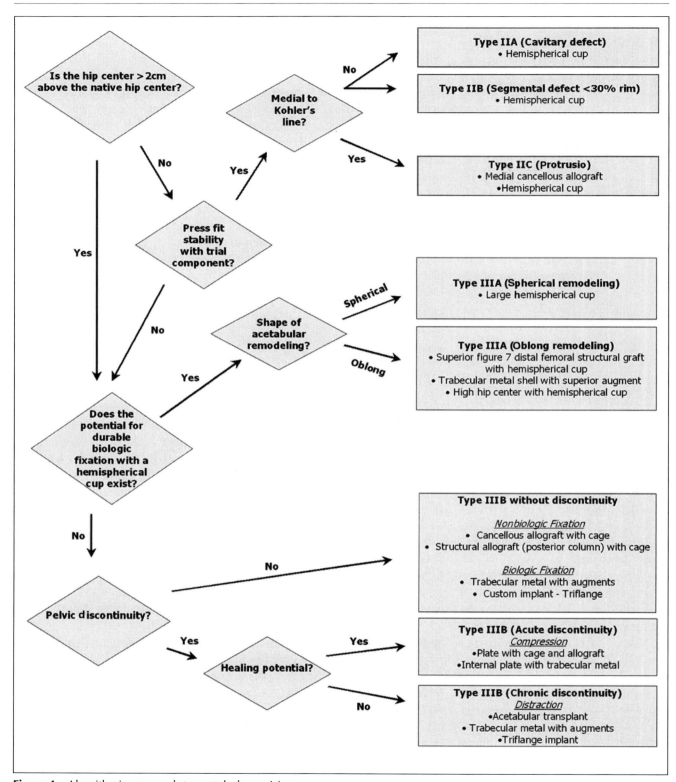

Figure 4 Algorithmic approach to acetabular revision.

bone graft into the defect. The initial stability of the structural graft or the modular reconstruction is greatly enhanced by distraction (as opposed to compression, with which there is little chance for the host bone to bring about healing of the discontinuity).

Techniques
General Principles
Preoperative planning based on the aforementioned classification system is critical so that the appropriate grafting material, tools for implant removal, and components are available at the time of surgery. If there has been extensive medial migration, imaging (angiography or CT scanning with intravascular infusion of contrast medium) and possibly intrapelvic mobilization of vascular structures should be considered.

The patient must be positioned carefully, with particular attention paid to the orientation of the pelvis and torso relative to the floor, as internal landmarks often are distorted in the setting of revision surgery. A posterolateral approach is used. Extensile exposures often are necessary, with the incision extending toward the posterior superior iliac spine. The plane between the iliotibial band and the underlying vastus lateralis and the abductors (often scarred to the iliotibial band) is redeveloped. After the borders of the gluteus medius and gluteus minimus have been identified, the plane between the gluteus minimus and the capsule is identified and the abductors are mobilized anteriorly. We do not routinely expose the sciatic nerve unless dissection through heterotopic ossification is necessary. A posterior capsular flap is developed off of the greater trochanter subperiosteally and is extended to the superior aspect of the acetabulum and

then continued distally along the proximal part of the femur in a subperiosteal fashion. Intraoperative evaluations (a cell count and analysis of frozen sections) are done to rule out infection. We assume that a white blood cell count of $< 3,000/\mu L$ (3.0×10^9/L) indicates the absence of infection and a count of $> 10,000/\mu L$ (10.0×10^9/L) indicates the presence of an infection. When the cell count is between 3,000 and $10,000/\mu L$, we base our decision on the C-reactive protein level and on the findings of the analysis of frozen sections.

The posterior flap is retracted, and an anterior capsulectomy is done. If the femoral component is to be retained, an anterior pouch is developed for placement of the retained component during retraction. The superior aspect of the ilium and the posterior column are dissected in the subperiosteal plane to obtain the necessary exposure. An extended trochanteric osteotomy may be needed, depending on the visualization and the anticipated reconstruction of the femur. After the removal of the existing components, a systematic débridement of granulation tissue and interface membrane is performed to assess the entire remaining acetabular bone stock and to rule out the possibility of a pelvic discontinuity.

Type IIC Defects
In most type IIC defects, particulate graft is placed medially. If the medial membrane is not a sufficient buttress for the particulate graft, a femoral head cut into a wafer, with the diameter of the wafer greater than the diameter of the medial bone defect, can be used as a buttress for the particulate graft. Use of acetabular reamers in reverse impacts the cancellous allograft medially and recre-

ates the hemispherical shape of the socket. As more cancellous allograft is added medially, the reamer begins to translate laterally and to catch on the rim. The reamers (used in reverse) disengage from the reamer drive shaft as they come into contact with the host bone rim. At this point, sufficient graft has been placed medially.

Type IIIA Defects
Distal Femoral Structural Allograft With a Cementless Acetabular Component To optimize the outcome, an appropriate graft must be selected to match the mechanical demands of the proposed reconstruction. We do not use a femoral head allograft when the graft is to serve a structurally supportive role. Instead, we use a fresh-frozen distal femoral or proximal tibial allograft. The trabecular patterns of the graft are oriented parallel to the direction of load to optimize stress transfer. The graft is contoured to maximize the contact surface area between it and the host bone, to optimize the chance of union. The allograft should be fixed to the host bone with 6.5-mm screws oriented parallel with one another in the direction of loading, without interfering with placement or fixation of the component. If there is pelvic discontinuity, fixation with a posterior column plate should be performed before proceeding with the allografting. The fixation of the acetabular component to the host bone-allograft reconstruction is separate from the fixation of the allograft to the host bone.

The goal of acetabular reconstruction with the use of a structural allograft is to obtain a stable construct with the hip center of rotation positioned at the level of the native acetabulum. The desired hip center

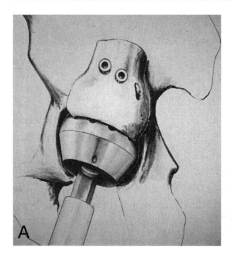
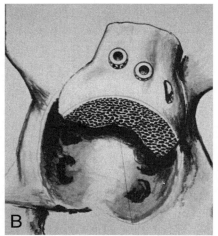
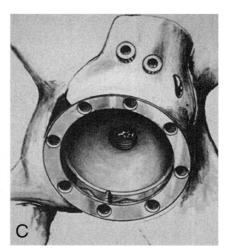

Figure 5 The surgical technique used to reconstruct a type IIIA acetabular defect with a distal femoral allograft. (Reproduced with permission from: Sporer SM, O'Rourke M, Chong P, Paprosky WG: The use of structural distal femoral allografts for acetabular reconstruction: Average ten-year follow-up. *J Bone Joint Surg Am* 2005;87:761.) **A,** Allograft bone is secured to the superior dome with multiple 6.5-mm cancellous screws. **B,** Allograft is reamed until the host anterior and posterior columns are engaged. **C,** A cementless hemispherical shell is inserted and is secured with multiple screws.

is identified, and acetabular reamers are used to size and shape the acetabulum for a hemispherical cementless implant. After it is ascertained that adequate host bone is available to come into contact with the implant, a trial component is placed to determine areas of contact, inherent stability, and the location of segmental loss.

Preparation of the distal femoral allograft begins with trimming of the epicondyles so that the medial-to-lateral dimension of the allograft matches the diameter of the acetabular cavity. A female reamer that is about 1 to 2 mm larger than the acetabular cavity is then used to ream the distal aspect of the allograft in slight flexion, to avoid notching of the anterior cortex of the graft and so that the reamed condyles will be directed into the acetabular cavity. The metaphyseal portion of the allograft is then cut in the coronal plane to create the shape of the number 7, with the anterior aspect of the metadiaphyseal bone left in continuity with the distal condyles.

The superior aspect of the allograft (the anterior cortex) is generally approximately 5 to 6 cm in length.

The angle between the condyles and the anterior cortex on the posterior aspect of the allograft is contoured with a burr to optimize the contact between the allograft and the host ilium. If a ledge of bone is present between the lateral margin of the ilium and the depth of the acetabular cavity at the site of the defect, the allograft should be cut at a more acute angle. This "tongue-in-groove" effect will provide tremendous stability at the graft-host junction.

The superior limb of the allograft is contoured to the lateral aspect of the ilium and is secured provisionally with Steinmann pins. It is important to tap the allograft screw-holes, to minimize the risk of fracture, before placing four parallel 6.5-mm cancellous screws with washers. The screws should be oriented obliquely into the ilium in the direction of loading to compress the graft against the remaining ilium. The acetabular

cavity then can be reamed to contour the portion of the graft that will be in contact with the component. Smaller reamers initially are used, and then the reamers are sequentially increased in size to obtain the dimensions of the desired acetabular cavity. Care must be taken to prevent removal of additional host bone or inadequate reaming of the allograft that can cause failure of contact between the remaining host bone and the component. Remaining voids are filled with particulate allograft, and a cementless cup is impacted into the newly sculpted acetabular cavity and fixed with multiple screws for adjunctive fixation (Figure 5).

Modular Trabecular Metal System
Treatment of a type IIIA defect with a modular trabecular metal system begins with use of acetabular reamers to identify the desired location for the cup placement and to determine the location of all remaining supportive host bone (which is usually anterior-superior and posterior-inferior). Progressive reaming is performed to en-

gage the bone of the anterior and posterior columns to achieve partial inherent stability of the trial acetabular component. With the trial component in the appropriate amount of version and abduction, the posterior-superior augment is placed against the host bone. The augment can be placed in any position or orientation to improve the initial stability, and the bone or the augment can be contoured with a barrel burr to optimize the surface contact area. With the trial component in place, the augment is secured to the host bone with screws. The augment is then packed with bone graft, leaving the portion facing the cup exposed. Polymethylmethacrylate cement is placed directly onto the trabecular metal revision cup but only in the areas mating with the augment. The acetabular component is then firmly impacted to achieve a press-fit against the host bone. We recommend the placement of multiple screws for initial fixation. If the liner is cemented, one should consider placing bone wax into the end of the screws to facilitate removal if needed.

Type IIIB Defects

Total Acetabular Transplant With a Cage Acetabular reamers are used to size the acetabular cavity and to identify the location of all remaining bone to support the allograft. The ledge of bone on the superior aspect of the ilium that will abut against the allograft should be identified. The acetabulum of the allograft is reamed on the back table, with care taken not to weaken it by excessive reaming. A cage is sized to the allograft before placement. The allograft hemipelvis is cut in a curvilinear fashion from the greater sciatic notch to the anterior superior iliac spine to maintain a portion of the ilium attached to the acetabulum. The pubic and ischial portions of the allograft are cut distal to the confluence of the acetabulum with enough length to accommodate the inferior defects. One should avoid leaving excessive inferior bone on the allograft that prevents optimal medialization of the inferior aspect of the graft as this can result in vertical cup placement and lateralization of the hip center. Medialization of the hip center is desired.

A female reamer, 1 to 2 mm larger than the acetabular reamer used to size the acetabulum, can be used to mark and shape the medial aspect of the graft to fit the defect. A groove is made in the superior aspect of the ilium of the allograft to correspond to the ledge of bone along the superior aspect of the native acetabulum. This tongue-and-groove junction provides a stable buttress between the host and the allograft. A burr is used to debulk the inner table of the ilium on the allograft and to maintain a shelf distally that will fill the acetabular defect. The allograft should be press-fit and then secured with Steinmann pins provisionally. It is then fixed with four 6.5-mm partially threaded screws with washers directed obliquely into the ilium from both the intra-articular and the lateral iliac aspects of the graft. A pelvic reconstruction plate is then contoured to the posterior column, ideally with three screws in the native ilium and ischium. It is recommended that a cage, secured with cage-host bone screws as well as cage-allograft bone screws, be used to protect all transplants. If possible, the inferior flange of the cage is inserted into a slot in the ischium for fixation. A metal shell or a polyethylene liner is then cemented into the cage-allograft composite, with the surgeon avoiding the tendency to place the component in a vertical and/or retroverted position.

Modular Trabecular Metal System

When a type IIIB defect is treated with a modular trabecular metal system, the acetabular defect is sized with reamers in the desired location to find the dimension of the cavity until two points of fixation are achieved (anterior to posterior, anterior-inferior to posterior-inferior, or posterior-superior to anterior-inferior). Augments are used to decrease acetabular volume and to restore a rim to support a revision cup. The location and orientation of the augments are highly variable, depending on the bone loss pattern. Augments are often placed on the medial aspect of the ilium or they may be stacked. It is more common to use the augments with the wide base placed laterally and the apex placed medially, which is the opposite of how the augments are often used in type IIIA defects. The revision cup will have direct contact with the augments, which will be necessary to achieve a press-fit. As is done for a type IIIA defect, the augments are initially secured to the host bone with the use of multiple screws. Portions of the augments may need to be removed with a burr or a reamer to optimize the surface area contact between them and the revision shell. Particulate bone graft is then placed into any remaining cavities before the hemispherical revision shell is impacted into place. As is done for a type IIIA defect, the interfaces between the revision shell and the augments are cemented. (These interfaces should be in compression.) Multiple screw fixation is used through the revision shell.

Outcomes of Revision

Several authors have reported durable results at a minimum of 10 years following acetabular revision with the use of a hemispherical ce-

Table 1
Clinical Results of Cementless Acetabular Revision

Author	Year	No. of Hips	Mean Duration (Range) of Follow-up (years)	Results
Templeton et al[1]	2001	61	12.9 (11.5-14.3)	3.5% radiographically loose
Leopold et al[8]	1999	138	10.5 (7-14)	1.8% radiographically loose
Silverton et al[9]	1995	138	8.3 (7-11)	0.7% failure
Garcia-Cimbrelo[10]	1999	65	8.3 (6-11)	10.8% failure; 28% loose
Whaley et al[11]	2001	89	7.2 (5-11.3)	4.5% failure
Lachiewicz and Poon[12]	1998	57	7 (5-12)	No failures
Dearborn and Harris[13]	2000	24	7 (5-10.3)	No failures
Weber et al[14]	1996	61	6.5 (5-8)	1.6% radiographically loose
Chareancholvanich et al[15]	1999	40	8 (5-11)	12.5% failure
Paprosky et al[7]	1994	147	5.7 (3-9)	4.1% failure
Lachiewicz and Hussamy[16]	1994	60	5 (2-8)	No failures
Tanzer et al[17]	1992	140	3.7 (2-5.5)	1.4% failure
Padgett et al[18]	1993	138	3.6 (3-6)	No failures
Moskal et al[19]	1997	32	4.8 (3-9.5)	6.3% failure
Jasty[20]	1998	19	10 (8-11)	No failures due to loosening

mentless socket [1,8-20](Table 1). Because of these predictable clinical results, hemispherical cementless sockets are now used for almost all type I and II acetabular defects. Type IIIA acetabular defects can be treated with a distal femoral allograft, a bilobed implant, or a trabecular metal acetabular component with a superiorly placed trabecular metal augment. The long-term clinical results of acetabular reconstruction with the use of a trabecular metal system are currently unknown. However, trabecular metal appears to allow extensive bone ingrowth and is associated with high initial frictional resistance.

The midterm results of revisions with bilobed acetabular components have been disappointing. These implants were designed to lower the hip center of rotation and to obtain fixation, both in the true acetabulum and in the ilium. Chen and associates[21] reported a 24% failure rate in 37 hips followed for an average of 41 months postoperatively. In contrast, the midterm results of revisions with a distal femoral allograft and a hemispherical cementless acetabular component have been acceptable. After a minimum of 7 years and an average of 10 years of follow-up of 22 hips, 17 hips were found to be functioning well without loosening, and only 4 had been revised (at an average of 5.5 years postoperatively).

Treatment of type IIIB acetabular defects with an acetabular transplant and a cemented acetabular component (without a cage) has had poor clinical results. According to the senior author (WGP) 16 patients were followed for a minimum of 8 years (average, 18 years); and found that 6 hips were functioning without loosening, 6 had been revised because of aseptic loosening at an average of 2.9 years, and an additional 4 had radiographic evidence of loosening. Because of these poor results

following use of an unsupported structural allograft, we began to use reconstruction cages. At 2 to 8 years following use of such a cage in 48 hips with a type III defect, 20 hips were functioning without loosening, 9 had been revised because of aseptic loosening, and an additional 9 had radiographic evidence of loosening.

The poor clinical results observed after treatment of type IIIB defects recently prompted us to use a trabecular metal acetabular component with one or two augments in most type IIIB defects. Modular trabecular metal revision systems have not been used long enough for us to report follow-up results at the present time; however, we are encouraged by the early outcomes.

Summary

The increasing prevalence of arthroplasties and the younger age and greater life expectancy of the patients who receive them promises a continued need for solutions for patients requiring acetabular revision in the face of severe bone loss. The algorithmic approach outlined allows the surgeon to predict the findings in the operating room, plan the treatment of expected bone loss patterns, and make appropriate judgments regarding the reconstructive technique that will achieve the best possible results. Our preference is to achieve cementless fixation when possible and to use alternative solutions when initial stability cannot be obtained.

References

1. Templeton JE, Callaghan JJ, Goetz DD, Sullivan PM, Johnston RC: Revision of a cemented acetabular component to a cementless acetabular component: A ten to fourteen-year follow-up study. *J Bone Joint Surg Am* 2001;83:1706-1711.

2. Gaffey JL, Callaghan JJ, Pedersen DR, Goetz DD, Sullivan PM, Johnston RC: Cementless acetabular fixation at fifteen years: A comparison with the same surgeon's results following acetabular fixation with cement. *J Bone Joint Surg Am* 2004;86:257-261.

3. Della Valle CJ, Berger RA, Rosenberg AG, Galante JO: Cementless acetabular reconstruction in revision total hip arthroplasty. *Clin Orthop Relat Res* 2004;420:96-100.

4. Hallstrom BR, Golladay GJ, Vittetoe DA, Harris WH: Cementless acetabular revision with the Harris-Galante porous prosthesis: Results after a minimum of ten years of follow-up. *J Bone Joint Surg Am* 2004;86:1007-1011.

5. D'Antonio JA: Periprosthetic bone loss of the acetabulum: Classification and management. *Orthop Clin North Am* 1992;23:279-290.

6. D'Antonio JA, Capello WN, Borden LS, et al: Classification and management of acetabular abnormalities in total hip arthroplasty. *Clin Orthop Relat Res* 1989;243:126-137.

7. Paprosky WG, Perona PG, Lawrence JM: Acetabular defect classification and surgical reconstruction in revision arthroplasty: A 6-year follow-up evaluation. *J Arthroplasty* 1994;9:33-44.

8. Leopold SS, Rosenberg AG, Bhatt RD, Sheinkop MB, Quigley LR, Galante JO: Cementless acetabular revision: Evaluation at an average of 10.5 years. *Clin Orthop Relat Res* 1999;369:179-186.

9. Silverton CD, Rosenberg AG, Sheinkop MB, Kull LR, Galante JO: Revision total hip arthroplasty using a cementless acetabular component: Technique and results. *Clin Orthop Relat Res* 1995;319:201-208.

10. Garcia-Cimbrelo E: Porous-coated cementless acetabular cups in revision surgery: A 6- to 11-year follow-up study. *J Arthroplasty* 1999;14:397-406.

11. Whaley AL, Berry DJ, Harmsen WS: Extra-large uncemented hemispherical acetabular components for revision total hip arthroplasty. *J Bone Joint Surg Am* 2001;83:1352-1357.

12. Lachiewicz PF, Poon ED: Revision of a total hip arthroplasty with a Harris-Galante porous-coated acetabular component inserted without cement. A follow-up note on the results at five to twelve years. *J Bone Joint Surg Am* 1998;80:980-984.

13. Dearborn JT, Harris WH: Acetabular revision arthroplasty using so-called jumbo cementless components: An average 7-year follow-up study. *J Arthroplasty* 2000;15:8-15.

14. Weber KL, Callaghan JJ, Goetz DD, Johnston RC: Revision of a failed cemented total hip prosthesis with insertion of an acetabular component without cement and a femoral component with cement: A five to eight-year follow-up study. *J Bone Joint Surg Am* 1996;78:982-994.

15. Chareancholvanich K, Tanchuling A, Seki T, Gustilo RB: Cementless acetabular revision for aseptic failure of cemented hip arthroplasty. *Clin Orthop Relat Res* 1999;361:140-149.

16. Lachiewicz PF, Hussamy OD: Revision of the acetabulum without cement with use of the Harris-Galante porous-coated implant: Two to eight-year results. *J Bone Joint Surg Am* 1994;76:1834-1839.

17. Tanzer M, Drucker D, Jasty M, McDonald M, Harris WH: Revision of the acetabular component with an uncemented Harris-Galante porous-coated prosthesis. *J Bone Joint Surg Am* 1992;74:987-994.

18. Padgett DE, Kull L, Rosenberg A, Sumner DR, Galante JO: Revision of the acetabular component without cement after total hip arthroplasty: Three to six-year follow-up. *J Bone Joint Surg Am* 1993;75:663-673.

19. Moskal JT, Danisa OA, Shaffrey CI: Isolated revision acetabuloplasty using a porous-coated cementless acetabular component without removal of a well-fixed femoral component: A 3- to 9-year follow-up study. *J Arthroplasty* 1997;12:719-727.

20. Jasty M: Jumbo cups and morsalized graft. *Orthop Clin North Am* 1998;29:249-254.

21. Chen WM, Engh CA Jr, Hopper RH Jr, McAuley JP, Engh CA: Acetabular revision with use of a bilobed component inserted without cement in patients who have acetabular bone-stock deficiency. *J Bone Joint Surg Am* 2000; 82:197-206.

Index

Page numbers with *f* indicate figures
Page numbers with *t* indicate tables

Crescent sign, 48, 48f
Crossfire gamma-cross-linked and annealed polyethylene, 91, 107
Cross-linked polyethylene acetabular bearings, 104, 105–108, 106f
C-sign, 5–6
Cushing's disease, 46

D

Débridement
    arthroscopic, 8, 10f
    of labral lesions, 8
Degenerative disease, 8–9, 10f
Delayed-type hypersensitivity, 111–112, 112
Dental infection in revision total hip arthroplasty, 224
Dermal hypersensitivity to metal, 146
Developmental hip dysplasia, 20, 99, 142
Dislocations, 145, 146–147
    anterior, 177
    diagnosis of, 177
    following total hip arthroplasty, 164–165
    posterior, 177
    recurrent, 164–165
Distal femoral structural allograft with cementless acetabular component, 263–264, 264f
Dorsal subluxation of femoral head, 18
Double innominate osteotomy, 26
Dropkick test, 130
Durasul electron beam-cross-linked and remelted polyethylene, 88f, 91, 107
Durasul process, 91
Dysbaric osteonecrosis, 46
Dysbarisms, 46
Dysplasia, 4

E

Ehlers-Danlos syndrome, 11
Electron beam irradiation, 105
Elevated acetabular rim liners, effect on hip stability, 169
Embolic phenomena, risk of, 188
Epidural anesthesia and analgesia for total joint arthroplasty, (TJA), 134
Epidural opioids, 134
Extended-release epidural morphine (EREM), 135
    for total joint arthroplasty (TJA), 135, 135f, 136f
Extensively coated stems, removal of, 238f, 241–243, 241f, 242f, 243f

F

Factor V, 47
Fatigue, 83, 104
Femoral component, 128–129
    role in hip dislocation risk, 168
    rotation of, in dislocation, 179

Femoral heads
    ceramic, 109
    dorsal subluxation of, 18
    insufficiency fracture in, 3
    lateralization of, 15
    osteonecrosis of, 149
    penetration of, into acetabular polyethylene, 107
Femoral neck
    fixation in osteoporotic bone, 71–74, 72f, 73f
    fracture of, 65, 145–146, 145f (See also Osteoporotic femoral neck fractures) treated with bipolar arthro plasty, 169
    medializing, 125–126
Femoral nerve
    injury to, in hip dislocation, 190, 191f
    risk factors for palsy, 190
Femoral offset, 169
    increasing, 125–126
    restoration in soft-tissue balancing of hip, 121–130, 122f
        acetabular component, 127–128
        biomechanical principles, 122, 122f, 123f
        clinical implications, 123–124, 124f
        component, 125–126, 125f, 126f, 127f, 128–129
        effects on prosthesis, 124–125
        femoral offset, 123
        implications with regard to implant design, 124
        increasing offset, 125
        intraoperative measurements, 128f, 129–130
        limb length, 127, 127f
        method of, 126–127
        theoretic considerations, 123
Femoral osteotomy, 31
    combined pelvic and, 33, 33f
    valgus intertrochanteric, 31–33, 32f
    varus intertrochanteric, 31
Femoroacetabular clearance, 4
Femoroacetabular impingement, 2, 3, 4, 37–38
    cam, 38
    pincer, 38
Femoroacetabular impingement osteoplasty, 42–43, 42f, 43f
Femur
    bone stock deficiency of, 246
    cortical strut allografts, 253–254, 254f
        in reconstruction of, 205–206
    exposure of shaft, for removing extensively porous-coated stems, 237, 238f
    structural femoral allografts, 250–253, 251f
    treating fractured, during and after total hip arthroplasty, 195–207
        intraoperative fractures, 195–199, 196f, 197f
        postoperative fractures, 199–207

M

N

O